Serono Symposia Publications from Raven Press
Volume 28

RECENT ADVANCES IN PRIMARY
AND ACQUIRED IMMUNODEFICIENCIES

Serono Symposia Publications from Raven Press

Serono Symposia Publications from Raven Press
Volume 28

Recent Advances in Primary and Acquired Immunodeficiencies

Editors

F. Aiuti
*Department of Allergy and Clinical
Immunology
University of Rome
«La Sapienza»
Rome, Italy*

F. Rosen
*The Children's Hospital
Medical Center
Boston, Massachusetts, USA*

M.D. Cooper
*Tumor Institute
Birmingham, Alabama, USA*

Raven Press ■ New York

Raven Press, 1140 Avenue of the Americas, New York, New York 10036

Recent Advances in Primary and Acquired Immunodeficiencies
(Serono Symposia Publications from Raven Press; v. 28)

International Standard Book Number 0-88167-196-7
Library of Congress Catalog Number 85-043491

The material contained in this volume was submitted as previously unpublished material, except in the instances in which credit has been given to the source from which some of the illustrative material was derived. The views expressed and the general style adopted remain, however, the responsibility of the named authors. Great care has been taken to maintain the accuracy of the information contained in the volume. However, neither Raven Press, Serono Symposia, nor the editors can be held responsible for errors or for any consequences arising from the use of information contained herein.

The use in this book of particular designations of countries or territories does not imply any judgment by the publisher or editors as to the legal status of such countries or territories, of their authorities or institutions or of the delimitation of their boundaries.

Some of the names of products referred to in this book may be registered trademarks or proprietary names, although specific reference to this fact may not be made; however, the use of a name with designation is not to be construed as a representation by the publisher or editors that it is in the public domain. In addition, the mention of specific companies or of their products or proprietary names does not imply any endorsement or recommendation on the part of the publisher or editors.

Authors were themselves responsible for obtaining the necessary permission to reproduce copyright material from other sources. With respect to the publisher's copyright, material appearing in this book prepared by individuals as part of their official duties as government employees is only covered by this copyright to the extent permitted by the appropriate national regulations.

Printed in Rome, Italy
by Christengraf

Contents

Section III. Membrane defects

Section IV. Immunobiology of immunodeficiencies

Section V. Acquired Immunodeficiency Syndrome

List of Contributors

Aiuti F.
Dept. of Allergy and Clinical Immunology
University of Rome «La Sapienza»
Viale dell'Università, 37
00161 Rome, Italy

Beckmann R.
Children Hospital Matildenstr. 1
D-7800 Freiburg
W. Germany

Carbonara A.O.
Istituto di Genetica Medica
Università di Torino
Via Santena, 19
10126 Torino, Italy

Carbonari M.
Dept. of Allergy and Clinical Immunology
University of Rome «La Sapienza»
Viale dell'Università, 37
00161 Rome, Italy

Cooper M.D.
Tumor Institute
University of Alabama in Birmingham
Birmingham, Ala. 35294, USA

Cunningham-Rundles S.
Memorial Sloan-Kettering Institute
1275 York Avenue
10021 New York, NY, USA

Davis M.
Dept. of Medical Microbiology
Stanford University Medical Center
Palo Alto, CA, USA

De Weck A.
Institute of Clinical Immunology
Inserspital
University of Bern
3010 Bern, Switzerland

Dianzani F.
Cattedra di Virologia
University of Rome «La Sapienza»
00161 Rome, Italy

Doria G.
Laboratory of Pathology
C.R.E. Casaccia
C.P. 2400
00100 Rome, Italy

Drexhage H.A.
Lab. for Clinical Immunology
Dept. of Pathology
Free University Hospital
De Boellan, 1117 - 1007
MB Amsterdam, NL

Ebbesen P.
Institute of Cancer Research
Radium Stationen
DK-8000 Aarhus, Denmark

Eibl M.
Inst. fur Immunologie
University Wien
Borschke G BA 1090
Vienna, Austria

Fauci A.
National Institute of Allergy and Infectious Diseases
National Institutes of Health
Bethesda, MD 20205, USA

Fiorilli M.
Dept. of Allergy and Clinical
Immunology
University of Rome «La Sapienza»
Viale dell'Università, 37
00161 Rome, Italy

Gatti R.A.
Department of Pathology
Center of Health Sciences
University of Los Angeles
Los Angeles, CA, 90024, USA

Gelfand E.W.
Department of Immunology
Hospital for Sick Children
Toronto, Ontario M5G 1X8 Canada

Gilman S.
Wyeth Labs
P.O. Box 8299
Philadelphia, PA 19101, USA

Good R.
Cancer Research Program
Oklahoma Medical Research
Foundation
825 Northeast 13th Street
Oklahoma City, OK 73104, USA

Griscelli C.
Groupe Hospitalier Necker Enfants
Malades
149 Rue des Sevres
75730 Paris, Cedex 15

Gupta S.
Department of Medicine Med. Sci.
1 C264A
University of California
Irvine, 92717 CA, USA

Hayward A.
Department of Pediatrics
University of Colorado Medical Center
4200 East Ninth Avenue
Denver, CO 80262, USA

Lucivero M.
Clinica Medica II
Policlinico di Bari
Bari, Italy

Markham P.
Laboratory of Tumor Cell Biology
National Institute of Health
NCI
Bethesda, MD 20205, USA

Melchers F.
Basel Institute of Immunology
Postfach CH-4005
Basel 5, Switzerland

Neumuller J.
Ludwig Boltzmann.
Institute of Rheumatology and
Balneology
Vienna - Oberlaa - Austria

Niethammer D.
Abteilung für Padiatrische Hamatologie
Univ. Kinderlink
D-7400 Tubingen 1, Germany - FRG

Quinti I.
Dept. of Allergy and Clinical
Immunology
Viale dell'Università, 37
00161 Rome, Italy

Rosen F.
The Children's Hospital Medical Center
300 Longwood Avenue
Boston, MA 02119, USA

Ross G.
Department of Microbiology
University of North Carolina
Chapel Hill, NC, USA

Schlossman S.
Harvard Medical School
Dana-Farber Cancer Institute
44 Binney Street
Boston, MA 02115, USA

Schuff-Werner P.
University Clinics Department of
Internal Medicine Division Hematology
and Oncology
Robert Koch str. 40
D-3400 Gottingen FRG

Seligmann M.
Hospital St. Louis
Batiment Inserm
2, Place Dr. A. Fournier
75016 Paris, France

Shoham J.
Dept. of Life Sciences
Bar-Ilan University
52100 Ramat Gan, Israel

Springer T.
Dana-Farber Cancer Institute
JFB 424
44 Binney Street
Boston, MA 02115, USA

Ugazio A.
Cattedra di Puericultura
Clinica Pediatrica
University of Pavia
Pavia, Italy

Umetsu D.
Division of Allergy
The Children's Hospital Medical Center
300 Longwood Avenue
Boston, MA 02115, USA

Waldmann A.T.
National Center Institute,
Bethesda, MD.20892, USA

Wedgwood R.J.
Department of Pediatrics RD-20
University of Washington
Seattle, WA 98195, USA

Wigzell H.
Karolinska Institutet
Dept. of Immunology
Solnavagen 1
S-104 Stockholm, Sweden

SECTION I
ONTOGENY AND ACTIVATION
OF T AND B CELLS

Ontogeny of Human T Cells: Acquisition of a Functional Program

Marie Luise Blue and Stuart F. Schlossman

Division of Tumor Immunology, Dana-Farber Cancer Institute and the Department of Medicine, Harvard Medical School, Boston, MA 02115, USA

The thymus plays a central role in the development of an effective immune system. Profound changes in cell surface antigens mark the various stages of thymic T cell differentiation in mice (15,3) and humans (7,11,12). These stages of differentiation can be compartmentalized into cortical and medullary locations. Although still controversial, it is generally believed that functionally and phenotypically immature T cells are confined to the cortex and maturation of thymocytes is accompanied by migration to the medulla. Cortical thymocytes are distinguished by their ability to bind the peanut agglutinin lectin (PNA) with high affinity, while medullary thymocytes lack PNA reactivity. In humans, monoclonal antibodies to distinct T cell surface antigens have permitted phenotypic characterization of thymocytes and their separation into three discrete stages of intrathymic differentiation (12). Stage I thymocytes lack most mature T cell antigens except T11 (E-rosette receptor) but do express a series of activation antigens including T10 and T9 (transferrin receptor), which are not restricted to the T cell lineage. The latter thymocytes account for approximately 10% of the thymic population and are mainly cortical in location. The majority of cortical thymocytes (60-80%) are T4+T8+T6+T11+ and represent the stage II of differentiation. Stage III defines medullary thymocytes which lack T6, do not coexpress T4 and T8, and are functionally more mature cells (12,16,5,17).

The great number of monoclonal antibodies to human T cell surfaces antigens has allowed the further characterization of thymic subpopulations and the demonstration of extensive heterogeneity of subgroups within the cortex. This heterogeneity may represent various stages of activation and differentiation of cortical cells (16,5), or alternatively cells with aberrant phenotype destined for intra-thymic death. So far, a direct precursor-product relationship between these cortical thymic subpopulations as well as between cortical and medullary thymocytes has not been demonstrated.

Recent studies have shown a correlation between full surface expression of the T cell antigen receptor (Ti) and the associated T3 molecule on thymocytes and the acquistion of immunocompetence (16,5,17). Analysis of Tiβ gene rearrangement has shown that stage I thymocytes (T11+T6+T3−) do not have their β gene rearranged, while stage II thymocytes which lack full Ti/T3 surface expression have rearranged β genes (14). Since the majority of stage II thymocytes are immunoincompetent, this result emphasize the importance of the steps leading to gene activation and expression of the rearranged β genes as well as other genes governing the T cell receptor and associated molecules.

In order to study in detail the sequential steps in the activation and surface expression of thymic gene products leading to the acquisition of immunocompetence, we developed a system for activating and growing human thymocytes in vitro. Using two color fluorescence flow cytometry and other techniques, we were able to demonstrate that the T4+T8+ thymocyte (stage II) can be activated in vitro and gives rise to T4+T8− cells. The functional capacities expressed by the in vitro generated T4+T8− and T8+T4− thymocytes are characteristic but not identical to those of the corresponding peripheral blood T cell phenotypes. Our studies have shown that a series of growth related surface antigens are expressed prior to full expression of the T cell receptor associated T3 molecule. Furthermore, surface expression of antigen receptor-associated T3 precedes loss of T4 and T8 coexpression.

Proliferation of thymocytes in vitro

Incubation of thymocytes for 2 days in media containing Con A and TCGF, followed by growth in media supplemented with TCGF but without Con A, generally showed > 80% viability for the first 3 days and > 95% viability thereafter. Proliferation and DNA synthesis was virtually absent during the first 2 days of Con A activation. By day 3, cells enlarged and the majority of thymic samples proliferated extremely well, while some samples, although exhibiting similar overall patterns of activation and growth, grew slower. Regardless of the extent of later proliferation, tritiated thymidine incorporation in all thymic samples was near background levels for the first 2 days and increased at day 3. Thymocytes grew extremely well for 3 1/2 - 4 weeks provided they were supplied with fresh media and TCGF every 3 or 4 days.

Discrete stages of thymic activation and maturation defined by surface antigens

During activation and growth of thymic samples, there is both an appearance and loss of various surface antigens. The activation antigens, $IL-2R_1$ (IL-2 receptor) and T9 (transferrin receptor) are the earliest induced antigens. The number of IL-2 receptors and T9 molecules per cell are greatest for both on day 3. On this day, virtually all thymic cells react with anti-$IL-2R_1$ and anti-T9. The thymocyte antigen, T6 (7,11) becomes virtually undetectable on day 3 and remains undetectable from that point.

Freshly isolated thymocytes are composed of 3 subpopulations with regard to T3 expression; a T3 negative population generally comprising about 20-40% of cells, a population with low T3 and one with high T3 density. The proportion of low T3 and high T3 thymocytes varied with different thymic samples. Since T3 is known to be part of the T cell antigen receptor complex (8,13,9), its presence and induction on thymocytes suggests that these cells are maturing. For the first two days in culture, there is very little change in the thymic T3 surface density. The density of thymic T3 antigen expression appears maximal on day 7 when «in vitro» matured thymocytes begin to take on the phenotypic «look» of peripheral T cells, i.e. high T3 density and absence of T6.

Early stages of thymic activation detected by perpendicular light scatter analysis

Microscopic examination and forward angle light scatter profiles of thymocytes indicated no significant changes in thymic cell size until day 3, when cells become very large. Subsequently, there is a gradual reduction in cell size until by day 7, the majority of thymocytes have reached a size very similar to that of peripheral blood T cells. Forward angle light scatter primarily measures cell volume, however, perpendicular (log 90°) light scatter is thought to measure nuclear morphology and internal structures (1,2). Log 90° light scatter analysis revealed striking changes during the first 2 days of thymic activation; up to 50% of thymocytes clearly had larger scatter profiles. These results suggest that log 90°, but not forward angle light scatter, correlates with the induction of activation antigens. In Fig. 1, log 90° light scatter profiles illustrate thymic stages of activation.

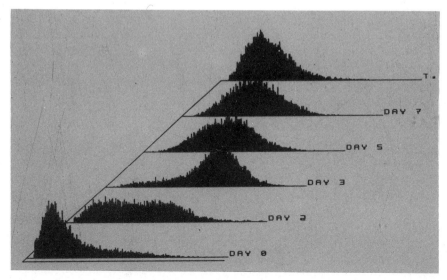

FIG. 1 Log 90° scatter histograms of developing thymocytes.

To demonstrate the association between log 90° light scatter and activation the distribution and expression of various surface antigens on small and large log 90° cells at day 2 were compared. The IL-2 receptor (IL-2R$_1$) and transferrin receptor (T9) were almost exclusively found on the large log 90° cells (Table 1). These activation antigens were also found at a much higher number

TABLE 1. *Antigen Expression on Small and Large Log 90° Scatter Gated Thymocytes at Day2*

Antigen	Percent Positive					
	Small Cells			Large Cells		
	Exp. 1	Exp. 2	Exp. 3	Exp. 1	Exp. 2	Exp. 3
T3	9	65	53	68	92	89
T6	32	43	45	24	19	13
IL-2R	2	n.d.[a]	24	70	n.d.	93
T9	0.9	n.d.	7	58	n.d.	83

[a] n.d. = not determined

per cell on large than on small log 90° cells. T9 molecules were 2 to 3 times and IL-2 receptors more than 10 times more numerous on large log 90° cells. Most of the large log 90° cells were T3 positive (Table 1) and expressed this antigen in 2-4 times higher amounts than the small log 90° cells that were T3 positive. The reverse held for T6. A larger portion of the T6 positive cells had a small log 90° scatter profile and the number of T6 molecules on small and large 90° cells were similar as judged by fluorescence intensity measurements.

Activation and maturation of the T4+T8+ thymocyte

Thymic T4 and T8 antigens were analyzed by two color fluorescence flow cytometry. Fig. 2 shows a typical T4, T8 profile of freshly isolated thymocytes. Panel A shows control staining, while panel B shows staining with conjugated anti-T8 (y-axis) and anti-T4 (x-axis) monoclonal antibodies.

After 2 days of in vitro Con A activation, there is a change in T4, T8 profile; all thymocytes are T4+T8+ or more fequently show mixed populations of T4+T8+ and T8+T4− cells. The small T4+T8− population seen at day 0 appears to be absent. Since there is no proliferation for the first 2 days, either T4+T8− cells selectively died or lost T4 antigen and have become T4−T8− cells. Alternatively, T4+T8− cells may have aquired detectable T8 antigen and are now found among the T4+T8+ population. We only have evidence to support the latter possibility. Freshly isolated thymocytes have lower numbers of T8 molecules per cell than normal T8+ peripheral T cells, however when cultured in vitro or activated with Con A, the number of T8 molecules

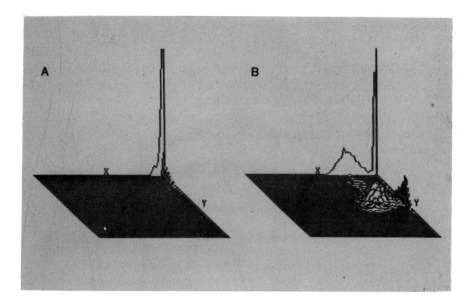

FIG. 2 T4 and T8 expression on freshly isolated thymocytes. Thymocytes were stained with mouse IgG/FITC and Texas Red avidin (panel A). The same cells as in panel A were stained for T4, T8 fluorescence with anti-T4 biotin/Texas ed avidin and anti-T8 FITC (panel B). Log red fluorescence is shown along the x-axis and log green fluorescence along the y-axis. Cell number is represented on the vertical axis.

but not T4 molecules increases within 24 hours to levels comparable to those found on peripheral blood T cells, which represents a 2 fold increase in T8 antigenic sites per cell. Regardless of what the small T4+T8− population found on day 0 may represent, we were able to generate large numbers of T4+T8− thymocytes with hight T4 fluorescence from a T4+T8+ (or T4+T8+ and T8+T4−) population.

Using anti-T3 biotin with Texas Red in conjunction with either anti-T8 FITC or anti-T4 FITC, we found that all T3+ cells at day 2 (generally about 65%) were also T8+. No T3+T8− cells were detectable on day 2, indicating the absence of mature T4+ cells with a T3+T4+T8− phenotype. However, some T8+T3− cells (12-21%) were present at this time.

Analysis of fluorescence on small log 90° (not activated) and large log 90° (activated) day 2 thymocytes, showed that the majority of higher T8 and T3 antigen density was found on the larger log 90° thymocytes, suggesting that an increase in numbers of T8 molecules is associated with activation in this system.

Sorted T4+T8+ thymocytes, like unfractionated thymocytes, can be activated by Con A treatment. Both sorted and unfractionated thymocytes display very similar log 90° scatter histograms. About 50% of both day 2 unfractionated and sorted T4+T8+ cells had larger log 90° scatter profiles as compared to their day 0 log 90° scatters. That it is the T4+T8+ thymocyte which is activated and not just a minor mature thymic population is also indicated by the fact that on day 3 where the T4, T8 fluorescence profile shows very little change as compared to day 2 of activation, the IL-2 and transferrin receptor as well as T3 are expressed on 94-98% of thymocytes. These data further suggest that acquisition of T3 precedes the generation of T4+T8− thymocytes.

Cytotoxic activity of in vitro generated T4+T8− and T8+T4− thymocytes

The cytotoxic potential of thymocytes at various stages of thymic in vitro maturation was assayed utilizing lectin approximation (18) and the standard ^{51}Cr release assay (6). The Epstein Barr virus transformed cell line, Laz 509, and Daudi, a Burkitt lymphoma derived cell line were used as target cells. Con A approximation was used to measure the ability of thymocytes and T cells to kill. In the absence of Con A, there was little cytotoxicity even at a 60:1 effector to target ratio. The presence of Con A (25 μg/ml) increased the cytotoxicity of thymocytes as well as T cells. These concentrations of Con A had no effect on spontaneous ^{51}Cr release. Table 2 shows little cytotoxic

TABLE 2.   *Thymocyte Cytotoxicity Against Daudi*

	Percent ^{51}Cr Release			
Effector: Target	60:1	30:1	15:1	7.5:1
day 0/−Con A	4 ± 2	1 ± 1	0	2 ± 1
day 0/+Con A	9[a]	10 ± 7	7 ± 5	2
day 2/+Con A[b]	3 ± 3	2 ± 3	3 ± 3	2 ± 2
day 3/−Con A	0.5 ± 0.6	0.8 ± 0.6	0.3 ± 0.3	0.3 ± 0.3
day 3/+Con A	1 ± 1	0.7 ± 0.8	1 ±1	0.3 ± 0.4
day 5/−Con A	3 ± 0.9	2 ± 1	1 ± 0.4	1 ± 0.7
day 5/+Con A	33 ± 7	26 ± 7	22 ± 4	18 ± 5
day 7/−Con A	6 ± 3	4 ± 3	2 ± 2	1 ± 0.8
day 7/+Con A	35 ± 21	31 ± 20	30 ± 17	22 ± 15
T cells/−Con A	11	10	6 ± 1	4 ± 0
T cells/+Con A	21	21	17 ± 6	13 ± 5

[a] Values for which no S.E.M. values are given represent 1 or 2 different experiments only.
[b] Day 2 thymocytes usually had nearly as high a killer activity in the absence as in the presence of Con A (25 μg/ml), therefore, only cytotoxicity in the presence of Con A is given.

activity against Daudi by day 0, day 2, and day 3 thymocytes, but high rates of cytotoxicity at day 5 and day 7. The onset of cytotoxicity against Laz 509 was also confined to day 5 and day 7 thymocytes, which consisted mainly of T8+T4− and T4+T8− cells. To test for subset restriction of cytotoxicity; day 5 thymocytes were sorted into T4+T8− and T8+T4− cells and the sorted cells were assayed for cytotoxic potential. The results demonstrated that the bulk of the cytotoxic activity against Laz 509 was associated with the T8+T4− population with very little cytotoxic activity residing in the T4+T8− subset.

Similarly, the T8+T4− population was cytotoxic for Daudi in the presence of Con A, but there was virtually no cytotoxicity shown by the T4+T8− thymocytes for this cell line.

Induction of Ig secretion

T cells can be induced to provide help for Ig secretion by allogeneic B cells either by addition of antibodies against the T cell antigen receptor (Ti), or against surface antigens T3, or T11 (alternate pathway, ref. 17). We used anti-T11$_2$ and anti-T11$_3$ (17) to assay for the ability of thymocytes to provide help for IgG and IgM secretion. Whether we tested day 0, day 5, or day 7 cultured thymocytes, we could not detect IgG above background levels in cultures of B cells and thymocytes activated with anti-T11$_2$ and anti-T11$_3$. In contrast, peripheral blood T cells induced IgG secretion quite well under the same conditions. However, thymocytes clearly provided help for IgM production. Day 0 and in vitro matured day 5 or day 7 thymocytes provided similar degrees of help after activation with anti-T11$_2$ and anti-T11$_3$. This result is not surprising since thymic activation and differentiation may have occurred in day 0 cultures during the 7 day assay in response to anti-T11$_2$ and anti-T11$_3$ (4). Although thymocytes could provide help for IgM production, this help was generally substantially lower than that provided by peripheral T cells under the same circumstances. To test whether help analogous to that in peripheral blood was confined to T4+T8− thymocytes, we sorted day 5 thymocytes in T4+T8− and T8+T4− cells and assayed for IgM secretion as described. Table 3 shows one representative experiment which suggests that the T4+T8− thymocyte population is more effective than the T8+T4− thymocyte subset in inducing IgM secretion.

TABLE 3. *Induction of IgM Secretion by Thymocyte Subpopulations*

Thymocyte Population	IgM (ng/ml)[a]	
	−anti-T11$_2$/T11$_3$	+anti-T11$_2$/T11$_3$
Unfractionated/day 0	40	345
Unfractionated/day 5	0	383
T4+T8−/day 5	0	385
T8+T4−/day 5	0	95

[a] Values for IgM secretion are given after subtraction of values for spontaneous IgM secretion by B lymphocytes incubated without thymocytes. The values shown for IgM secretion in the absence of anti-T11$_2$ and anti-T11$_3$ are zero for some samples because spontaneous IgM secretion by B cells was slightly higher than that seen upon the addition of thymocytes. Spontaneous IgM secretion by B cells was generally below 100 ng/ml.

CONCLUSION

We have defined three sequential stages in the in vitro activation and maturation of human thymocytes. The earliest stage is marked by the induction of the IL-2 and transferrin receptors and by increased expression of the T8 antigen. The second stage is distinguished by the loss of T6 and the gradual acquisition of the T3 antigen complex. During the third stage of activation, thymocytes maximally express the T3 antigen receptor complex and lose T4, T8 coexpression. The in vitro generated T4+T8− and T8+T4− thymocytes display detectable functional capacities associated with mature peripheral blood T cell subsets. The results of our studies suggest that this in vitro system can be used to study human thymocyte maturation.

Acknowledgements

This work was supported by grant AI12069 from the National Institutes of Health.

REFERENCES

1. Benson, M.C., McDougal, D.C. and Coffey, D.S. (1984): The application of perpendicular and forward light scatter to assess nuclear and cellular morphology. *Cytometry* 5:515-522.
2. Brunsting, A. and Mullaney, P.F. (1974): Differential light scattering from spherical mammalian cells. *Biophys. J.* 14:439-453.
3. Ceredig, R., MacDonald, H.R. and Jenkinson, E.Y. (1983): Flow microfluorometric analysis of mouse thymus development in vivo and in vitro. *Eur. J. Immunol.* 13:185-190.
4. Fox, D.A., Hussey, R.E., Fitzgerald, K.A., Bensussn, A., Daley, J.F., Schlossman, S.F. and Reinherz, E.L. (1985): Activation of human thymocytes via the 50 KD T11 sheep erythrocyte binding protein induces the expression of interleukin 2 receptors on both T3+ and T3− populations. *J. Immunol.* 134:330-335.
5. Gelin, C., Boumsell, L., Dausset, J. and Bernard, A. (1984): The heterogeneity and functional capacity of human thymocyte subpopulations. *Proc. Natl. Acad. Sci. USA* 81:4912-4916.
6. Hercend, T., Meuer, S.C., Reinherz, E.L., Schlossman, S.F. and Ritz, J. (1982): Generation of a cloned NK cell line derived from the «null cell» fraction of human peripheral blood., *J. Immunol.* 129:A1299-1305.
7. McMichael, A.J., Pilch, J.R., Galfre, G., Mason, G., Fabre, D.Y., and Milstein, J.W. (1979): A human thymocyte antigen defined by a hybrid myeloma monoclonal antibody. *Eur. J. Immunol.* 9:205-210.
8. Meuer, S.C., Acuto, O., Hussey, R.E., Hodgdon, J.C., Fitzgerald, K.A., Schlossman, S.F. and Reinherz, E.L. (1983): Evidence for the T3-associated 90K heterodimer as the T-cell antigen receptor. *Nature* 303:808-810.
9. Meuer, S.C., Fitzgerald, K.A., Hussey, R.E., Hodgdon, J.C., Schlossman, S.F. and Reinherz, E.L. (1983): Clonotypic structures involved in antigen specific human T cell function: Relationship to the T3 molecular complex. *J. Exp. Med.* 157:705-719.
10. Meuer, S.C., Hussey, R.E., Fabbi, M., Fox, D.A., Acuto, O., Fitzgerald, K.A., Hodgdon, J.C., Protentis, J.P., Schlossman, S.F. and Reinherz, E.L. (1984): An alternative pathway of T cell activation: A functional role for the 50 KD T11 sheep erythrocyte receptor protein. *Cell* 36:897-906.
11. Reinherz, E.L., Kung, P.C., Goldstein, G., Levey, R.H. and Schlossman, S.F. (1980): Discrete stages of human intrathymic differentiation. Analysis of normal thymocytes and leukemic lymphoblasts of T cell lineage. *Proc. Natl. Acad. Sci. USA* 77:1588-1592.
12. Reinherz, E.L. and Schlossman, S.F. (1980): The differentiation and function of human T lymphocytes. *Cell* 19:821-827.

13. Reinherz, E.L., Meuer, S., Fitzgerald, K.A., Hussey, R.E., Levine, H. and Schlossman, S.F. (1982): Antigen recognition by human T lymphocytes is limited to surface expression of the T3 molecular complex. *Cell* 30:735-743.
14. Royer, H.-D., Acuto, O., Fabbi, M., Tizard, R., Ramachandran, K., Smart, J.E. and Reinherz, E.L. (1984): Genes encoding the Ti β subunit of the antigen/MHC receptor undergo rearrangement during intrathymic ontogeny prior to surface T3-Ti expression. *Cell* 39:261-266.
15. Scollay, R. and Shortman, K. (1983): Thymocyte subpopulations: and experimental review, including flow cytometric cross-correlations between the major murine thymocyte markers. *Thymus* 5:245-295.
16. Umiel, T., Daley, J.F., Bhan, A.K., Levey, R.H., Schlossman, S.F. and Reinherz, E.L. (1982): Acquisition of immune competence by a subset of human cortical thymocytes expressing mature T cell antigens. *J. Immunol.* 129:1054-1060.
17. Van Agthoven, A., Terhorst, C., Reinherz, E.L. and Schlossman, S.F. (1981): Characterization of T cell surface glycoproteins T1 and T3 present on all human peripheral T lymphocytes and functionally mature thymocytes. *Eur. J. Immunol.* 11:18-21.
18. Van Boehmer, H. and Haas, W. (1981): H-2 restricted cytotoxic and noncytolytic T cell clones: isolation, specificity and functional analysis. *Immunol. Rev.* 54:27-56.

Activation and Regulation of T Lymphocytes in Vivo

Hans Wigzell

Department of Immunology, Karolinska Institute, 10401 Stockholm, Sweden

INTRODUCTION

Detailed studies on T cells can nowadays be made in vitro allowing fine analysis as to individual lymphocyte functions previously impossible to carry out under in vivo conditions. Despite the obvious positive sides of such an in vitro development there exist certain dangers insofar as in vitro results may too readily be interpreted to indicate that the very same conditions prevail in vivo. This may not be true resulting in a twarted concept as to which factors are of biological relevance both with regard to quantity and quality in the normal immune response in vivo. Likewise, it is of interest to analyze to what degree lymphokines known to act during an immune response in vitro do function under normal and immune situations in vivo. Finally, some comments will also be made in relation to the regulation of fine specificity interactions between T and B cells as appearant by genetic restriction of idiotype expression. The article should be read as a personal view and is not intendend by any means to convey a complete picture in a review-like manner.

Activation of T cells in vivo versus in vitro

Ample data exist showing that in vivo B cells proliferate and are selected for high affinity antibody production with switched isotypes of immunoglobulins as immunization proceeds with time. It is not as clearcut, however, when it comes to clonal expansion and proliferation of T cells in vivo following immunization. It is well established in animal systems that introduction of lymphocytes into irradiated recipients or in situations where graft-versus-host reactions of severe nature will be induced will result in T cell proliferation and the appearance of blasts of T cell types in vivo. However, in the intact individual it does seem likely from several points of evidence that proliferation of T cells may not play such an important part during induction of immunity but this may rather occur via a change in the regulation of activity of T cell function. Thus, in vivo induction of T helper cell immunity would thus seem to take place via a change in suppression resulting in a release of previously inhibited T helper cells rather than through an increase in actual physical numbers of helper lymphocytes (5). Similar results were also obtained by these workers with regard to precursor frequencies for cytotoxic cells, that is multiple suppressor cells were considered to exist normally inhibiting killer precursor cells in the unimmunized individual. In agreement with such a concept are also the observations that in vivo activation of killer T cells in intact animals against alloantigens do seem to occur in the absence of significant proliferation as measured both by lack of changes in cell size and density and failure to incorporate tritiated thymidine (6).

Here it would seem clear that less than 5% of all killer T cells induced by allogeneic immunization using intact mice and followed over a 10 day period did arise from recently dividing cells. Killer T cells could thus in this system be shown to arise in an efficient manner in vivo in the absence of significant proliferation but rather through a combination of activation and relocalization. In the human systems results available may be used to argue in a similar manner. In active rheumatoid synovia the T cells accumulating showed significant signs of activation as indicated by the presence of receptors for IL-2 and of HLA-D molecules but again virtually all of these «activated» lymphocytes were small lymphocytes (2). Yet, if extracted from the tissues and placed in presence of IL-2 in vitro they could clearly become blasts and proliferate in the «conventional» manner. Similarly, in a minority of tumor patients it is possible to demonstrate the existance in the patients of specific killer T cells with seemingly exquisite specificity for the autotochtonous cances cells (13). These specific cytotoxic T cells are also always found to be small lymphocytes with high density again emphasizing the ability to in vivo activated effector T cells to express their full function in absence of proliferation. Thus, it is not farfetched to argue and suggest that possibly a sizeable part or even the absolute dominating majority of T cells being activated in vivo during immunization are induced to effector function in the absence of clonal expansion and proliferation. This is not merely a point of theoretical interest but of obvious relevance when considering drugs for interference or elimination of T lymphocytes during immune situations. At the same time it is as always wise to consider the situation in vivo not to be as distinct as black versus white in relation to T cell proliferation. It is clear that T lymphocytes obviously can proliferate in vivo such as in the post-thymic expansion phase and in situations where the immune system has been damaged from for instance ionizing radiation this proliferative capacity is a major factor to replace lost cells.

Is the main function of IL-2 in vivo to cause T cell division?

One question arising from the above chapter is the «true» function of IL-2 under normal conditions in vivo. It is already documented beyond doubt that IL-2 indeed can function as a most powerful T cell growth hormone in vitro and removal of IL-2 will cause a major halt to most T cell activation in vitro.

Likewise, administration of large amounts of IL-2 in vivo will not only allow inoculated T blasts to continue to be active but they can also be maintained in a proliferative mood by the repeated inoculations of the interleukin (3). However, whilst proving that IL-2 can act in vivo in a proliferative promoting manner for T cells such results do not exclude that IL-2 may have highly significant activities at lower molar concentrations which afflict T cell functions without evoking cellular division. It is here thoughtprovoking to consider the situation of gamma-interferon, which despite its name is a relatively poor interferon at low concentrations where its capacity to change other immunological parameters such as MHC expression is already very impressive (15). In line with such a reasoning are the previously discussed findings in human rheumatoid arthritis where activated T cells in synovial tissue express receptors for IL-2 (= are «activated and IL-2 responsive) yet do not proliferate in a situation where immune T cell reactivity is clearly indicated by other parameters.

What is frequently overlooked with regard to IL-2 function is the capacity of this lymphokine to induce activation of lymphocyte function (T and/or B) without having to resort to proliferation. IL-2 is thus for instance a very active inducer of cytotoxic T cell function and will do this in the absence of proliferation and measurable gamma-interferon induction in vitro (8). In their system killer T memory cells were induced to cytotoxic capacity by IL-2 in the presence or absence of anti-proliferative drugs. No differences in the generation of killer capacity were noted between the various IL-2 treated cells within the first 24 hours whereafter in the absence of the drug a further increase in cytolytic potential was generated via proliferation as well. It is thus quite possible that IL-2 in vivo may have activating capacity for T cell functions in manners which do not require any T cell proliferation at all. At the same time in other maybe rather special circumstances may IL-2 function in vivo as well as a true T cell growth stimulator under normal conditions.

Is IL-1 or IL-2 used in vivo during thymocyte proliferation?

In the absence of added extraneous antigen there is one place within the body, the thymus, where a rapid proliferation of cells restricted to the T cell lineage is taking place. During this proliferation we now know that maturation into immunocompetence does take place which is paralleled by a selection for cells with the best «fit» for function in the individual. It would thus seem likely that the thymic environment may be one such «special circumstance» as speculated above for IL-2 to have a function under the normal, proliferating T cell conditions. However, the interleukin known to have some unique active in relation to thymocytes as compared to peripheral mature T cells is IL-1, where the classical way to measure IL-1 is to use PHA and thymocytes and add the presumed IL-1 containing medium. Presence of IL-1 is here observed as induction of thymocyte proliferation. Mitogens such as PHA are presumed to have the ability to function as opening signals for T cells but do require

additional helping factors to induce T cell proliferation, in the case of thymocytes this is provided for by IL-1. But the thymus is considered to function as
a selective breeding ground for self-MHC restricted T cells, in particular for
MHC molecules of the class II type (14). Indications that IL-1 has the potential
power to function as an internal proliferative stimulus under these self-MHC
selecting conditions have recently come from the observations that thymocytes
but not peripheral T cells can be induced to efficient proliferation when
confronted in vitro with syngeneic cells with high density of class II MHC
antigens *if* IL-1 is present in the medium (11). The fact that accessory cells
from the thymus were excellent presenters of class II MHC antigens in these
studies are thus well in line with the possibility that IL-1 or an IL-1 related
molecule may act to drive the thymocytes to via anti-self-MHC recognition
achieve the optimal response patterns in relation to the individual's own MHC
antigens.

But are there any data to support a similar function in vivo for IL-2 and
thymocytes? Intrathymic T stem cells have been reported to express IL-2
receptors whilst being unresponsive per se to IL-2 as measured by proliferation
in vitro (9). However, the addition of a second signal in the form of Con A
does allow IL-2 to drive thymocytes into proliferation. As PHA is known to
require MHC recognition by T cells to achieve optimal mitogenic activity, the
argument would here be that thymocytes can obtain functional IL-2 receptors
(= allowing IL-2 to induce proliferation) provided they receive proper,
specific signals. That this select stimulation may occur whithin the thymus is
now well documented in the murine systems using soluble protein antigens (7)
and would support the possibility that a similar pathway could be used by
normal thymocytes during a certain stage of differentiation with reactions to
self-MHC with or without additional antigens. If significant, elimination or
reduction of IL-1 and/or IL-2 would here result in a significant reduction in
intrathymic proliferation.

T cell specificity patterns: Influence by B cell products?

To further discuss normally occuring regulatory events afflicting T cells in
vivo one can also turn to the relationship between B and T cell specificity
patterns. When studies on T cell receptors began using the anti-idiotypic
approach which eventually led to the physical isolation of T cell receptors for
antigen it was relatively soon discovered that the inheritance pattern of T cell
idiotypes behaved like being genetically linked to the heavy chain Ig locus (1,
10). This was initially interpreted to most likely mean that structural variable
genes for T cell receptors were linked to the heavy chain Ig locus as well or,
alternatively, that the same variable genes were used for both T and B cells
at this locus. The second alternative explanation, that B cell products regulated the specificity pattern of T cells thus producing this linkage in a non-struc-
tural manner was discarded by myself due to the fact that the degree of
idiotypic pattern inheritance was so dominant affecting more than 85% of

specific total T cell reactivity in our antigenic system (= allo-MHC). From the genetic analysis at the chromosomal level we now know that seemingly no T cell receptor variable genes are to be found on chromosome 12, where the heavy chain Ig genes are located in the mouse. How could one then explain the linkage pattern of T cell specificity and idiotypes so clearly seen by several groups in the rodent systems? All immune systems of higher animals do have as a normal hall mark that they will develop during ontogeny in the presence of specific B cell molecules, that is immunoglobulin from the mother. It is well known from animal systems that idiotypic antibodies may have a significant and sometimes long-lasting impact in an active manner on the subsequent immune capacity of the offspring (Rubinstein et al., 1983). It is also known since long that particular in rabbits it is possible to transfer a state of active immunity from the mother to the foetus via placental transfer (= most likely antibodies) which will change the ability of the offsping for life as far as allotype producing ability is concerned (4). One can thus say that maybe for the first time a true Lamarckian phenomenon is observed, albeit acting in a Darwinian set-up; that is maternal antibodies may evoke an active immunity in the offspring leaving the immune system of the newborn in an actively induced state of reactivity dependant on the previous immune experience of the mother.

Experience is now gathering indicating that a similar phenomenon may also be responsible for the linkage phenomenon observed between T cell idiotypes and heavy chain Ig loci. Thus, removal at will from the developing immune system of circulating immunoglobulins by inoculation of anti-IgM antibodies will for instance change the T cell circuitry involved idiotypic-anti-idiotypic reactions and suppressor T cell generation. Here, absence of B cell Ig molecules from the mother or endogenously produced will release the T cell system from its heavy Ig chain locus restriction, thus proving that this restriction is indeed a result of educating T cells by B cell-derived antibody molecules (12). From this we may then conclude that in the ontogeny of the B and T cell systems it is easy to consider the T cells to be the dominating cell types in their relationship (B cells frequently requiring T cell help etc.). This is however probably an error as indicated by the above discussion where immunoglobulins can be shown to have a dramatic, significant impact on T cell behaviour as far as specificity and regulation is concerned. Such data do also suggest that in the future one would expect a further usage of immunoglobulins as active immune regulators not only in adults but also in utero allowing specific, active manipulation of T and B cell specific immunity.

REFERENCES

1. Binz, H., Wigzell, H., and Bazin, H., (1976), T cell idiotypes are linked to immunoglobulin heavy chain genes. *Nature*, 264:639-642.
2. Burmester, G.R., Jahn, B., Gramatzki, M., Zacher, J., and Kalden, J.R., (1984), Activated

T cells in vivo and in vitro: Divergence of expression of Tac and Ia antigens in the nonblastoid small T cells of inflammation and normal T cells activated in vitro. *J. Immunol.*: 133:1230-1234.

3. Cheever, M.A., Greenberg, P.D., Irle, C., Thompson, J.A., Urdal, D.L., Mochizuki, D.Y., Henney, C.S., and Gillis, S., (1984), Interleukin 2 administered in vivo induces the growth of cultured T cells in vivo *J. Immunol.* 132:2259-2266.

4. Dubiski, S. (1967) Synthesis of allotypically defined immunoglobulins in rabbits. *Cold Spring Harb. Symp. Quant. Biol.*, 32:311-316.

5. Fey, K., Melchers, I., and Eichmann, K., (1983), Quantitative studies on T cell diversity. IV. Mathematical analysis of multiple limiting populations of effector and suppressor T cells. *J. Exp., Med.*, 158: 40-52.

6. Kimura, A.K., and Wigzell, H., (1983), Development and function of cytotoxic T lymphocytes. I. In vivo maturation of CTL precursors in the absence of detectable proliferation. *J. Immunol.*, , 130:2056-2061.

7. Kyewski, B.A., Fathman, C.G., and Kaplan, H.S. (1984) Intrathymic presentation of circulating non-major histocompatibility complex antigens. *Nature*, 308:196-199.

8. Lefrancois, L., Kelin, J.R., Paetkau, V., and Bevan, M.J. (1984) Antigen-independent activation of memory cytotoxic T cells by IL-2. *J. Immunol.*, 133:1845-1850.

Ontogeny of B cells, and their Abnormal Development in Immunodeficiency Diseases

Max D. Cooper[1], Peter D. Burrows[2] and Hiromi Kubagawa[3]

Cellular Immunobiology Unit of the Tumor Institute, Departments of Pediatrics[1], Microbiology[1,2], and Pathology[3] and The Comprehensive Cancer Center, University of Alabama at Birmingham, Birmingham, Alabama 35294, USA

A fairly comprehensive, albeit still incomplete, picture of the life history of B lineage cells is now available. Some of the key steps in this process are depicted in Figure 1, which outlines the generation of IgM-producing members of a B cell clone. When multipotent hemopoietic stem cells migrate from the yolk sac into the embryonic liver, some of their progeny begin differentiation along the B cell pathway; later this process continues in the bone marrow.

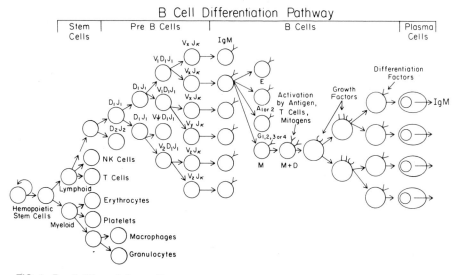

FIG. 1. B cell differentiation pathway.

Development along the B cell pathway can be divided into two discontinuous phases of population growth and cell differentiation. The initial phase concerns the generation of large numbers of clonally diverse B cells via a series of immunoglobulin gene rearrangements that occur in cascade fashion in a fixed order. The second phase concerns the growth and differentiation of selected clones of B cells that can be induced by antigen or mitogens, with the help of activated T cells and their soluble growth-and differentiation-promoting factors.

Differentiation of B lineage cells is also featured by a changing array of cell surface molecules. While membrane-bound immunoglobulins are expressed by B cells from the moment of their birth in hemopoietic tissues until terminal plasma cell differentiation, the pattern of immunoglobulin isotypes which B cells express changes during their maturation. Likewise, some non-immunoglobulin molecules are expressed only on immature B cells, whereas other are expressed in increasing amounts as a function of maturation. Receptors for growth and differentiation factors are expressed following B cell activation.

This differentiation scheme can be used as a map to chart the progression of B cells and some of the defects of B cell differentiation that result in antibody deficiency diseases. In this paper, we will briefly discuss some new information about B cell differentiation, controversies and gaps in our knowledge about this process, and efforts to define the differentiation abnormality for certain antibody deficiency diseases.

Orderly rearrangement and unexpected expression of immunoglobulin genes during B cell ontogeny

It is well established that heavy chain genes are rearranged and expressed before the light chain gene loci are (7,20,34, reviewed in refs. 17 and 53), and that attempts to achieve a productive $V-J_L$ rearrangement usually begin in the kappa gene family (26). $D-J_H$ rearrangements preceed $V-DJ_H$ rerrangement (4), the success of which allows transcription and processing of complete μ chain mRNA.

It comes as a surprise that $DJ_H-C\mu$ transcripts are generated, and may be translated along with a leader-like sequence (45). Even more surprising is recently obtained evidence suggesting that V_H genes may be transcribed in their germline configuration, even before the $D-J_H$ rearrangement process begins (57). This raises the question of the role of these gene products. One idea is that V_H and $DJ-C\mu$ products may be involved in clonal selection during the pre-B cell stage. This seems an unlikely possibility in view of the failure to find $DJ-C\mu$ or V_H gene products on the surface of pre-B cells (17,20,34; our unpublished observations). Alternatively, V_H and $DJ-C\mu$ transcripts or products could serve as signals for the initiation of the next step in the cascade of Ig gene rearrangements. So far there is no experimental data, nor indeed a clear hypothesis, concerning the mechanism(s) underlying the orderly sequence of immunoglobulin gene rearrangements and expression that is so evident during ontogeny (17).

Productive VDJ_H or VJ_L rearrangements on one chromosome appear rarely to be followed by additional rearrangement events on the homologous chromosomes (see refs. 4 and 53). Thus the pre-B cell apparently can sense the successful rearrangement events. This has lead to the idea that either the transcripts or the complete heavy and light chain products may in some way suppress further V gene rearrangements and this could explain *the* allelic exclusion phenomenon (e.g. 2,54).

The unresolved puzzle of heavy chain class switching

Many features of isotype switching are now well recognized. Immature B cells all express IgM. During clonal development, either before or after IgD expression, some IgM^+ B cells begin to express one of the γ, α or ε C_H genes (reviewed in ref 16) which are located on chromosome 14 in the following order: $C\mu$, $C\delta$, $C\gamma_3$, $C\gamma_1$, $C\psi\varepsilon$, $C\alpha_1$, $C\psi\gamma$, $C\gamma_2$, $C\gamma_4$, $C\varepsilon$, $C\alpha_2$ (5,18,41). Each of these C_H genes, except for $C\delta$, is preceded by a switch region composed of repetitive nucleotide sequences. Isotype switching is accomplished by cutting and splicing of the switch region of μ with the switch region 5' of the downstream heavy chain gene to be expressed next (reviewed in ref. 10). In order to switch from IgM to IgG_1 for example, the intervening DNA, including the $C\mu$, $C\delta$ and $C\gamma_3$ genes, would be deleted, thus bringing the $C\gamma_1$ gene next in line for transcription with the VDJ complex. It is *somewhat* surprising that this rearrangement process can be highly variable for the non-productive C_H gene locus on the homologous chromosome: the occurrence of deletion or persistence of 5' C_H genes, combinations of deletion and duplication of 5' genes, and deletions extending 3' of the expressed C_H gene (56) suggests that isotype-specific recombinases are probably not used by the B cell to switch its Ig isotype. Whatever the initiating mechanism, isotype switching can occur by DNA deletion in both normal and neoplastic B cells, and has even been observed in transformed pre-B cell clones undergoing an isotype switch (9). It is also noteworthy that isotype switching is not a random process. For example, neoplastic clones are preprogrammed for the isotype which they will express on switching (3,8,35,40,50).

In order to explain the simultaneous expression of membrane-bound IgM and an IgG or IgA isotype, several investigators have proposed that the initial B cell switch may involve differential processing of a long nuclear transcript extending from 5' of VDJ through all or most of the C_H gene loci (3,27,44). Much of the earlier evidence favoring this idea, however, has not been substantiated in subsequent studies (9,30). Although this remains a viable issue, it seems more likely that B cells may express multiple isotypes (e.g., IgM, IgD and IgG_1) simply because of temporary persistence of μ/δ mRNA and heavy chain products following the switch by DNA deletion.

Another unresolved issue is the role that T cells play in isotype switching. One view is that isotype switches occur as an integral part of the cascade of Ig gene rearrangements, beginning soon after completion of a productive VJ_L rearrangement (10,17). In support of this idea, immature B cells have been shown to undergo isotype switching in the absence of T cells (1,11). According to this hypothesis, the istoype-committed B cells can then be *selected* for preferential help by T cells and their soluble factors to undergo clonal expansion and differentiation (cf. 32, 33). A popular alternate view is that T cells produce «switch factors» which *instruct* B cells to undergo isotype switches. In support of the latter hypothesis, T cell clones and soluble factors have been identified which promote differentiation of IgM bearing cells into plasma cells producing IgG or IgA (29, 31, 39). In one such model system (29), however, $BCDF\gamma_1$ was found to activate a subpopulation of isotype-precommitted B cells (37). Thus the argument about whether T cells govern the isotypes produced in an antibody response through instruction or selective induction continues to rage.

The pathways which B cells take during isotype switching are also still debated. Evidence exists in support of sequential B cell switching in the 5' to 3' order of the C_H genes (21, 42), while other data suggest that direct switches from $C\mu$ to each of the downstream C_H genes is the usual rule for normal B cells (1, 36, 55). The resolution of these outstanding issues will require more precise information on the regulatory mechanisms involved in istoype switching.

What causes X-linked agammaglobulinemia (XLA)?

The study of immunodeficiency diseases began around 30 years ago with the discovery of XLA (6). This disease is characterized by a severe deficit in plasma cells and their secreted antibody products (23, 25) due to a paucity of precursor B cells (15). Although circulating B cells are reduced by approximately 100-fold, normal numbers of pre-B cells appear to be generated in the bone marrow of affected boys (43). Thus, it has been concluded that XLA represents a differentiation arrest in B cell development, and the search for the nature of the genetic defect has centered around the pre-B to B cell transition.

The results of one elegant series of studies led Schwaber and his coworkers to conclude that XLA pre-B cells produce short μ heavy chains lacking the V_H gene-encoded segment (47). The experimental approach involved rescue of pre-B cells in bone marrow samples from 3 XLA patients by hybridizing them with a «non-producer» human hybridoma cell line (LSM 2.7) established in culture (49). The hybridomas were shown to produce truncated μmRNA and μ chain products. Similarly, truncated μmRNA and μ chains were produced by a hybridoma which was formed by fusing normal fetal liver cells with the LSM 1.7 cells. The latter was thought to reflect fusion of cell belonging to a subpopulation of pre-B cells in fetal liver that failed to react with the polyclonal anti-V_H reagent used in this study.

Studies in our laboratory have reached a different conclusion. A panel of monoclonal anti-V_H antibodies made against $V\mu$ fragments from IgM parapro-teins and shown to react with different V_H subgroups, were found to react with pre-B cells in both normal and XLA bone marrow samples. However, the low frequencies of V_H^+ cells and the limited amounts of μ chains in both instances precluded detailed biochemical analysis. To circumvent this prob-lem, XLA and normal pre-B cells were transformed by Epstein-Barr virus (EBV), as accomplished previously by Fu *et al.* (19), and the μ chain products analyzed by immunochemical procedures. Pre-B cell lines from three XLA patients were found to produce μ chains of normal size and glycosylation characteristics (Fig. 2). Normal sized μ chains could also be immunoprecipi-tated by the anti-V_H antibody (MH44), and J_H rearrangement patterns could be demonstrated by use of a J_H probe for restriction fragment analysis of DNA from these pre-B cell cultures (our unpublished observations). Thus our data suggest that the heavy chain genes in pre-B cells of XLA patients undergo normal rearrangement and expression.

These results are not easily reconciled with those of Schwaber and his coworkers. One possible explanation is that we have examined different genetic forms of XLA. This can be resolved by exchanging patient-derived samples of pre-B cells. Another possibility is that EBV-transformation and cell fusion select different subpopulations of pre-B cells for study. However, in one case the XLA pre-B cells were EBV-transformed before fusion with LSM 2.7 cells for study (47). Finally, a trivial explanation could be the derivation and unusual characteristics of the LSM 2.7 fusion partner used for constructing pre-B cell hybridomas. The LSM 2.7 cell line was originally derived from fusion of normal blood mononuclear cells with a 6-thioguanine (6-TG)-resistant, Ig non-producing variant of an IgG_k human myeloma cell line, and subsequently reselected for resistance to 6-TG (49). Since it has been *stated* (48) that the LSM 2.7 cell line does not produce Ig, lacks detectable mRNA for Igs and has deleted *the Cμ* genes, the short μmRNA and μ chains found in the pre-B hybridomas (47) probably are not merely products of the LSM 2.7 fusion partner. One of the unusual characteristics of this partner cell line was that all hybridis between LSM 2.7 cell line and human splenic or blood cells ceased to secrete Ig molecules 28 to 42 days post-fusion (49). *Thus it could be helpful in resolving this issue to compare the μmRNA and μ chain products of hybridomas formed by fusions of LSM 2.7 and XLA pre-B cells with those by LSM 2.7 x normal pre-B cell fusions..*

It is noteworthy that XLA patients consistently produce a limited number of B cells which express complete IgM and IgD molecules in their membrane (14, 52). Moreover, these B cells can be induced to divide and differentiate into antibody secreting plasma cells of all major isotypes, albeit in highly variable numbers even in the same family (24). These results suggest that all of the normal immunoglobulin gene rearrangements can take place in XLA

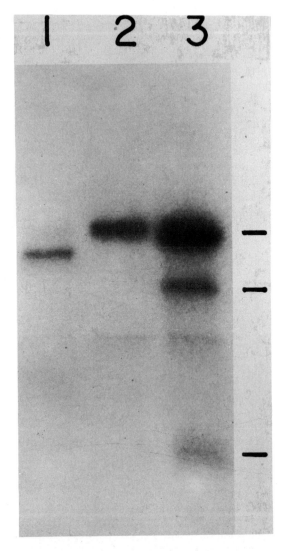

FIG. 2. Immunoglobulin biosynthesis by EBV-transformed pre-B cells from a patient with XLA. *Lane 1:* 69 kd unglycosylated μ chains produced by XLA pre-B cells. *Lane 2:* 74 kd glycosylated μ chains produced by XLA per-B cells. *Lane 3:* Normal μ (74 kd), α (59 kd) and light (23 kd) chains produced by EBV-transformed B cells from a normal individual.

B lineage cells, but do not exclude a rate limiting step in the cascade. For example, a rate-limiting defect in V-J_L rearrangement process could be postulated.

We have used a panel of monoclonal anti-B cell antibodies to examine the circulating B cells in boys with XLA (52). The results of these studies and the similar studies of Conley (14), reveal a striking level of immaturity of the XLA B cells in comparison with the B cell populations in both normal individuals and those affected with a variety of other antibody deficiency diseases. For example, most of the circulating B cells in XLA patients do not express sufficient levels of the C3d/EBV receptor to be detected with the HB5 antibody and, like normal immature B cells, express detectable levels of the HB7 (T10) antigen. Thus another possible explanation for the B cell deficit in XLA is that the X chromosomal defect retards maturation in a way that impedes survival of the B cells in affected boys.

An interesting and unexpected finding in our analysis of XLA patients was an indication that the population of circulating T cells is also relatively immature. The HB10 antibody, which reacts with virgin T cells and not activated or *memory* T cells (51), was found to be expressed by approximately 90% of the circulating T cells of XLA patients as compared with around 50% of the T cells in normal individuals. This could be explained as a secondary consequence of the T cell deficit, assuming that B cells may play an even more important role in T cell antigen presentation and activation than would be expected (For review, see ref. 28). Alternatively, the X gene defect could affect both B and T cell development, albeit in different degrees. This hypothesis is rendered more attractive by the recent discovery of a family of genes on the X chromosome which may be expressed in both T and B cells and a defect of which may account for an X-linked immunodeficiency in inbred mice (12, 13). The identification of a family of comparable genes on the X chromosome in humans may thus provide greater insight into the genetic basis of XLA.

Hyper-IgM immunodeficiency: An intrinsic B cell or switch T cell defect?

The production of elevated levels of IgM in the face of very low or undetectable IgG has also been seen in females and as an acquired disorder (see review in ref. 46). Impaired isotype switching is not simply due to the deletion of Cγ or Cα genes (Gary V. Borzillo, unpublished results) and appears to be the basic biological abnormality in these patients, a conclusion that is supported by studies of the *immunocompetent* cells from affected individuals (22, 38). Two pathogenetic mechanism have been proposed for this switch defect. The first hypothesis is that the switch defect operates at the level of the B cell. This idea is supported by the following observations in affected boys: 1) absence of B cells and plasma cells expressing IgG or IgA isotypes, 2) inability to induce their B cells to express IgG or IgA isotypes following mitogen stimulation in the presence of normal T cells or following EBV transformation, and

3) the ability of their T cells to normally enhance IgG and IgA responses of normal B cells (38). Thus the defect could be one of a switch enzyme gene on the X chromosome.

An alternate hypothesis is that the hyper IgM syndrome may reflect an impairment of switch T cells. This idea is supported by the suppression of IgM and induction of IgG production when B cells from an affected individual were cultured with leukemic «switch» T cells (39). (The latter were Sezary cells that could support IgG and IgA responses of IgM$^+$ tonsillar B cells). Thus, it has been suggested that T cells may secrete a switch recombinase activator (39). Presumably the signaling activity of these factors would require complementary receptors on the B cell surface.

Since the hyper-IgM immunodeficiency is a genetically polymorphic disorder, it is likely of course that multiple pathogenetic mechanisms may be operative. Thus each affected individual must be analyzed as a separate experiment of nature.

In an attempt to determine whether the isotype switch failure is due to an inherent abnormality of the B cell, we have examined the B cells from the mother of an affected boy (A.C., in ref. 38). The mother was selected for study because she proved to be heterozygous for the X gene encoded glucose-6-phosphate dehydrogenase (G6PD) isoenzyme. Her G6PD phenotype was A/B, whereas the son with the isotype switch defect was A. Theoretically, this could provide an opportunity to determine which X chromosome can be utilized by switched maternal B cells. To examine this, the mother's B cells were transformed by EBV infection and then cloned. Clones of her B cells which were producing either IgM, IgG or IgA were then selected and the G6PD isoenzyme determined. If all of the IgG and IgA producing clones had utilized the X chromosome carrying the G6PD type B gene, this would have supported the idea of an inherent B cell defect. Instead we found both clones of type A and ones of type B among the IgM, IgG and IgA clones. This result might be interpreted as an argument against the idea of an intrinsic abnormality of the B cell. However, we have since learned that the mother's brother, who also has the G6PD type A isoenzyme, does not share the switch defect with his nephew. Thus the gene defect in this boy could represent either a spontaneous new mutation of an X gene or an inherited autosomal gene abnormality. Additional studies are clearly needed of this and other families with affected individuals to *elucidate* the genetic mechanism(s) involved in regulation of isotype switching.

Acknowledgements

This work was supported by grants CA 16673 and CA 13148, awarded by the National Institutes of Health. We thank C. Tate Holbrook, Gary V. Borzillo, and Nancy C. Martin for providing patient materials and unpublished data and excellent technical assistance, respectively, and E. Ann Brookshire for preparing the manuscript.

REFERENCES

1. Abney, E.R., Cooper, M.D., Kearney, J.F., Lawton, A.R., and Parkhouse, R.M.E. (1978): Sequential development of immunoglobulin on developing mouse B lymphocytes: a systematic survey that suggest a model for the generation of immunoglobulin isotype diversity *J. Immunol.*, 120:2041-2049.
2. Alt, F.W., Rosenberg, N., Enea, V., Siden, E., and Baltimore, D. (1982): Multiple immunoglobulin heavy chain gene transcripts in Abelson murine leukemia virus-transformed lymphoid cell lines. *Mol. Cell. Biol.*, 2:386-400.
3. Alt, F.W., Rosenberg, N., Casanova, R.J., Thomas E., and Baltimore D. (1982): Immunoglobulin heavy chain expression and class switching in a murine leukemia cell line. *Nature*, 296:325-331.
4. Alt, F.W., Yancopoulos, G.D., Blackwell, T.K., Wood, C., Thomas, E., Boss, M., Coffman, R., Rosenberg, N., Tonegawa, S., and Baltimore D. (1984): Ordered rearrangement of immunoglobuline heavy chain variable region segments. *EMBO J.*, 3:1209-1219.
5. Bech-Hansen, N.T., Linsley, P.S., and Cox, D.W. (1983): Restriction fragment length polymorphisms associated with immunoglobulin C genes reveal linkage disequilibrium and genomic organization. *Proc. Natl. Acad. Sci. U.S.A.*, 80:6952-6956.
6. Bruton, O.C. (1952): Agammaglobulinemia. *Pediatrics*, 9:722-728.
7. Burrows, P.D., LeJeune, M., and Kearney, J.F. (1979): Evidence that murine pre-B cells synthesize μ heavy chains but not light chains. *Nature*, 280:838-841.
8. Burrows, P.D., Beck, G.B., and Wabl, ML.R. (1981): Expression of μ and γ immunoglobulin heavy chains in different cells of a cloned mouse lymphoid line. *Proc. Natl. Acad. Sci. U.S.A.*, 78:564-568.
9. Burrows, P.D., Beck-Engese, G.B., and Wabl, M.R. (1983): Immunoglobulin heavy-chain class switching in a pre-B cell line is accompanied by DNA rearrangement. *Nature*, 306:243-246.
10. Burrows, P.D. and Cooper, M.D. (1984): The immunoglobulin heavy chain class switch. *Mol. Cell. Biochem.*, 63:97-113.
11. Calvert, J.E., Kim, M.F., Gathings, W.E., and Cooper, M.D. (1983): Differentiation of B lineage cells from liver of neonatal mice. Generation of immunoglobulin isotype diversity *in vitro. J. Immunol.*, 131:1693-1697.
12. Cohen, D.E., Hedrich, S.M., Nielsen, E.A., D'Eustachio, P., Ruddle, F., Steinberg, A.D., Paul, W.E., and Davis, M.M. (1985): Isolation of a cDNA clone corresponding to an X-linked gene family (XLR) closely linked to the murine immunodeficiency disorder *xid. Nature*, 314:369-372.
13. Cohen, D.I., Steinberg, A.D., Paul, W.E., and Davis, M.M. (1985): Expression of an X-linked gene family (XLR) in late stage B cells and its alteration by the *xid* mutation. *Nature*, 314:372-374.
14. Conley, M.E. (1985): B cells in patients with X-linked agammaglobulinemia. *J. Immunol.*, 134:2070-2074.
15. Cooper, M.D., Lawton, A.R., and Bockman, D.E. (1971): Agammaglobulinemia with B lymphocytes: Specific defect of plasma cell differentiation. *Lancet*, ii:791-795.
16. Cooper, M.D., Kearney, J.F., Gathings, W.E., and Lawton, A.R. (1980): Effects of anti-Ig antibodies on the development and differentiation of B cells. *Immunol. Rev.*, 52:29-54.
17. Cooper, M.D., Velardi, A., Calvert, J.E., Gathings, W.E. and Kubagawa, H. (1983): Generation of B cell clones during ontogeny. In: *Progress in Immunology, V*, edited by Y. Yamamura and T. Tada, pp. 603-612. Academic Press, Japan, Inc.
18. Flanagan, J.G., and Rabbitts, T.H. (1982): Arrangement of human immunoglobulin heavy chain constant region genes implies evolutionary duplication of a segment containing γ, ε and α genes. *Nature*, 300:709-713.
19. Fu, S.M., Hurley, J.N., McCune, J.M., Kunkel, H.G. and Good, R.A. (1980): Pre-B cells and other possible precursor lymphoid cell lines derived from patients with X-linked agammaglobulinemia. *J. Exp. Med.*, 152:1519-1526.
20. Gathings, W.E., Mage, R.G., Cooper, M.D., and Young-Cooper, G.O. (1982): A subpopulation of small pre-B cells in rabbit bone marrow expresses k light chains and exhibits allelic exclusion of b locus allotypes. *Eur. J. Immunol.*, 12:76-81.
21. Gearhart, P.J., Hurwitz, J.L., and Cebra, J.J. (1980): Successive switching of antibody isotypes expressed within the lines of a B-cell clone. *Proc. Natl. Acad. Sci. U.S.A.*, 77:5424-5428.
22. Geha, R.S., Hyslop, N., Alami, S., Farah, F., Scheneeberger, E.E., and Rosen, F.S. (1979):

Hyper immunoglobulin M immunodeficiency (dysgammaglobulinemia): Presence of im-munoglobulin M-secreting plasmacytoid cells in peripheral blood and failure of immunog-lobulin M-immunoglobulin G switch in B-cell differentiation. *J. Clin. Invest.*, 64:385-391.

23. Gitlin, D. (1955): Low resistance to infection: relationship to abnormalities in gammaglobu-lin. *Bull. New York Acad. Med.*, 31:359-365.

24. Goldblum, R.M., Lord, R.A., Cooper, M.D., Gathings, W.E., and Goldman, A.S. (1974): X-linked B lymphocyte deficiency. I. Panhypo-γ-globulinemia and dys-γ-globulinemia in siblings. *J. Pediatr.*, 83:188-191.

25. Good, R.A. (1955): Studies on agammaglobulinemia. II. Failure of plasma cell formation in the bone marrow and lymph nodes of patients with agammalobulinemia. *J. Lab. Clin. Med.*, 46:167-181.

26. Hieter, P.A., Korsemeyer, S.J., Waldmann, T.A., and Leder, P. (1981): Human immunog-lobulin k light-chain genes are deleted or rearranged in λ-producing B cells. *Nature*, 290:368-372.

27. Honjo, T. (1982) The molecular mechanism of the immunoglobulin class switch. *Immunol. Today*, 3:214-217.

28. Howard, J.C., (1985) Immunological help at last. *Nature*, 312:494-495.

29. Isakson, P.C., Pure, E., Vitetta, E.S., and Krammer, P.H. (1982): T cell-derived B cell differentiation factor(s): Effect on the isotype switch on murine B cells. *J. Exp. Med.*, 155:734-748.

30. Katona, I.M., Urban, J.F., and Finkelman, F.D. (1985): B cells that simultaneously express surface IgM and IgE in *Nippostrongylus brasiliensis*-infected SJA19 mice do not provide evidence for isotype switching without gene deletion. *Proc. Natl. Acad. Sci. U.S.A.*, 82:511-515.

31. Kawanishi, H., Galtzman, L.E., and Strober, W. (1983): Mechanisms regulating IgA class-specific immunoglobulin production in murine gut-associated lymphoid tissues. I. T cells derived from Peyer's patches that switch IgM B cells to IgA B cells *in vitro. J. Exp. Med.*, 158: 649-669.

32. Kiyono, H., Cooper, M.D., Kearney, J.F., Mosteller, L.M., Michalek, S.M., Koopman, W.J., and McGhee, J.R. (1984): Isotype-specificity of helper T cell clones: Peyer's patch Th cell preferentially collaborate with mature IgA B cells in IgA responses. *J. Exp. Med.*, 159:798-811.

33. Kiyono, H., Mosteller-Barnum, L.M., Pitts, A.M., Williamson, S., Michalek, S.M., and McGhee, J.R. (1985): Isotype-specific immuno-regulation: Ig binding factors produced by Fcα receptor-positive T cell hybridomas regulate IgA response. *J. Exp. Med.*, 161:731-747.

34. Kubagawa, H., Gathings, W.E., Levitt, D., Kearney, J.F., and Cooper, M.D. (1982): Immunoglobulin isotype expression of normal pre-B cells as determined by immunofluores-cence. *J. Clin. Immunol.*, 2:264-269.

35. Kubagawa, H., Mayumi, M., Crist, W.M., and Cooper, M.D. (1983): Immunoglobulin heavy chain switching in pre-B leukemias. *Nature*, 301:340-342.

36. Kuritani, T. and Cooper, M.D. (1982): Human B cell differentiation. I. Analysis of immunog-lobulin heavy chain switching using monoclonal anti-immunoglobulin M, G, and A antibodies and pokeweed mitogen-induced plasma cell differentiation. *J. Exp. Med.*, 155:839-851.

37. Layton, J.E., Vitetta, E.S., Uhr, J.W., and Krammer, P.H. (1984): Clonal analysis of B cells induced to secrete IgG by T cell derived lymphokines. *J. Exp. Med.*, 60:1850-1863.

38. Levitt, D., Haber, P., Rich, K., and Cooper, M.D. (1983): Hyper IgM immunodeficiency: A primary dysfunction of B lymphocyte isotype switching. *J. Clin. Invest.*, 72:1650-1657.

39. Mayer, L., Posnett, D.N, and Kunkel, H.G. (1985): Human malignant T cells capable of inducing an immunoglobulin class switch. *J. Exp. Med.*, 161:134-144.

40. Mayumi, M., Kubagawa, H., Omura, G.A., Gathings, W.E., Kearney, J. F., and Cooper, M.D. (1982): Studies on the clonal origin of human B cell leukemia using monoclonal anti-idiotype antibodies. *J. Immunol.*, 129:904-910.

41. Migone, N., Oliviero, S., DeLange, G., Delacroix, D.L., Boschis, D., Altruda, F., Silengo, L., DeMarchi, M., and Carbonara, A.O. (1984): Multiple gene deletions within the human immunoglobulin heavy-chain cluster. *Proc. Natl. Acad. Sci. U.S.A.*, 81:5811-5815.

42. Mongini, P., Paul, W.E., and Metcalf, E.S. (1982): T cell regulation of immunoglobulin class expression in the antibody response to trinitrophenol-Ficoll: evidence for T cell enhancement of the immuno-globulin class switch. *J. Exp. Med.*, 155:884-902.

43. Pearl, E.R., Vogler, L.B., Okos, A.J., Crist, W.M., Lawton, A.R., and Cooper, M.D. (1978): B lymphocyte precursors in human bone marrow. An analysis of normal individuals and patients with antibody-deficiency states. *J. Immunol.*, 120:1169-75.

44. Perlmutter, A.P. and Gilbert, W. (1984): Antibodies of the secondary response can be expressed without switch recombination in normal mouse B cells. *Proc. Natl. Acad. Sci. U.S.A.*, 81:7189-7193.
45. Reth, M.G. and Alt, F.W. (1984): Novel immunoglobulin heavy chains are produced from DJ$_H$ gene segment rearrangements in lymphoid cells. *Nature*, 312:418-423.
46. Rosen, F.S. and Janeway, C.A. (1966): The gamma globulins. III. The antibody deficiency syndromes. *New Engl. J. Med.*, 275:769-775.
47. Schwaber, J., Molgaard, H., Orkin, S.H., Gould, H.J., and Rosen, F.S. (1983): Early pre-B cells from normal and X-linked agammaglobulinemia produce C µ without an attached V$_H$ region. *Nature*, 304:355-358.
48. Schwaber, J. (1983): Pre-B cells in X-linked agammaglobulinemia. In: *Primary Immunodeficiency Disease*, edited by R.J. Wedgwood, F.S. Rosen and N.W. Paul, pp. 177-182. March of Dimes Birth Defects Foundation, Alan R. Lis, Inc., New York.
49. Schwaber, J.F., Posner, M.R., Schlossman, S.F., and Lazarus, H. (1984): Human-human hybrids secreting pneumococcal antibodies. *Hum. Immunol.*, 9:137-143.
50. Stavnezer, J., Sirlin, S., and Abbott, J. (1985): Induction of immunoglobulin isotype swithing in cultured 1.29 B lymphoma cells: Characterization of the accompanying rearrangements of heavy chain genes. *J. Exp. Med.*, 161:577-601.
51. Tedder, T.F., Clement, L.T., and Cooper, M.D., (1985): Human lymphocyte differentiation antigens HB-10 and HB-11. I. Ontogeny of antigen expression. *J. Immunol.*, 134:2983-2988.
52. Tedder, T.F., Crain, M.J., Kubagawa, H., Clement, L.T., and Cooper, M.D. Evaluation of lymphocyte differentiation in primary and secondary immunodeficiency disease. (Submitted for publication).
53. Tonegawa, S. (1983): Somatic generation of antibody diversity. *Nature*, 302:575-581.
54. Wable, M. and Steinberg, S. (1982): A theory of allelic and isotypic exclusion for immunoglobulin genes. *Proc. Natl. Acad. Sci. U.S.A.*, 79:6976-6978.
55. Webb, C.F., Gathings, W.E., and Cooper, M.D. (1983): Effect of anti-3 antibodies on immunoglobulin isotype expression in lipopolysaccharide-stimulated cultures of mouse spleen cells. *Eur. J. Immunol.*, 13:556-559.
56. Webb, C.F., Cooper, M.D., Burrows, P.D., and Griffin, J.A. (1985): Immunoglobulin gene rearrangements and deletions in human EBV-transformed cell lines producing different IgG and IgA subclasses. *Proc. Natl. Acad. Sci. U.S.A.* (in press).
57. Yancopoulos, G.D. and Alt, F.W. (19859: Developmentally controlled and tissue-specific expression of unrearranged V$_H$ gene segments *Cell*, 40:271-281.

Regulation of B Cell Responses

F. Melchers

Basel Institute of Immunology, Basel Switzerland

«In vitro» analysis of B lymphocyte proliferation and differentiation has given insights into the mechanism of cellular cooperations and molecular activities which control these processes. In this paper I present a summary of our current knowledge that has previously been published in papers and review articles (10, 6, 11, 12, 13,14). This knowledge should enable a through investigation into the possible deregulations of these processes that might contribute to immnodeficiency syndromes.

The majority of B lymphocytes in the immune system are resting cells, arresting in the Go phase of the cell cycle. When antigen enters the system it stimulates to proliferation and maturation to immunoglobulin (Ig) secretion those B cells which possess antigen-binding Ig molecules on their surface. One B cell produces only one specificity of Ig, though in many copies; a wide variety of Ig molecules with different binding capacities is produced by a wide variety of different B cells. B cells can also be stimulated in polyclonal ways, e.g. by the binding of antibodies with specificities for constant regions of Ig, i.e. of light or μ-heavy chains (7, 18). Polyclonal activation such as lipopolysaccharides (LPS) or lipoproteins even circumvent this binding to surface-bound Ig, when they stimulate B cells polyclonally (1, 8).

Although the selection of B cells for activation is initiated by the binding of either antigen or Ig-specific antibodies to surface Ig, or by the binding of polyclonal activators to B cells, neither of these binding reactivities to B cells is sufficient to trigger them to proliferation and for maturation to Ig secretion. Other cells must cooperate (15, 16). In T-cell dependent responses of B cells helper T cells and accessory cells (A cells) cooperate, while in T-cell independent responses only A cells appear to be needed. The cooperation is needed on two levels: for one, helper T cells and A cells each provide a set of growth and maturation factors, often also called lymphokines, which act on B cells; for the other helper T cells interact with B cells and antigen in major histocompatibility comples (MHC) antigen-restricted ways to control the cell cycle of B cells.

T cell-dependent B cell responses

Growth and maturation factors for B cells are produced by the endocrine system of helper T cells and A cells, in which A cells (usually macrophages or monocytes, or dendritic cells) take up and process antigen to represent it on their surface. This processed antigen is then recognized together with MHC-class II-antigens on the surface of A cells by the antigen-specific, MHC-class II antigen-restricted T cell receptor of helper T cells. This recognition leads to the activation of A- and T cells and to the production and secretion of lymphokines. We have called the B cell-active lymphokines produced by A cells α-factors, those produced by helper T cells β factors. The most purified model cells for A cells are macrophage colonies grown in the presence of colony-stimulatory factors in semi-solid media, or the P388Dl macrophage line. Model cells for helper T cells are the cloned, long-term growing helper T cells which show specificity for a given antigen and are restricted by a given MHC antigen. T-cell independent activation of these model A cells can be achieved by polyanions such as dextransulfate, agar mitogen, LPS or lipoprotein at low concentrations (4, 5), while cloned helper T cells can be activated antigen- and A-cell-independently by Concanavalin A. These conditions for activation yield conditioned media, which are sources for α- and β factors, that can further be enriched by biochemical purification procedures.

The action of lymphokines on resting B cells

Neither α- or β-factors alone, nor the combination of both, induce proliferation in resting, G_o-phase B cells. Maturation to Ig secretion, however, occurs, with much the same kinetics that are customary for proliferation-dependent maturation of the same cells. This maturation without proliferation, in fact, leads to the inability of the maturing B cells to subsequently respond to proliferation-inducing signals (9).

Therefore, resting B cells have to be excited to become susceptible to the action of α- and β factors. In T-cell dependent responses excitation occurs when helper T cells interact via their antigen-specific, MHC-restricted receptors with B cells that either have bound antigen via surface Ig or have processed antigen in ways similar to A cells, and that present antigen in the context of MHC-class II antigens. T cell-dependent excitation of B cells, in the specificity and restriction of interaction, therefore, closely resembles the interaction of T cells with A cells which lead to α- and B-factor production. It becomes evident that only antigen-specific B cells only with the right class II-MHC antigens on their surface are excited. This guarantees the antigen specificity of a B cell response in the immune system.

Polyclonal activation by Ig-specific antibodies

Antibodies with specificities for constant regions of light or μ-heavy chains can excite B cells from their resting state. This has recently been shown to be true for monoclonal antibodies specific for either one of the four constant region domains of the murine μ-H chain (7). Crosslinking of surface Ig on the B cells appears to be mandatory, as most antibodies must be presented to the B cells in immobilized, i.e. probably repetitively binding, forms (18). Here, excitation is not MHC-class II-antigen-restricted, as B cells of different MHC haplotypes can be excited. Proliferation of B cells, however, needs the activity of α- and β-factors. Purified, particularly A-cell depleted, B cell populations do not initiate DNA replication and do not go through mitosis when exposed to immobilized Ig-specific antibodies alone.

Polyclonal activation by polyclonal activators such as LPS

Mitogens such as LPS excite B cells of different MHC haplotypes poly-clonally. They, therefore, circumvent the requirements of occupancy of either surface Ig or surface class II antigens. Again, A-cell depleted B cell popula-tions do not initiate DNA replication and do not divided when excited by LPS (4). In contrast to Ig-specific antibodies, however, only α-factors produced by A cells, but not β factors, are needed to do so after excitation. LPS, therefore, replaces the action of β factors in the cell cycle.

Polyclonal activation of B cells by Ig-specific antibodies resembles the antigen-specific activation by T-cell independent antigens of type II, while activation by LPS resembles that by T-independent antigens of Type I (17). Again, both T-independent antigens of Type I and of Type II are usually structured as repetitive antigenic determinants, that may allow crosslinking of surface Ig on B cells.

Not all B cells are activated, even by the polyclonal activators, to enter cell cycle and divide. This strongly suggests, but does not prove, differently reac-tive B cell subpopulations. In studies with murine B cells mostly newly gener-ated, relatively immature, primary B cells appear to be mainly studied, while in the human case peripheral blood B cells may be enriched for longer-lived, memory-type B cells. This may in part explain the discrepancies that have been observed in the mechanisms of proliferation control between murine and human B cell populations.

Cell cycle control

Resting B cells are activated asynchronously from their resting state into the cell cycle. Remarkable is the discrepancy between this asynchronous entry into DNA replication and mitosis on the one side, and the synchrony in early changes after excitation, that lead to depolarization of the membrane, Ca^{++} uptake, activation of phosphatidylinositol metabolism, expression of myc-and fosproto oncogenes and many other biochemical parameter (3, 10). Once in cell cycle, remarkable synchrony for several divisions has been observed for single clones of B cells (2). We have recently succeeded in synchronity polyc-lonally activated, A-cell depleted B cell populations by size selection through velocity sedimentation (12, 13). In the presence of either Ig-specific antibodies, α- and β factors, or of LPS and α-factors these synchronized B cells continue to divide synchronously every 20 hours at 37°C for at least the next five divisions. Neither of the stimuli alone are sufficient to stimulate even one further round of division. In the presence of α- and β-factors, but in the absence of Ig-specific antibodies, cells undergo one more cycle and then stop. This indicates, that Ig-specific antibodies (and in T cell-dependent, antigen-specific, MHC-class II-restricted B cell responses: antigen and the T cell-receptor) are needed at the beginning of each cell cycle to excite B cells to susceptibility for α- and β-factors. Controlled addition and removal of α- and β-factors, and of Ig-specific antibodies during the B cell cycle have shown that the cell cycle is controlled by three restriction points.

The first restriction point occurs directly after mitosis and is controlled by the occupancy of surface Ig. The second is observed around four to six hours after mitosis in the G1 phase of the cell cycle, i.e. before DNA replication. This restriction point is controlled by α-factors produced by macrophages. We have recently found that crosslinked C3b and C3d replaces the action of α factors at this point in the cell cycle (13). In contrast, soluble C3d inhibits the action of α-factors at this point. This indicates that the C3d-specific complement receptor CR2, specifically expressed on B cells, controls this cell cycle point. It further suggest, that this receptor signals differently to B cells depending on its state of crosslinking and/or up- and down regulation. C3d, in summary, controls the B cell cycle at a point where epidermal growth factor controls fibroblast growth, and where nerve growth factor controls nerve cell growth. It is, therefore, all the more interesting that a comparison of the recently published cDNA sequence of murine C3d reveals weak, though significant homology with those of murine EGF, NGF and IGF-II. It indicates, that an insulin-like growth factor could be the active principle of α-factors produced by macrophages (13).

The third restriction point occurs in the G2 phase, two to four hours before mitosis, and is controlled by β factors produced by helper T cells. It is interesting to recall that it is at this late point in G2 that sister chromatids could undergo unequal crossing over. This mechanism has been implied in heavy chain class switching that, in turn, has been suggested to be controlled by helper T cells. A prolonged stay at this point in the cell cycle, controlled by *lack* of help, i.e. of β factors, would increase the probability for such unequal crossing-over, and, thus, maybe of class switching. The structure of B-factors, and of their corresponding receptors on B cells, remain to be elucidated.

Possible immunodeficiencies of the B cell cycle

A series of factors and receptors and their functioning in the control of the B cell cycle can now be assayed for in the known cases of murine immunodeficiencies. These assays should include tests for α-factor production by A cells, β-factors production by T cells, excitation of B cells and B cell cycle control by α- and β-factors. These functional assays should be useful correlates to the assays that eventually will probe the expression of the genes for the factors and receptors involved in B cell cycle control. If they can be established also for human B cells, a much wider variety of documented immunodeficiencies in the human will become amenable for the same analysis.

Acknowledgements

The Basel Institute for Immunology was founded and is supported by F. Hoffmann-La Roche & Co. Ltd.

REFERENCES

1. Andersson, J., Sjöberg, O. and Möller, G. (1972). Induction of immunoglobulin and antibody synthesis *in vitro* by lipopolysaccharide. *Eur. J. Immunol.* 2: 349:353.
2. Andersson, J., Coutinho, A., Lernhardt, W. and Melchers, F. (1977). Clonal growth and maturation to immunoglobulin secretion *in vitro* of every growth-inducible B lymphocyte. *Cell 10:* 27-34.
3. Cambier, J.C., Monroe, J.G., Coggeshall, K.M. and Ransom, J.T. (1985). On the biochemical basis of transmembrane signaling by B lymphocyte surface immunoglobulin. *Immunology Today,* in press.
4. Corbel, C. and Melchers, F. (1983). Requirement for macrophages or for macrophage - or T cell - derived factors in the mitogenic stimulation of murine B-lymphocytes by lipopolysaccharides. *Eur. J. Immunol. 13:* 528-533.
5. Corbel, C. and Melchers, F. (1984). The synergism of accessory cells and of solube α-factors derived from them in the activation of B cells to proliferation. *Immunol. Rev.*
6. Howard, M. and Paul, W.E. (1983). Regulation of B cell growth and differentiation by soluble factors. *Rev. Immunol. 1:* 307-333.
7. Leptin, M., Potash, M.H., Grützmann, R., Heusser, C., Shulman, M., Köhler, G. and Melchers, F. (1984). Monoclonal antibodies specific for murine IgM I. Characterization of antigenic determinants on the four constant domains of the μ-heavy chain. *Eur. J. Immunol. 14:* 534-542.
8. Melchers, F., Braun, V. and Galanos, C. (1975). The lipoprotein of the outer membrane of Escherichia coli: a B lymphocyte mitogen. *J. Exp. Med. 142:* 473-482.
9. Melchers, F., Andersson, J., Lernhardt, W. and Schreier, M.A. (1980). H-2 unrestricted polyclonal maturation without replicaton of small B cells induced by antigen-activated T cell help factors. *Eur. J. Immunol. 10:* 679-685.
10. Melchers, F., Andersson, J., Corbel, C., Leptin, M., Lernhardt, W., Gerhard, W. and Zeuthen, J. (1982). Regulation of B lymphocyte replication and maturation. *J. Cell. Biochem. 19:* 315:332.
11. Melchers, F. and Andersson, J. (1984). B cell activation: Three steps and their variations. *Cells 37:* 715-720.
12. Melchers, F. and Lernhardt, W. (1985). Three restriction points in the cell cycle of activated murine B lymphocytes. *Proc. Natl. Acad. Sci. US,* in press.
13. Melchers, F., Erdei, A., Schulz, Th. and Dierich, M. (1985). Growth control of activated, synchronized murine B cells by the C3d fragments of human complement. *Nature,* in press.
14. Melchers, F., Corbel, C., Leptin, M. and Lernhardt, W (1985). B cell activation and cell cycle control. *J. Cell Science,* in press.
15. Miller, J.F.A.P. and Mitchell, G.F. (1967). The thymus and the precursors of antigen-reactive cells. *Nature 216:* 659.
16. Mosier, D.E. (1967). A requirement for three cell types for antibody formation *in vitro*. *Science 158:* 1573.
17. Mosier, D.H. and Subbarao, B. (1982). Thymus-independent antigens: complexity of B lymphcyte activation revealed. *Immunology Today 3:* 217-222.
18. Parker, D.C. (1975). Stimulation of mouse lymphocytes by insoluble anti-mouse immunoglobulins. *Nature 258:* 365.

A New, X-chromosomal Gene Family (XLR) Expressed in Mature Lymphoid Cells

Mark M. Davis and David I. Cohen

Department of Medical Microbiology School of Medicine
Stanford University - Stanford, CA 94305
Laboratory of Immunology
National Institute of Allergy and Infectious Diseases
National Institutes of Health - Bethesda, MD 20205, USA

INTRODUCTION

For some years it has been noted that a somewhat surprising number of distinct immunodeficiency disorders map to the X chromosome in the human and murine systems. These disorders span a range of developmental defects (references 6, 11, 12, 13 14, summarized in Table 1) from the apparent stem cell deficiency of SCID patients to more subtle B cell maturation and switching disorders. One explanation for this large number of different syndromes occuring on the X chromosome is that there are an unusual number of genes there responsible for immune function. An alternative possibility is that these defects have made themselves more apparent on the X chromosome and less so on autosomes because of the ease with which X chromosomal recessive mutations would show up in males. While this may very well be true for the human disorders. which are very rare, this does not seem to be the case for those in the mouse, since both of the mutant strians, CBA/N and DBA/2H, arose within inbred colonies of mice and both sexes were tested randomly. That is, they were not revealed through and agressive mutagenesis and screening of male progeny comparable to the self-screening that the human population undergoes. In any event, these deficiencies afford us a unique opportunity to correlate some of the B and T cell specific genes of unknown function that we have been isolating over the years (3, 4, 5, 9) with mutations which might help to reveal their particular function. With the possibility of such a correlation in mind, and in collaboration with Drs. P. D'Eustachio and F. Ruddle, we screened a set of 15 Mouse B and T cell specific cDNA clones for X-linkage, using a series of mouse-hamster somatic cell hybrids. One of these cDNA clones, pX 310, hybridizes to a group of 8-10 bands on a southern blot (1) all of which are on the X chromosome. We have designated this family «XLR» for X-linked, lymphocyte-regulated. This gene family has an interesting pattern of expression in B and T cell lymphomas and plasmacytomas and is very likely defective in the xid mutation of the CBA/N mouse (1, 2). It also seems likely that its human equivalent will be involved in one or more of the human disorders outlined in Table 1.

TABLE 1.   *X-Linked Immunodeficiency Diseas*

Human	Cells Affected (ref.)
Severe Combined Immunodeficiency (SCID)	T,B (13)
Wiskott-Aldrich	T,B. Platlets (13)
Bruton's Agammaglobulinemia	pre-B (13)
Agammaglobulinemia with growth hormone deficiency	pre-B (6)
Lymphoproliferative Syndrome	B (1)
Hyper IgM, reduced IgG, IgA	Plasma Cells (13)
Hyper IgM, IgG, reduced IgA	Plasma Cells (14)
Murine Defects	
CBA/N (xid)	B(11)
DBA/2Ha	B (12)

The XLR locus is expressed in both T and B lymphocytes

Analysis of RNA preparations indicates that members of the XLR family are expressed in both B and T cell tumor lines (2). Although the precise pattern of T cell expression is not yet clear, a survey of a large number of different B lineage murine tumors (Table 2) indicate that XLR is only expressed in very late stage B cells. In particular, only cells at the pre-secretory and secretory stages express any detectable message from this family. This characteristically takes the form of a 1200 nt species in the pre-secretory cells and a 1150 nt and 1050 nt doublet in the plasma cells and hybridomas (2). We have even seen this difference in a situation from a plasma cell line as a non-secret-

TABLE 2.   *XLR Expression (from ref. 2)*

Stage	Ig	J	14G8	XLR
pre-B	cyto μ	−	+	−(1/9)
early B	mIgM	−	+	−(0/2)
inter B	mIgM mIgD	−	+	−(0/3)
Late B	mIgM	−/+	−	+(3/3)
Plasma Cell (wt)	sIg	+	−	++12/12)
(.xid)	sIg	+	N.D.	−(0/3)

ory variant (M315P and M315J, ref. 2, 7). This indicates a remarkable plasticity in the expression of this locus and a close correspondence to the phenotype of the cell. We do not yet know how many distinct species might underlie these specific molecular weight RNAs nor whether those expressed in the different B cells stages are the same as those observed in various T cell tumors and hybrids. These studies are currently underway. One may conclude, however, that XLR has a very interesting pattern of expression, that it is helpful in defining the later stages of B cell maturation, and that various proteins in this family are shared between specific B and T cell subpopulations.

Correlation of XLR with the xid Defect

Three principle lines of evidence indicate an association between at least some members of the XLR family and the *xid* defect. The first of these is the fact that the *xid* defect alters the usual pattern of XLR expression in plasmacytomas. Specifically, of 12 wild plasmacytomas assayed, all 12 transcribed XLR mRNA, whereas none of the three *xid* mutant plasmacytomas did (as summarized in table 2). Secondly, the B cell tumors which transcribe XLR have caracteristics of those B cells which are absent from the spleens of mice with the *xid* defect (8, 10). In particular, the spleens of *xid* mice have very few mature B cells lacking the 14G8 marker (10) and these are precisely the B cell tumors which transcribe XLR. This interesting inverse correlation between 14G8 and XLR is also shown in table 2. Therefore the expression of XLR in B cells correlates exactly with one aspect of the *xid* phenotype (high incidence of 14G8 expression). Finally, Southern analysis of the DNA of mice congenic for the *xid* trait revealed restriction fragment length polymorphisms in the XLR family derived from the *xid* background (12). Since these congenic mice should have only 5-10 centimorgans of DNA surround *xid* from the *xid* background, this shows that at least some membrs of the XLR family are closely linked to *xid*. Thus, both linkage and expression studies suggest a close relationship between the XLR gene family and the *xid* defect.

Properties of the XLR Protein

The translated sequences of full-length XLR cDNA clones contain an open reading frame of 208 amino acids encoding a protein of 24 kilodaltons. This protein is strikingly hydrophilic, and is overall somewhat acidic. Since it possesses no leader peptide or transmembrane sequence, the protein is unlikely to be membrane-associated, but may instead be cytoplasmic or nuclear. No N-linked glycosylation sites are found. Interestingly, the amino and carboxy termini are quite acidic, while a central core is highly basic. In addition, this basic central core is flanked on both sides by lys-arg residues, which are sites for potential proteolytic cleavage. Whether this protein possess DNA binding properties or is subject to proteolytic cleavage and where it is located in normal cells is currently under investigation.

CONCLUSION

In these studies, we have characterized a new X-linked gene family. In doing so, we have defined a new problem and a new family of proteins by first isolating a cDNA clone encoding one of these proteins. This reverses the usual procedure in which definition of the protein typically permits isolation of the gene. Current data suggests very strongly that this gene family is involved in the B cell defect of the *xid* mouse. In addition, the human equivalents of these genes may very well be involved in some of the many human X-linked immunodeficiencies. The recent finding that a human B cell tumor line transcribes RNA homologous to XLR means that the human probes may soon be in hand to address this question.

REFERENCES

1. Cohen, D.I., Hedrick, S.M., Nielsen, E.A., D'Eustachio, P., Ruddle, F., Steinberg, A.D., Paul, W.E., and Davis, M.M. (1985). Isolation of a cDNA clone corresponding to an X-linked gene family (XLR) closely linked to the murine immunodeficiency disorder *xid. Nature* 314:372-374.
2. Cohen, D.I., Steinberg, A.D., Paul, W.E., and Davis, M.M. (1985). Expression of an X-linked gene family (XLR) in late-stage B cells and its alteration by the *xid* mutation. *Nature* 314:369-372.
3. Davis, M.M., Cohen, D.I., Nielsen, E., DeFranco, A.L., and Paul, W.E. (19829: The isolation of B and T cell specific genes. In: *B and T Cell Tumors: Biological and Clinical Aspects.* Vitetta, E., and Fox, C.F. (Eds.), UCLA Symposium, Vol. XXIV, Academic Press, New York.
4. Davis, M.M., Cohen, D.I., Nielson, E.A., Steinmetz, M., Paul, W.E. and Hood, L. (1984). Cell-type-specific cDNA probes and the murine I region: the localization and orientation of A_α. *Proc. Natl. Acad. Sci. USA* 81:2194-2198.
5. Davis, M.M., Chien, Y., Gascoigne, N.R.J., and Hedrick, S.M. (1984). A murine T cell receptor gene complex: isolation, structure and rearrangement. *Immunol. Rev.* 81:234-257.
6. Fleisher, T.A., White, R.M., Broder, S., Nissley, S.P., Blaese, R.M., Mulvihill, J.J., Olive, G., and Waldmann, T.A. (1980). X-linked hypogammaglobulinemia and associated growth hormone deficiency. *New Engl. J. Med.* 302:1429-1434.
7. Gebel, H.M., Autry, J.R., Rohrer, M., and Lynch, R.G. (1979). In vitro and in vivo studies of a TNP-binding IgA lymphoma isolated from MOPC-315, a TNP-binding IgA plasmacytoma of BALB/C mice. *J. Natl. Cancer Inst.* 62:201-212.
8. Hardy, R.R., Hayakawa, K., Parks, D.R., Herzenberg, L.A., and Herzenberg, L.A. (1984). Murine B cell differentiation lineages. *J. Exp. Med.* 159:1169-1188.
9. Hedrick, S.M., Cohen, D.I., Nielsen, E.A., and Davis, M.M. (1984). The isolation of cDNA clones encoding T cell-specific, membrane-associated proteins. *Nature* 308:149-153.
10. Kung, J.T., Sharrow, S.O., Ahmed, A., Habbersett, R., Scher, I., and Paul, W.E. (1982). B lymphocyte subpopulations defined by a rat monoclonal antibody, 14G8. *J. Immunol.* 128:2049-2056.
11. Scher, I., (1982). The CBA/N mouse strain: an experimental model illustrating the influence of the X-chromosome on immunity. *Adv. Immunol.* 33:2-71.
12. Takatsu, K., and Hamaoka, T. (1982) DBA/2Ha mice as a model of an X-linked immunodeficiency which is defective in the expression of TRF-acceptor site(s) on B lymphocytes. *Immunol. Rev.* 64:35-55.
13. Waldmann, T.A., Stober, W. and Blaese, R.M. (1980). T and B cell immunodeficiency diseases. in *Clinical Immunology.* edited by C.W. Parker, Vol. 1, pp. 314-375, W.B. Saunders, New York.
14. Waldmann, T.A. Personal communication.

Role of Ion Channels in the Activation of T Lymphocytes

Sudhir Gupta

Division of Basic and Clinical Immunology
University of California, Irvine, CA 92717, USA

INTRODUCTION

Ion channels are essential for the function of excitable cells, (e.g. nerve and muscle) in a number of species, including humans. It is well established that ion fluxes across the membrane of lymphocytes play an important role in triggering the immune response. The evidence has primarily come from tracer studies and from the use of dyes as indicators of changes in membrane potential or internal ion concentrations (19, 41, 49). Until recently direct measurement of ion currents in lymphocytes was impossible because of their small size (5-10 μM). However, the gigaohm seal patch clamp technique has permitted the study of ion currents in T lymphocytes, myeloma cells and macrophages (9-11, 13-17, 20-22, 35, 50). In this paper I will review the role of ion channels in T cell activation, proliferation, in response to mitogens, alloantigens, autoantigens and T cell receptor-complex, production of interleukins, and cytotoxic effector T cell functions.

MATERIAL AND METHODS

Peripheral blood mononuclear cells and T cells (purified by rosetting with sheep red blood cells) were obtained from healthy volunteers.

Ion Channel Blockers: 4-aminopyridine (4-AP, K^+ channel blocker), tetraethylamonium (TEA) and Quinine (both "maxi" K^+ channel blockers), verapamil and diltiazem (both Ca^{2+} channel blockers), and tetrodotoxin (specific Na channel blocker) were used.

Proliferative responses: Response to phytohemagglutinin (PHA) and in the autologous mixed lymphocyte reaction (MLR) were performed by a standard microtiter culture technique.

IL-2 Production: IL-2 production in response to PHA was measured on IL-2 dependent CTLL cell line (10).

IL-2 Receptor Expression: Purified T cells activated with PHA were examined for the expression of IL-2 receptor, using monoclonal anti-Tac antibody and FACS analyzer.

Cytotoxic T lymphocytes (CTL): CTL were generated in the MLR and tested against blast cells from stimulator.

Gigaohm seal recording technique: T cells were studied at 20-24°C using the gigaohm seal recording technique in whole cell or outside-out patch conformation (9). The method requires the formation of a very tight seal, greater than 5 gigaohm (1 gigaohm = 10^9 ohms) between a clean glass fire polished pipette (housing a micro-electrode) and the cell membrane. The high electrical resistance of the seal enables current flowing through single channel to be recorded against a low background noise level, it also allows the potential across the patch of membrane to be varied in a controlled manner (voltage-clamped). In the outside-out patch recording the external surface of the patch of membrane is exposed to bathing solution. Isolated patch allows the properties of the single ion channel to be studied under controlled ionic conditions. In the whole cell recording configuration the patch of membrane under the pipette is ruptured by applying strong suction giving access to cell interior. It is possible to control the membrane potential of the cell and record whole cell currents. As a result of the rupture of the cell membrane the solution in the pipette exchanges with the cytosol of the cell so that one can modify the intracellular ion concentrations.

RESULTS AND DISCUSSION

Ion Channels in T Lymphocytes

The predominant ion channel in human T cells is a voltage-gated K^+ channel (9, 10, 11, 13, 15, 36). Lymphocyte K^+ currents turn on with a sigmoid time course upon depolarization and then inactivated completely, with voltage dependence and kinetics that closely resemble delayed rectified K^+ channels of muscle and nerve. K^+ channels in human T lymphocytes can be blocked by 4-aminophyridine, (4-AP) and tetraethylamonium (TEA) with one to one drug molecule, channel stoicheiometri (15). K^+ currents were also blocked by non-specific Ca^{2+} activated K^+ channel blockers and by Ca^{2+} channel blockers, virapamil and diltiazem (15). The mean K^+ conductance in human T lymphocytes is 4.2 nS (9). The estimate number of K^+ channels per cell is 400, corresponding to approximately 3 channels/μm^2 membrane area. The gating kinetics of K^+ channels depend on permeant cations present in the external solution. This would suggest interactions between permeant ions and the gating apparatus of the channel. Increasing the external K^+ concentration from 4.5 mM to 160 mM shows the deactivation time constant about 2 folds, whereas replacing Rb^+ Ringer for K^+ ringer slows deactivation about 5 fold. These effects of external K^+ and Rb^+ ions upon K^+ channel gating kinetics of human T cells are more pronounced than in nerve and muscle (4, 5,8,48). The voltage dependence of activation and deactivation kinetics and the peak conductance of voltage-gated K^+ channel in human T cells (9) resembles qualitatively with the delayed rectifer K^+ currents in squid axon (28), myelinated nerve (4), skeletal muscle fiber (6, 42, 47) or in frog skeletal muscle fibers (42, 47); however K^+ channels in T lymphocytes close about 10 times slower than do K^+ channels in skeletal muscle fibers (9). The inactivation of K^+ currents upon maintained depolarization is several time slower in murine cytotoxic T cell clone (21) and in murine cultured macrophages (51) than in human peripheral blood T lymphocytes but the kinetics of recovery from inactivation are similar. Human T lymphocyte K^+ channels dispaly two amplitude of single channel current events, of 9 and 16 Ps conductance. Ypey and Clapham (51) have also observed 16 Ps of unitary conductance of K^+ channels in murine cultured macrophages.

At resting potential approximately 0.1 to 2 K^+ channels are open at a given time (9), the net K^+ efflux through a single open channel is estimated to be 100-200 attomoles/min/cell. The estimated totale efflux of K^+ would then be 10-400 attomoles (attomole = 10-18 moles) per min/cell. Resting Rb^+ or K^+ efflux measured in human lymphocytes is about 50-100 attomoles per min per cell (26, 45). We have demonstrated that PHA rapidly shifts the K^+ conductance voltage relationship to more negative potentials (15). Based on the conductance voltage curve measured before and after addition of PHA a shift of about -15 mV was observed. This should increase the K^+ efflus through an open K^+ channel approximately 5-10 fold. PHA has also been reported to increase K^+ or Rb^+ efflux in human T lymphocytes by 50-100% (26-29). Owens and Kaplan (41) have shown that suspensions of Balb/c splenic lymphocytes took up ^{86}Rb at net rate of 4.6 fmol per hour per cell before stimulation with Con A and of 8.5 fmol (100% increase influx) per hour per cell following stimulation. The net transport rates were of similar magnitude to those of resting and stimulated peripheral blood human lymphocytes. The only difference between human and mouse systems is the increased transport noted within minutes of stimulation in human and require approximately 6 hours in mouse lymphocytes. ^{86}Rb efflux from Con A -treated Balb/c splenocytes rise to a rate 40% higher than that from resting cells. This imbalance between the magnitude of increase in influx (100%) and efflux (40%) could account for the increased number of K^+ ions required to be transported into the cell water in order that concentration of K^+ ion be kept constant during the enormous expansion of cell volume characteristic of blastogenesis.

Several investigators have provided evidence to suggest an important role of passive influx of Ca^{2+} ions and an elevated levels of cytosolic free CA^{2+} in early stages of T cell activation, proliferation and interleukin 2 production upon stimulation with mitogens, and antibody against T cell differentiation antigen, the T3 and T3-Ti receptor complex (49, 19, 34, 54, 23, 38, 3, 40, 33, 52, 53, 29, 55, 37, 27, 18, 32, 1, 39, 35, 43). These data have led to the logical suggestion that the Ca^{2+} influx may be due to activation of Ca^{2+} selective channels. Oettgen et al (40) have present evidence to suggest that the T3-T receptor complex of human T lymphocytes may be an antigen-regulated Ca^{2+} channel, which indeed could be a K^+ channel. Although Ca^{2+} channels have been observed in murine myeloma cells (20) but no Ca^{2+} channel currents have been observed either in human T lymphocytes (9) or in murine cytotoxic T cell clones (21). We have observed that potassium channel blocker (4-AP) will inhibit PHA-induced increase in intracellular Ca^{2+} as demonstrated by Quin-2 dye. This would suggest that Ca^{2+} ions may pass through K^+ channels. Inoue (30) observed that delayed rectifier K^+ channels in squid axon are sparingly permiable to Ca^{2+}. This would also suggest that Ca^{2+} might enter T lymphocytes through the voltage gated K^+ channels. Based upon the Ca^{2+} permiability of K^+ channel in squid axon we estimated that about 4000 Ca^{2+} ions/second might enter the T cells through K^+ channel (9). Although this level of permiability to Ca^{2+} appears to be very low compared with that for K^+, the calculated current carried by Ca^{2+} through K^+ channel is only about an order of magnitude lower than the current carried by Ca^{2+} through Ca^{2+} channels at physiological levels of Ca^{2+}. If following T cell activation an additional K^+ channel is opened, the intracellular free Ca^{2+} concentration in the absence of buffering would double in about 3 second; however due to cytoplasmic buffering the free Ca^{2+} levels would rise more slowly. Therefore Ca^{2+} could enter the T cell through K^+ channel without depolarizing the membrane. Despite these observations, the existance of highly labile Ca^{2+} channels or of Ca^{2+} channels which are activated or maintained in a functional state by some normal cytoplasmic constituent cannot be ruled out.

Small Na^+ current have been observed in a subset of human T lymphocytes (9) and in 25% of T cells from MRL +/+ mice (16). Tetrodotoxin, a sodium channel blocker had no inhibitory effect on PHA induced ^3H thymidine incorporation by T lymphocytes (9). This could suggest that either the Na^+ channels are not required for T cell proliferation or alternatively Na^+ channels are necessary for mitogenesis or other functions in only a small subset of T lymphocytes.

Ion Channels and Immune Function Mitogenesis

We have examined the role of functional K^+ channels on ^3H thymidine incorporation and ^3H leucine incorporation by human peripheral blood T cells upon stimulation with PHA, using a number of chemically unrelated substances that are known to block K^+ currents and Ca^{2+} currents. Quinine, 4-AP and TEA inhibit PHA-induced ^3H thymidine incorporation in human T lymphocytes in a dose dependent manner with the similar potency sequence as for channel block (10). Verapamil and diltiazem, two organic calcium channel blockers also inhibit PHA-induced ^3H thymidine incorporation at concentrations similar to those required to block the T lymphocyte K^+ channel. 4-AP inhibited PHA-induced ^3H thymidine incorporation when added to the cultures during first 30 hours (10); however in the AMLR, the inhibitory effect of 4 AP, TEA, Verapamil and Quinine was observed when these agents were added as late as 3 days of cultures (unpublished data). This inhibitory effect was not due to nonspecific cytotoxicity. Tetramethylamonium (TMA), an analogue of TEA that do not block K^+ channel, did not inhibit PHA-induced ^3H thymidine incorporation. Human T lymphoblastoid cell line, CCRF-HSB2 lacks K^+ channels and 4-AP had no effect on ^3H thymidine incorporation by cells of these cell lines (10). All these observations support the specificity of the channel blockers and the role of K^+ channels in ^3H thymidine incorporation by T lymphocytes.

The effect of ion channel blockers was also examined on T cells activated in the AMLR and MLR. T cells stimulated in the AMLR were most sensitive, followed by T cells activated in MLR and then the PHA activated T cells (Table 1). Since the precursor frequency of T cells activated with PHA >

TABLE 1. *Relative Sensitivity of PHA−, MLR− and AMLR− activated T cells to Ion Channel Blockers*

Activated T Cells	Concentrations 4AP (mM)	Required for TEA (mM)	50% Bloc Q (μM)
PHA	2,1	13,0	33,0
MLR	< 1,0	6,0	25,0
AMLR	0,25	< 1,25	6,5
K Current	1,9	8,0	14,0

MLR > AMLR, it is likely that least number of T cells in the AMLR have open K^+ channels, whereas maximum number of PHA activated T cells have open channels and therefore, the differences in sensitivity to ion channel blockers.

We have also shown that Quinine, TEA and 4 AP also inhibit ^3H Leucine incorporation in PHA-activated T cells in the same potency sequence as for block of K^+ channel currents and inhibition of ^3H thymidine incorporation (10).

The proponent of Ca^{2+} channel theory have shown the influx of Ca^{2+} and increase in the free intracellular cytosolic Ca^{2+} levels following stimulation with mitogen or antigen, including antibodies against T cell antigen-receptor complex, (34, 54, 23, 38, 3, 40, 33, 52, 53, 29, 55, 37, 27, 18, 32, 1, 39, 35, 48). Since we did observe any Ca^{2+} channel in T lymphocytes, we believe that the rise in intracellular free cytosolic Ca^{2+} and influx of Ca^{2+} is via K^+ channels.

Interleukin Production and Interleukin-2 (IL-2) Receptor Expression

Interleukin 2 (IL-2) is an 15,000 dalton protein that is produced primarily by helper T cells (although suppressor T cells upon appropriate stimulation can also produce IL-2) and is required for T cell proliferation, differentiation of cytotoxic T lymphocytes (CTL), and enhances natural killer cell function (24). The production of IL-2 is dependent upon signal from macrophage that can be replaced by interleukin 1 (IL-1). IL-2 mediates its effects via its receptors on activated lymphocytes. IL-2 receptors are not presynthesized and require RNA and protein synthesis for its expression (24). We have examined the effect of 4-AP on IL-2 production by PHA-stimulated mononuclear cells. 4-AP at a concentration that completely inhibits ^{3}H thymidine incorporation inhibited the production of IL-2 (10). Since IL-1 is required for the production of IL-2 and because the macrophages have voltage-gated K^+ channels, we examined the effect of ion channel blockers on IL-1 production by lipopolysaccharide activated human peripheral blood monocytes and mouse macrophage cell line (P-338D). K^+ channel blockers markedly inhibited IL-1 production by activated macrophages (25, 50). Therefore ion channel blockers mediated inhibiton of IL-2 production by mononuclear cells could be due to their effects on both T cells and macrophages.

Because ion channel blockers block the PHA-induced protein synthesis, we expected that the ion channel blockers will also inhibit the expression of IL-2 receptors. However, we did not observe any effect of 4 AP, TEA and Quinine on IL-2 receptor expression on PHA-activated T cells (10). This would suggest that IL-2 receptor expression does not require K^+ channels. Recently Mills et al (38) have also reported that Ca^{2+} fluxes and increased intracellular free Ca^{2+} are required for IL-2 production but not for the IL-2 receptor expression. However, Birx et al (7) have reported decreased IL-2 receptor expression on Con A activated T cells in the presence of Ca^{2+} channel blockers. The reason for this discrepancy is unclear at the present time. Johnson et al (31) have shown that IL-2 helper signal for γ-interferon production is Ca^{2+} dependent. We have demonstrated that exogenous purified IL-2 will overcome the block of 4 AP (at low concentration) on PHA induced ^{3}H thymidine incorporation (10). Recently we have examined the effect of recombinant IL-2 on 4 AP, Quinine, Verapamil and TEA induced inhibition of ^{3}H thymidine incorporation in the AMLR (AMLR is a very sensitive system to examine the effect of ion blockers and growth factor, unpublished observations). IL-2 (20-40 unit) overcome the 90% block of various in channel blockers (Fig. 1). These results will be consistent with our observations that channel blockers inhibit IL-2 production and not the IL-2 receptor expression as well as the observations of Mills et al (39) that IL-2 induced proliferation is independent of increases in free intracellular cytoplasmic Ca^{2+}.

Cytotoxic T Lymphocyte (CTL) Function

Fukushima et al (21) have reported the presence of voltage-gated K^+ channels in murine cytotoxic T cell clone. Conjugation of cytotoxic T cells with target cells during the lethal hit phase is accompanied by increase in K^+ conductance and ^{86}Rb efflux. We have investigated the role of K^+ channels in the generation of cytotoxic T lymphocytes (afferent phase) and in the

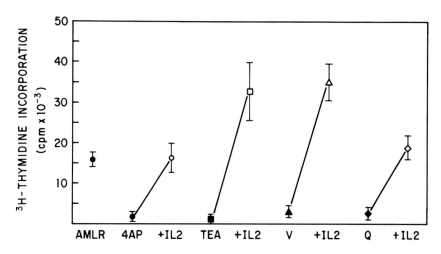

FIG. 1. The in vitro effect of recombinant interleukin 2(IL-2) to override the 4-aminopryidine (4-AP), tetraethylamonium (TEA), Verapamil (V) and Quinine (0) on PHA-induced T cell proliferation. IL-2 was used at 20 units/ml.

effector cytotoxic function (efferent phase). K^+ channel blockers inhibited the generation of CTL in a dose dependent manner (unpublished observations). The differentiation of precursor CTL to effector CTL requires IL-2. Therefore, it would be of interest to know whether IL-2 will override the block and will reconstitute the CTL generation in the presence of ion channel blockers. We also examined the effect of 4-AP and TEA on target cell killing by $T4^+$ and $T8^+$ T cells (as CTL effectors) generated in the MLR (12). Both blockers reversibly inhibited CTL-mediated target cell lysis in a dose dependent manner. TMA neither blocked the channel nor inhibited target cell lysis. 4 AP and TEA did not cause any cytotoxicity to effector or target cells. These experiments demonstrate the role of K^+ channels during killing however do not segregate whether the channel blockers, (during lethal hit phase), are acting on effector cells or target cells or both.

SUMMARY

In this paper I have reviewed our work and those of others with regard to role of ion channels in T cell functions. Gigaohm seal recording data provided direct evidence of existance of only voltage-gated K^+ channels in T lymphocytes. Investigation are in progress to examine the role of functional K^+ channels in early events of cells activation e.g. phosphorylation of membrane, induction of c-fos, c-myc, and cMyb cellular genes, the expression of cyclic nucleotides and the expression of protein kinases etc. The electrophysiological, immunological and molecular approaches together should be instrumental in clarifying the role of ion channel in the transmission of signals from membrane to the cell nucleus.

Acknowledgement

Part of work cited here was supproted by USPHS grants: AI-21808, A1-20717 and AG-04361.

REFERENCES

1. Abboud C.N., Scully S.P., Lichtman A.H., Brennan J.K. and Segel G.B. (1985). The requirements for ionized calcium and magnesium in lymphocyte proliferation. *J. Cell Physiol.* 122:64-72.
2. Adrian R.H., Chandler W.K. and Hodgkin A.L. (1970). Voltage-clamp experiments in striated muscle fibers. *J. Physiol.* 208:607-644.
3. Altwood G., Asherson G.L., Jean Davey M. and Goodford P.J. (1971). The early uptake of radioactive calcium by human lymphocytes treated with phytohemagglutinin. *Immunology* 21:509-516.
4. Arhem P. (1980). Effects of rubidium, calcium, strontium, barium and lanthanum on ionic currents in myetinated nerve fibers from xenopus laevis. *Acta. Physiol. Scand.* 108:7-16.
5. Beam K.G. and Donaldosn P.L. (1983). Slow components of potassium tail currents in rat skeletal muscle. *J. General Physiol.* 81:513-530.
6. Beam K.G. and Donaldson P.L. (1983). A quantitative study of K^+ channel kinetics in rat skeletal muscle from 1 to 37°C. *J. General Physiol.* 81:485-512.
7. Birx D.L., Berger M. and Fleisher T.A. (1984). The interference of T cell activation by calcium channel blocking agent. *J. Immunol.* 133:2904-2909.
8. Cahalan M.D. and Pappone P.A. (1983). Chemical modification of potassium channel gating in frog myelinated nerve by trinitrobenzene sulphonic acid. *J. Physiol.* 342:119-143.
9. Cahalan M.D., Chandy K.G., DeCoursey T.E. and Gupta S. (1985). A voltage-gated potassium channel in human T lymphocytes. *J. Physiol.* 358:197-237.
10. Chandy K.G., DeCoursey T.E., Cahalan M.D., McLaughlin C. and Gupta S. (1984). Voltage-gated potassium channels are required for human T lymphocyte activation. *J. Exp. Med.* 160:369-385.
11. Chandy K.G., DeCoursey T.E., Cahalan M.D. and Gupta S. (1985). Ion channels in lymphocytes. *J. Clin. Immunol.* 5:1-6.
12. Chandy K.G., Sharma B., DeCoursey T.E., Cahalan M.D. and Gupta S. (1985). K channel requirement in human T cell-mediated cytotoxicity. *J. Allergy Clin. Immunol.* 75:187-192.
13. Chandy K.G., De Coursey T.E., Cahalan M.D. and Gupta S. (1985). Electroimmunology: The physiological role of ion channels in the immune system. *J. Immunol.* (In Press).
14. DeCoursey T.E., Chandy K.G., Fishbach M., Talal N., Cahalan M.D. and Gupta S. (1984). Differences in ion channel expression in T lymphocytes from MRL−lpr and MRL−+/+ mice. *Fed. Proc.* 43:1736.
15. DeCoursey T.E., Chandy K.G., Gupta S. and Cahalan M.D. (1984). Voltage-gated K^+ channels in human T lymphocytes: a role in mitogenesis? *Nature* 307:465-468.
16. DeCoursey T.E., Chandy K.G., Fishbach M., Talal N., Gupta S. and Cahalan M.D. (1985). Potassium channel expression in proliferating murine T lymphocytes. *Fed. Proc.* 44:1310-1315.
17. DeCoursey T.E., Chandy K.G., Fishbach M., Talal N., Gupta S. and Cahalan M.D. (1985). Two type of K channels in T lymphocytes from MRL mice. *Biophys. J.* 44:1861-1865.
18. Deutsch C. and Price M.A. (1982). Cell calcium in human peripheral blood lymphocytes and the effect of mitogen. *Biochimica et Biophysica Acta.* 687:211-218.
19. Freedman M.H., Raff M.C. and Gomperts B. (1975). Induction of calcium uptake in mouse T lymphocytes by concanavalin A and its modulation by cyclic nucleotides. *Nature* 255:378-383.
20. Fukushima Y. and Hagiwara S. (1983). Voltage gated Ca^{2+} channel in mouse myeloma cells. *Proc. Natl. Acad. Sci. (USA)* 80:2240-2242.
21. Fukushima Y., Hagiwara S. and Henkart M. (1984). Potassium current in clonal cytotoxic T lymphocytes from the mouse. *J. Physiol.* 351:645-656.
22. Gallin E.K. (1984). Calcium-and voltage-activated potassium channels in human macrophages. *Biophys. J.* 46:821-825.
23. Gelfand E.W., Cheung R.K. and Grinstein S. (1984). Role of membrane potential in the regulation of lectin-induced calcium uptake. *J. Cell Physiol.,* 121:533:539.
24. Gupta S. (1985). Interleukins: Molecular and biological characteristics. In *Immunology of Rheumatic Disesaes* Edited by S. Gupta and N. Talal, in press, Plenum Press, New York.

25. Gupta S., Chandy K.G., Vayuvegula B., Ruhling M.L., DeCoursey T.E. and Cahalan M.D. (1985). Role of potassium channels in interleukin 1 and interleukin 2 synthesis and IL-2 receptor expression. In. *Cellular and molecular biology of lymphokines.* Edited by C. Sorg and A. Schimple, in press, Academic Press, N.Y.
26. Hamilton L.J. and Kaplan J.G. (1977). Flux of $^{86}Rb^+$ in activated human lymphocytes. *Canad. J. Biochem.* 55:774-778.
27. Hesketh T.R., Bavetta S., Smith G.A. and Metcalfe J.C. (1983). Duration of the calcium signal in the mitogenic stimulation of thymoctyes. *Biochem. J.* 214:575-579.
28. Hodgkin A.L. and Huxley A.F. (1952). A quantitative description of membrane current and its application to conductance and excitation in nerve. *J. Physiol.* 117:500-544.
29. Imboden J.B., Weiss A. and Stobo J.D. (1985). The antigen receptor on a human T cell line initiates activation by increasing cytoplasmic free calcium. *J. Immunol.* 134:663-665.
30. Inoune I. (1981). Activation-inactivation of potassium channels and development of the potassium-channel spike in internally perfused squid giant axon. *J. General Physiol.* 78:43-61.
31. Johnson H.M., Vassallo T. and Torres B.A. (1985). Interleukin 2-mediated events in γ-interferon production are calcium dependent at more than one site. *J. Immunol.* 134:967-970.
32. Kaibuchi K., Takai Y. and Nishizuka Y. (1985). Protein kinase C and calcium ion in mitogenic response of macrophage depleted human peripheral blood lymphocytes. *J. Biol. Chem.* 260:1366-1369.
33. Lederman H.M., Lee J.W.W., Cheung R.K., Grinstein S. and Gelfand E.W. (1984). Monocytes are required to trigger Ca^{2+} uptake in the proliferative response of human T lymphocytes to staphylococcus aureus protein A. *Proc. Natl. Acad. Sci. (USA)* 81:6827-6830.
34. Luckasen J.R., White J.G. and Kersey J.H. (1974). Mitogenic properties of a calcium inophore, A23187. *Proc. Natl. Acad. Sci. (USA)* 71:5088-5090.
35. Maino V.C., Green N.M. and Crumpton M.J. (1974). The role of calcium ions in initiating transformation of lymphocytes. *Nature* 251:324-327.
36. Matteson D.R. and Deutsch C. (1984). K channels in T lymphocytes: A patch clamp study using monoclonal antibody adhesion. *Nature* 307:468-471.
37. Metcalfe J.C., Pozzan T., Smith G.A. and Hesketh T.R. (1980). A calcium hypothesis for the control of cell growth. *Biochem. Soc. symp.* 14:1-26.
38. Mills G.B., Cheung R.K., Grinstein S. and Gelfand E.W. (1985). Increase in cytosolic free calcium concentration is an intracellular messenger for the production of interleukin 2 but not for expression of the interleukin 2 receptor. *J. Immunol.* 134:1640-1643.
39. Mills G.B., Cheung R.K., Grinstein S. and Gelfand E. (1985). Interleukin 2 induced lymphocyte proliferation is independent on increases in cytosolic-free calcium concentrations. *J. Immunol.* 134:2431-2435.
40. Oettgen H.C., Terhorst C., Cantley L.C. and Rosoff P.M. (1985). Stimulation of the T3 T cell receptor complex induces a membrane-potential-sensitive calcium influx. *Cell.* 44:583-590.
41. Owens T. and Kaplan J.G. (1980). Increased cationic fluxes in stimulated lymphocytes of the mouse response of enriched B- and T- cell subpopulations to B- and T- cell mitogens. *Canad. J. Biochem.* 58:831-839.
42. Pappone P. (1980). Voltage-clamp experiments in normal and denervated mammalian skeletal muscle fibers. *J. Physiol.* 306:377-410.
43. Parker C.W. (1974). Correlation between mitogenicity and stimulation of calcium uptake in human lymphocytes. *Biochem. Biophys. Res. Comm.* 61:1180-1186.
44. Segel G.B., Gordon B.R., Lichtman M.A., Hollander M.M. and Klemperer M.R. (1975). Exodus of $^{42}K^+$ and $^{86}Rb^+$ from rat thymic and human peripheral blood lymphocytes exposed to phytohemagglutinin. *J. Cell Physiol.* 87:337-344.
45. Segel G.B. and Lightman M.A. (1976). Potassium transport in human blood lymphocytes treated with phytohemagglutinin. *J. Clin. Invest.* 58:1358-1369.
46. Segel G.B., Simon W. and Lichtman M.A. (1979). Regulation of sodium and potassium transport in phytohemagglutinin stimulated human blood lymphocytes. *J. Clin. Invest.* 64:834-841.
47. Stanfield P.R. (1975). The effect of zinc ions on the gating of the delayed potassium conductance of frog sartorium muscle. *J. Physiol.* 251:711-735.
48. Swensen R.P. and Armstrong C.M. (1981). K^+ channels close move slowly in the presence of external K^+ and Rb^+. *Nature* 291:247-429.
49. Tsien R.Y., Pozzan T. and Rink T.J. (1982). T-cell mitogen cause early changes in cytoplasmic free Ca^{2+} and membrane potential in lymphocytes *Nature* 295:68-71.
50. Vayuvegula B., Butler G., Chandy K.G., Ruhling M.C. and Gupta S. (1985). Requirement of functional K^+ channel for interleukin 1 production. *Fed. Proc.* 44:1861.

Role of Calcium on Gamma Interferon Production

F. Dianzani, G. Antonelli and M.R. Capobianchi

Institute of Virology, University of Rome
Viale di Porta Tiburtina 28, 00185 Rome, Italy

Mitogenic, as well as antigenic, stimulation of gamma interferon (gamma IFN) production by human peripheral blood mononuclear cells (PBMC) occurs through oxidation of galactose residues on the cell membrane (3, 5, 7). A role for calcium was suggested by finding that gamma IFN production was stimulated by the calcium ionophores A23187 (4) and ionomycin (2) and was confirmed by observation that IFN production did not occur in the presence of the chelating agent ethylene glycol-bis (Beta-aminoethyl ether) -N, N-tetraacetic acid (EGTA) (7). Since these data indicated that activation of a calcium flux through the cell membrane could be a second specific event, after oxidation of membrane-bound galactose residues, leading to genetic derepression of gamma IFN locus, experiments were planned to explore the role of calcium in IFN induction by oxidizing agents, conventional mitogens, and specific antigens.

Role of calcium in IFN induction by mitogens

A first approach to test the role of calcium in IFN induction by mitogens and oxidizing agents was to stimulate Ficoll-Hypaque PBMC from healty human donors with various specific and nonspecific mitogens in the presence or absence of EGTA. The results are shown in Table 1.

It can be seen that IFN induction by all mitogens and oxidizing agents tested was prevented by calcium depletion. However it would also be possible, although unlikely, that calcium depletion by EGTA may block IFN induction nonspecifically by affecting some other cell function. To rule out this possibility IFN induction by calcium ionophore A23187 and staphylococcal enterotoxin B (SEB) was performed in the presence of calcium antagonists, whose action has been shown to be highly selective in blocking calcium entry through specific channels (8). The results are shown in Table 2.

TABLE 1.   *Effect of calcium depletion on gamma interferon induction*

Inducer	Gamma interferon production (I.U./ml)*	
	EGTA absent	EGTA present
Galactose oxidase	2000	< 10
Con A	300	< 10
PHA	160	< 10
Staphylococcal enterotoxin A	300	< 10

* No significant variation is observed in different experiments.

TABLE 2.   *Effect of calcium antagonists on gamma IFN production by staphylococcal enterotoxin B-treated peripheral blood mononuclear cells*

Compound	IFN yeld ($\log_{10}$) I.U./ml* in the presence of the compound at a concn of:				
	0	$10^{-3}M$	$10^{-4}M$	$10^{-5}M$	$10^{-6}M$
None (control)	2.8	—	—	—	—
Nitrendipine	—	< 0.5	< 0.5	2.3	2.7
Nitrendipine (photoinactivated)	—	N.D.**	2.4	2.8	3.0
Nisoldipine	—	< 0.5	< 0.5	1.5	2.8
Nimodipine	—	< 0.5	< 0.5	2.8	3.0
Diltiazem	—	N.D.	< 0.5	2.8	2.8
Verapamil	—	0.5	< 0.5	1.0	3.0
Trifluoperazine	—	0.5	< 0.5	1.0	3.0
$MnCl_2$	—	0.5	1.0	2.8	2.8

*   Inhibition of 0.5 $\log_{10}$ is significant ($P \leqslant 0.01$). No significant variation is observed in different experiments.
** ND, Not done.

It can be seen that IFN induction by the mitogen was completely abolished by specific calcium entry blockers (Nitrendipine, Nisoldipine, Nimodipine and Verapamil), by extracellular calcium antagonists ($MnCl_2$ and EGTA), and by an intracellular inhibitor of calmodulin function (trifluoperazine diihydrocloride) (13,14). On the other hand IFN induction by the calcium ionophore A23187 was prevented by calcium depletion (by EGTA and $MnCl_2$) but was not prevented by any of the specific blockers of calcium channels (not shown). This finding is not surprising, since ionophores are capable of causing calcium intake through the membrane bypassing regular calcium channels. Additional experiments (not shown) demonstrated that Procaine, a blocker of sodium channels and photoinactivated nitrendipine did not affect IFN induction (6); moreover simultaneous control experiments showed that the concentrations of the compounds which inhibited gamma IFN production did not have any effect on cell viability (95% survival), on protein synthesis (no significant difference of (^{35} S) methionine incorporation as compared to untreated controls), nor on alpha IFN production after induction with Newcastle disease virus.

Taken togheter these findings clearly show that activation of a calcium flux through specific channels of the cell membrane is indeed critical for mitogenic induction of gamma IFN production. This view is substantiated by the lack of inhibitory activity by specific calcium channel blockers on IFN induction by ionophore A23187, a compound capable of opening new channels through the lymphocyte membrane.

Role of calcium on IFN induction by specific antigens

Oxidation of membrane bound galactose and activation of a calcium flux through the membrane are required steps also in the induction of gamma IFN by antigens in specifically sensitized lymphocytes. In fact PBMC from: *a)* donors showing a strong positive reaction in a routine intradermal tuberculin test; *b)* adult vaccinated volonteers boosted with tetanus toxoid 10 days before blood collection; *c)* donors who in preliminary test had shown particularly strong and early reactivity in a conventional mixed lymphocyte reaction, did produce consistant IFN amount when stimulated with the appropriate antigen. However IFN induction was completely prevented by either enzymatic cleavage of terminal galactose residues or by calcium depletion with EGTA. These latter findings are shown in Table 3.

TABLE 3.   *Gamma IFN induction by antigens in sensitized human lymphocytes*

Inducer	Interferon yield (I.U./ml)* after treatment with:		
	None	B-galactosidase	EGTA
None	< 4	< 4	< 4
PPD	100	8	< 4
Tetanus toxoid	42	< 4	< 4
MLR	160	8	< 4
GO	2000	20	< 4
A23187	300	N.D.**	< 4

* No significant variation is observed in different experiments.
** N.D. not done.

Taken together the data show that oxidizing agents, conventional mitogens and specific antigens activate gamma IFN production through a common pathway, the oxidative alteration of galactose containing glycoprotein of the cell membrane, followed by the activation of a calcium flow across specific channels of the cell membrane.

Macrophages are not required for IFN induction by A23187 and ionomycine

The data do not help define whether the oxidative event occurs directly in the interferon producing cells or in some other type of precursor cell whose mediation is critical for interferon induction. The latter hypothesis is supported by data from our laboratory suggesting that the oxidative changes occur in macrophages (1), cells which have been shown to play a critical role in gamma IFN induction since the early, pioneering work by Epstein (9). It remains to be established, however, whether also the activation of a calcium flux occurs in effector or mediator cells. To test this hypothesis PBMC were depleted of macrophages by sequential adherence to plastic, followed by filtration through a nylon fibre column and the remaining cells were stimulated with mitogens and ionophores. The effectiveness of the procedure used to remove macrophages from the lymphocyte population was tested using monoclonal antibodies OKM_1 and OKT_3. After the depletion procedure the OKM_1 positive cells (macrophages and NK cells) were 4% and the OKT_3 positive cells (T lymphocytes) were 90%. The results are summarized in Table 4.

TABLE 4. *Gamma IFN production by normal and macrophage-depleted human peripheral blood mononuclear cells*

IFN inducers	Gamma IFN (I.U./ml)*	
	Normal	Macrophage-depleted
Staphylococcal enterotoxin B	1000	10
Galactose oxidase	300	< 10
Calcium ionophore	300	300
Ionomycin	300	300

* a three- fold difference in IFN titer is significant at $p \leq 0.05$.

It can be seen that the yield of gamma IFN induced by galactose oxidase and staphylococcal enterotoxin B was considerably diminished when the macrophages were eliminated from the cell population. In contrast, the calcium ionophores (A23187 and ionomycin) induced gamma IFN production whose yield was not affected by depletion of macrophages. These data confirm previous observations (2, 9) on the macrophage requirement for mitogenic activation of lymphocytes but clearly show that the co-operation of macrophages is not required by lymphocytes induced by calcium ionophores; this suggest that ionophores act at a level that is independent and probably subsequent to the event involving the macrophages. Since the A23187 calcium ionophore and ionomycin can bypass the macrophage requirement for gamma IFN production, it is tempting to speculate that a macrophage-derived signal may act through the opening of a calcium channel in T lymphocytes. This hypothesis is supported by the finding that IFN-gamma induction by mitogens and antigens is prevented by calcium depletion or by compounds capable of blocking calcium entry at the cell membrane (8).

Can defects of calcium intake be responsible of immunodeficiency?

Previous data indicate that PBMC from patients with immunoregulatory or lymphoproliferative T disorders exert an impaired gamma IFN production when stimulated *in vitro* with either conventional mitogens or the enzyme galactose oxidase (GO). The defect includes ataxia teleangectasia (AT), immunodeficiency (ID) with hyper-IgM, hyper-IgE syndrome, OKT_4 T-leukemia and occasional common variable immunodeficiency (CVI) patients (10-12).

Data reported in Table 5 and 6 indicate that treatment with the calcium

TABLE 5.   *Gamma IFN production by peripheral blood mononuclear cells from normal donors and OKT_4 T-leukemia patients induced with a conventional mitogen or with calcium ionophore A23187.*

Inducer	Interferon production (I.U./ml) by:			
	Normal donors*	Patients		
		case 1	case 2	case 3
None	< 3	< 3	< 3	< 3
Staphylococcal enterotoxin B	457 (100-500)	20	< 3	< 3
Calcium ionophore	345 (50-500)	100	100	300

* Mean and range of 12 different donors.

TABLE 6.   *Gamma IFN production by peripheral blood mononuclear cells from normal donors and immunodeficiency patients induced with a conventional mitogen or with calcium ionophore A23187.*

Inducer	Interferon production (I.U./ml) by:				
	Normal donors	Immunodeficiency patients			
		ID with Hyper-IgM	Hyper-IgE	CVI	AT case 1	case 2
None	< 3	< 3	< 3	< 3	< 3	< 3
Staphylococcal enterotoxin B	457 (100-50)	< 3	< 3	< 3	< 3	< 3
Calcium ionophore	345 (50-500)	20	30	10	5	20

* Mean and range of 12 different donors.

ionophore A23187 is capable of fully restore gamma IFN production in PBMC from OKT_4 T-leukemia, whereas very low levels of IFN were obtained in AT, ID with hyper-IgM, hyper IgE syndrome and CVI cases.

These results indicate that the defect observed in T-leukemia patients may lie on a stage of lymphocyte activation that preceeds calcium intake into the

T-lymphocyte. However, since the addition of normal macrophages is not capable of bypassing the block of gamma IFN production induced either with SEB or GO (12), it seems reliable that the affected stage is intermediate between the release of macrophage-derived signal and the subsequent activation of calcium flux in the IFN-producing lymphocyte. On the contrary, the impaired gamma IFN production in the other cases seems to be due to a block subsequent to the activation of calcium flux across the lymphocyte membrane.

ACKNOWLEDGMENTS

This work has been supported by grants from CNR, Progetti Finalizzati Controllo Malattie da Infezione n. 84.01849.52 and Oncologia n. 84.00563.44, and from Ministero della Pubblica Istruzione, progetto 40%.

REFERENCES

1. Antonelli, G., Amicucci, P., Codella, G. and Dianzani, F. (1984): Mechanism of induction of interferon gamma: the oxidative event required for induction occurs on macrophages rather than on lymphocytes. *Antiv. Res.* 3: 147.
2. Antonelli, G. and Dianzani, F. (1985): Induction of human interferon-gamma by calcium ionophores: lack of macrophage requirement. *IRCS Med. Sci.* 13: 59.
3. Dianzani, F., Monhahan, T.M., Scupham, A., and Zucca, M. (1979): Enzymatic induction of interferon production by galactose oxidase treatment of human lymphoid cells. *Infect Immun.* 26: 879-882.
4. Dianzani, F., Monahan, T.M., Georgiades, J. and Alperin, J.B. (1980): Human immune interferon: induction in lymphoid cells by a calcium ionophore. *Infect. Immun.* 29: 561-563.
5. Dianzani, F., Monahan, T.M. and Santiano, M. (1982): Membrane alteration responsible for the induction of gamma-interferon. *Infect. Immun.* 26:879-882.
6. Dianzani, F., Capobianchi, M.R. and Facchini, J. (1984): The role of calcium in gamma interferon induction: inhibition by calcium entry blockers. *J. Virol.* 50: 964-965.
7. Dianzani, F., Santiano, M., Ramenghi, U., Capobianchi, M.R. and Antonelli, G. (1985): Membrane events leading to interferon-gamma induction by antigens. *Proc. Soc. Exptl. Biol. Med.* 178: 139-143.
8. Dianzani, F., Antonelli, G. and Capobianchi, M.R. (1985): Induction of human immune interferon with ionophores. *Meth. Enzimol.:* in press.
9. Epstein, L.B.: (1982). The ability of macrophages to augment *in vitro* mitogen and antigen stimulated production of interferon and other mediators of cellular immunity by lymphocytes. In: *Immunobiology of the macrophage,* edited by D.S. Nelson, pp. 201-233 Academic Press, New York.
10. Matricardi, P.M., Capobianchi, M.R., Paganelli, R., Facchini, J. Sirianni, M.C., Seminara, R., Dianzani, F. and Aiuti, F. (1984): Interferon production in primary immunodeficiencies *J. Clin. Imunol.,* 4: 388-394.
11. Paganelli, R., Capobianchi, M.R., Matricardi, P., Cioè, L., Seminara, R., Dianzani, F. and Aiuti, F. (1984): Defective interferon gamma production in Ataxia-Teleangectasia. *J. Clin. Immunol. Immunopathol.,* 32: 387-391.
12. Pandolfi, F., Capobianchi, M.R., Matricardi, P., Facchini, J., Bonomo, G., De Rossi, G., Semenzato, G., Fiorilli, M., Dianzani, F. and Aiuti, F. (1985): Impaired gamma interferon production by cells from patients with lymphoproliferative disorders of mature T and NK cells. *Scand. J. Immunol.* 21, 315-320.
13. Smith, R.D. (1983): Calcium entry blockers: key issue. *Fed. Proc.* 201-206.
14. Weiss, B. and Levin, R.M. (1978): Mechanisms for selectively inhibiting the activation of cyclic nucleotide phosphodiesterase and adenylate cyclase by antipsychotic agents. *Adv. Cyclic Nucleotide Res.* 9: 285-303.

Requirements for the Human T Cell Response to Antigen

Dale T. Umetsu, David Katzen, and Raif S. Geha

From the Department of Medicine, Children's Hospital and the Department of Pediatrics, Harvard Medical School, Boston, MA 02115, USA

Antigen specific proliferation by T lymphocytes requires antigen presentation by accessory cells. The macrophage is the classic APC type and it possesses properties that are required the for activation of T cells. These qualities include the capacity to

1. take up antigen.
2. "process antigen".
3. recycle the antigen to the cell surface in association with Ia antigens.
4. secrete soluble factors such as Interleukin 1 which may be required to activate resting T cells.

There are several other cell types that have the capacity to activate T cells. These include dendritic cells, Langerhans' cells of the skin, and certain B lymphoma cells. Our laboratory has been involved in examining antigen presentation by 2 cell types:

1. Epstein Barr Virus transformed B cells, and
2. human dermal fibroblasts.

I shall present data showing that such cells can indeed present antigen and activate T cells, and I shall discuss how these cell types differ from calssical macrophages.

EBV transformed B cells activate T cells (3). B cells from healthy individuals were transformed with Epstein Barr virus and stable B cell lines were derived. Such EBV-B cells were as capable as monocytes in presenting TT antigen and activating T lymphocyte clones. The extent of T cell proliferation with EBV-B cells was equivalent to that seen in the presence of autologous monocytes. Further, EBV-B cells took up 125I-TT as effectively as did monocytes. In addition, antigen presentation by EBV-B cells appeared to be HLA-DR restricted. For example only HLA-DR3+ EBV-B cells presented antigen to DR3 restricted clones. Antigen presentation was inhibited by antisera to HLA-DR and not by antisera to B2microglobulin.

EBV-B cells do not present antigen to resting T cells (3). Since T cell clones are partially activated and may have less stringent requirements for activation, we next asked if resting T cells present in peripheral blood could be activated by EBV-B cells. Resting T cells were purified from the peripheral blood of three donors who had no detectable serum antibody titers against the EBV capsular antigen. The purification of T cells involved a 5 step procedure and resulted in T cells which were unable to respond to TT or to the mitogen phytohemagglutinin in the absence of added monocytes. In contrast to monocytes, irradiated EBV-B cells were unable to support the proliferation of autologous resting T cells to TT antigen. However, the EBV-B cells presented TT antigen to TT specific autologous T cell blasts, indicating that failure of EBV-B cells to present antigen to resting T cells was not caused by an inability of process TT. Furthermore, the unresponsiveness was not due to suppressive effects of the EBV-B cells. Addition of EBV-B cells to cultures of T cells plus optimal numbers of monocytes caused no decrease in the response. In fact EBV-B cells augmented the ability of suboptimal numbers of monocytes to present TT antigen to resting T cells.

Activation of resting T cells versus T cell clones (2). One possible explanation for the differential response of resting T cells versus T cell clones to antigen presented by EBV-B cells is that T cell clones do not require the soluble factors derived from macrophages, such as IL1. Indeed the proliferative response of resting T cells to antigen was inhibited by rabbit anti-IL 1, but not by normal rabbit serum. In contrast, the proliferative response of T cell blasts to TT presented by monocytes or EBV-B cells was not inhibited by rabbit antihuman IL 1. Furthermore, addition of 10 units/ml of IL 1 to cultures of resting T cells and EBV-B cells allowed the T cells to proliferate to TT antigen although to a lesser degree than in the presence of monocytes. These data suggest that the inability of EBV-B cells to trigger the proliferation of resting T cells to antigen may be due to the inability of the EBV-B cells to secrete IL 1. Direct examination of the capacity of EBV-B cells to secrete IL 1 in response to a variety of stimuli which included *Staph. epidermidis* and Concanavalin A revealed no biologically active IL 1 in the cell supernatants as assessed by a thymocyte costimulator assay.

Four conclusions can be derived from the above data.

1. EBV-B cells fail to trigger proliferation of resting T cells in response to antigen although they efficiently trigger the proliferation of antigen specific T cell blasts.

2. the failure of EBV-B cells to trigger the proliferation of resting T cells to antigen could be reversed by exogenous IL1.

3. EBV-B cells fail to secrete IL 1 under conditions which result in IL 1 release by monocytes.

4. IL 1 is required for the optimal proliferation of resting T cells, but not of activated T cells to antigen.

Antigen presentation by resting B cells. In contrast to EBV-B cells, highly purified irradiated peripheral blood B cells failed to present TT antigen to either resting T cells or T cell clone (1). The failure of resting B cells to present TT was not simply due to their poor capacity to take up antigen. If one managed to attach TT to the surface of resting B cells with a hybrid antibody, this with a rabbit antibody constructed with antibody to human IgM and with antibody to TT, B cells coated with this hybrid antibody and TT still failed to stimulate TT specific T cell clones. When resting B cells were preincubated with such a hybrid antibody, they took up as much 125I radiolabelled TT antigen as monocytes. Yet irradiated resting B cells coated with the hybrid antibody and TT were unable to activate TT specific T cell clones. This failure was not corrected by the addition of IL 1.

A possible explanation for this failure of irradiated resting B cells to present antigen was that these B cells did not generate the immunogenic complex recognized by the T cells. This was indirectly demonstrated by examining the capacity of TT pulsed monolayers of hybrid antibody coated B cells to specifically adsorb TT reactive T cells. As expected, when T cells were adsorbed over monolayers of monocytes pulsed with TT, the capacity of the T cells to respond to TT but not to diptheria toxoid was specifically adsorbed out. If the TT pulsed monocytes were replaced with TT pulsed hybrid coated resting B cells, there was no specific loss of responsiveness to TT. This suggests that irradiated resting B cells may not be able to generate an immunogenic moiety of antigen plus self Ia which is recognized and bound by T cells. In summary:

1. Irradiated resting B cells are unable to present antigen to TT specific T cell clones.
2. This failure is not corrected when B cells are allowed to take up adequate amounts of antigen via the use of a hybrid antibody to IgM and TT.
3. This failure is not corrected by the addition of purified IL1.
4. Irradiated resting B cells appear not to process bound antigen because they are not able to adsorb out TT specific T cells.

Antigen presentation by fibroblasts. There are multiple cell types that have been found to express HLA-DR antigens. These include myeloid cells, endothelial cells, melanocytes, and human dermal fibroblasts exposed to IFN-γ. The presence of HLA-DR antigens on fibroblasts suggested that somatic cell types might function as antigen presenting cells, and we therefore examined the capacity of human dermal fibroblasts to present antigen to T cells (5).

Human T cell clones were cultured with either irradiated fibroblasts, or monocytes as the antigen presenting cells, and proliferation was assessed by thymidine incorporation. Irradiated autologous monocytes, as expected, functioned well in presenting TT. IFN-γ treated fibroblasts were as efficient as monocytes in presenting TT to the clones. On the other hand, fibroblasts which were not treated with IFN, were unable to present TT to these clones. The proliferation of both clones F6 and G8 was antigen and accessory cell dependent, as it did not occur in the presence of TT alone nor in the presence of IFN-treated fibroblasts alone.

The role of HLA-DR antigen on IFN-γ pretreated fibroblasts in T cell proliferation in response to antigen was examined. First, a panel of HLA-DR typed fibroblasts was used to present antigen to Clone G8, which is DR5 restricted when proliferating to TT. HLA -DR5+ fibroblasts but not HLA-DR5– fibroblasts were capable of presenting TT to Clone G8.

Next we examined the effect of monoclonal antibodics to HLA-DR on antigen presentation by IFN treated fibroblast. Addition of monoclonal anti HLA-DR to the cultures abolished T cell proliferation when fibroblasts were the APC. In contrast, monoclonal anti HLA-A,B; monoclonal anti-DC; and an irrelevant monoclonal antibody did not inhibit T cell proliferation. The inhibition seen here with anti DR antibody was not due to binding of the antibody to T cells because proliferation of the T cells in response to IL-2 was not affected. These results taken together support the idea that IFN-γ induced HLA-DR antigens expressed by fibroblasts allows antigen specific IA restricted proliferation of T cell clones to occur.

We next asked if resting T cells could also be activated by IFN- treated fibroblasts. Highly purified peripheral blood T cells were depleted of monocytes. These cells failed to proliferate in response to TT or PHA unless reconstituted with autologous monocytes. Like EBV-B cells, IFN-γ treated fbroblasts failed to present TT antigen to resting T cells. However, fibroblasts enhanced the ability of small numbers of monocytes to present antigen to resting T cells to antigen. In summary:

1. IFN-γ pretreated human dermal fibroblast cultures can present tetanus toxoid antigen to tetanus specific autologous T helper/inducer cell clones.

2. Presentation by DR+ fibroblasts appears to be HLA-DR restricted and can be blocked by anti-DR but not by anti-HLA-A,B or anti-DC monoclonal antibodies.

3. IFN-γ pretreated fibroblast cultures fail to present antigen to highly purified resting T cells.

4. IFN-γ pretreated fibroblast cultures can augment the capacity of monocytes to present antigen to resting T cells.

5. Thus it appears that the requirements to activate a resting T cell may be best provided by a cell of the monocyte/macrophage lineage, but the requirements for activation of cloned T cells can be easily met by multiple IA+ cell types.

In vivo fibroblasts do not normally express surface Ia antigens. Modulation of Ia expression on fibroblasts may be a mechanism by which their antigen presenting activity is regulated as has been suggested for macrophages. We therefore do not suggest that fibroblasts play a primary role in antigen presentation in vivo. Rather they may serve to amplify in vivo immune responses, and allow the ubiquitous fibroblasts to participate in local immune responses.

Sustained Ia expression by dermal fibroblasts in tissues infiltrated by activated T cells may perpetuate the immune response and produce chronic inflamation and tissue injury, as perhaps is seen in contact dermatitis, GVH disease, and other connective tissue disease.

Activation of resting T cells in the absence of accessory cells. We have taken highly purified monocyte depleted resting T cells and asked under what circumstances can they be activated without accessory cells. PHA alone, IL 1 alone, or both in combination are unable to activate these T cells. However, we have found that the combination of recombinant IL 2 plus PHA together can activate these resting T cells to a degree similar to that seen with monocytes and PHA (4).

Since T cell proliferation requires the expression of receptors for IL2, we examined the ability of PHA and IL2 to induce expression of the IL2 receptor Tac. Indeed the combination of PHA and IL 2 induced Tac expression in 20-27% of T cells, similar to that seen with PHA and monocytes. Surprisingly we have found that there was no induction of endogenous IL2 synthesis. Indeed removal of exogenous IL2 up to 42 hours after initiation of cultures resulted in cessation of proliferation by T cells.

Failure of endogenous IL 2 secretion in cultures stimulated with IL2 and PHA was directly demonstrated by measuring the IL2 content of 24-48 hour culture supernatants of T cell cultures stimulated for 24 hours then washed. There was no demonstrable IL2 secretion by T cells stimulated with PHA and IL2. As expected there was vigorous IL2 secretion by T cells stimulated by PHA and macrophages. This secretion was not inhibited by the addition of exogenous IL2 to these cultures in the first 24 hours.

The results of these experiments show that:

1. PHA and IL 2 are sufficient signals to activate resting T cells.

2. In the presence of PHA, IL2 induces its own receptor.

3. PHA and IL2 are not sufficient to induce endogenous IL2 secretion

4. The latter may require cell to cell contact between T cell and antigen presenting cell.

REFERENCES

1. Brozek, C., Umetsu, D., Schneeberger, E., and Geha, RS. (1984): Mechanisms of the failure of resting B cells to present tetanus toxoid antigen to T cells. *J. Immunol.* 132:1144-1150.
2. Chu, E., Rosenwasser, LJ., Dinarello, A., Lareau, M., and Geha, RS. (1984): Role of interleukin 1 in antigen-specific T cell proliferation. *J. Immunol.* 132:1311-1316.
3. Chu, E., Lareau, M., Rosenwasser, LJ., Dinarello, CA., and Geha, RS. (1985): Antigen presentation by EBV-B cells to resting and activated T cells: role of interleukin 1. *J. Immunol.*, in press.
4. Katzen, D., Chu, E., Terhost, C., Gesner, M., Miller, RA., and Geha, RS. (1985) PHA and IL2 are sufficient for T cell proliferation but not IL2 secretion. *J. Immunol.*, in press.
5. Umetsu, DT., Pober, JS., Jabara, HH., Fiers, W., Yunis, EJ., Burakoff, SJ., Reiss, CS., and Geha, RS. (1985): Human dermal fibroblasts present tetanus toxoid to antigen specific T cell clones. *J. Clin. Inves.* in press.

SECTION II
LYMPHOKINES

Molecular Genetic Analysis of T-Cell Antigen and Interleukin-2 Receptors on Normal and Leukemic Lymphocytes

A. T. Waldmann

National Cancer Institute, National Institutes of Health
Bethesda, Maryland 20892, USA

INTRODUCTION

Within recent years investigators using recombinant DNA technology have provided insights into the processes by which the diversity of antibodies and antigen-specific T-cell receptors are generate (1-8). Furthermore, the analysis of immunoglobulin gene structure and arrangement has proven of value in the study of human lymphoid neoplasms. We and other have utilized rearrangements of immunoglobulin genes as DNA level clonal markers for neoplasms of B-cell lineage (9-13). All B-cell malignancies of mature phenotype had clonally rearranged heavy and light chain immunoglobulin genes, while the human T-cell neoplasms we examined uniformly retained germline (unrearranged) light chain genes and, in most instances (21 of 23), germline heavy chain genes as well (9, 10). Thus, the detection of both rearranged heavy and light chain genes within a neoplasm served as a clonal marker uniquely associated with B-cell lineage. This approach allowed the classification of neoplasms that were previously of uncertain lineage, aided in the diagnosis of clonal B-cell neoplasms, and defined the state of differentiation of B-cell precursor leukemia (9-13).

The recent molecular cloning of the genes encoding the T-cell antigen-specific receptor has provided definitive insights into the generation of the antigen-specific repertoire of T cells (3,5-7). Moreover, these genes are proving of clinical importance. Before their isolation there was no marker of T-cell clonality that was uniformly applicable in all T-cell neoplasms. Previously, the determination of clonality had been restricted to T cells displaying a consistent cytogenetic abnormality or to those that arose in patients with two distinguishable glucose-6-phosphate dehydrogenase isoenzymes. In the present study we have applied recombinant DNA technologies involving analysis of T-cell receptor gene arrangements to classify neoplasms that were of controversial lineage previously; to define the clonality of lymphoid proliferations; to assist in the diagnosis of neoplasms of the T-cell and B-cell series; and to monitor the therapy of lymphoid malignancies.

T-Cell Antigen Receptor Gene Rearrangements Serve as Specific T-cell Lineage and Clonal Markers in Human Lymphoid Neoplasms

The human antigen-specific T-cell receptor has been shown to be a polymorphic disulfide-linked heterodimer corresponding to a molecular weight (M_r) of about 90 Kd consisting of a 45-50 Kd α subunit and a 40-45 Kd β subunit (14-16). This receptor is associated with three or four 20-28 Kd nonpolymorphic peptide chains identified by the T3 monoclonal antibody. cDNA clone encoding the β and α chain of the T-cell receptor have been isolated (3-7). The human T_β chain genes in their germline form consist of multiple germline variable region genes (V_β) and duplicate sets of diversity, joining, and constant T_β gene segments. In the present study, we have used a cDNA clone that encodes the $C_{\beta 1}$ and $C_{\beta 2}$ genes to observe the arrangements of these T_β gene subsegments in human lymphoid neoplasms and germline tissues. The arrangement of the T_β gene in circulating white blood cells of normal individuals was analyzed using a cDNA clone that encodes the $C_{\beta 1}$ and $C_{\beta 2}$ genes to define the germline arrangement of this gene. In their germline form the gene segments encoding the two C_β genes were present on a single 24 kb BamHI fragment, on two EcoRI fragments of 4 and 11 kb, and on three HindIII fragments of 3.5, 6.5 and 8.0 kb. In only rare cases were polymorphisms observed in this gene pattern. The arrangement of the T_β genes was shown to be retained in the germline form in all nonlymphoid malignancies examined as well as in polyclonal populations of B cells and EBV transformed B-cell lines. In general, clonal B-cell populations derived from patients with Burkitt's lymphoma, B-cell precursor acute lymphocytic leukemia, or B-cell chronic lymphocytic leukemia manifested T_β genes in their germline configuration.

Normal polyclonal T cells presumably possess numerous different T_β gene rearrangements. Collectively, none of these gene rearrangements is detectable as a new band on Southern blot because they are below the threshold of sensitivity of this method. However, such polyclonal T cells have a marked diminution of the intensity of the 11 kb EcoRI band when compared to the 4 kb band defined by the T_β probe. The virtual loss of the 11 kb as compared to the 4 kb band in polyclonal T cells reflects the arrangement of the EcoRI endonuclease sites. The $C_{\beta 2}$ gene segment present on the 4 kb EcoRI fragment is flanked by EcoRI sites with an enzyme site between $C_{\beta 2}$ and $J_{\beta 2}$. Thus, the size of the EcoRI fragment bearing this gene is not altered by a VDJ rearrangement of this gene complex and the intensity of the band reflecting this gene segment is identical in all tissues. In contrast, the size of the EcoRI fragment bearing the $C_{\beta 1}$ gene (11 kb in germline tissues) is altered by virtually all rearrangements affecting V, D_1, or J_1. Thus, the marked diminution of the intensity of the 11 kb *Eco*RI band when compared to the 4 kb band in polyclonal T cells suggests that effective or aberrant rearrangements or deletions at least involving D_β and J_β elements have occurred for both T_β alleles in the majority of polyclonal T cells.

In contrast to the polyclonal T- and B-lymphocyte populations, all malignant expansions of T cells examined, including four leukemic populations from patients with the human T-cell leukemia/lymphoma virus (HTLV-I)-associated adult T-cell leukemia, five with Sezary leukemia, and five with acute lymphoblastic leukemia reactive with monoclonal antibodies to T cells, displayed an identifiable DNA rearrangement. In 13 of 14 cases, the leukemic cells manifested multiple (two or even three) rearrangements with loss of certain germline bands as assessed by Southern analysis, supporting the view that most T cells manifest an aberrant or effective rearrangement of both T_β alleles. The demonstration of nongermline bands on Southern analysis indicates that these T-leukemic populations represent clonal (mono- or at least oligoclonal) expansions of T lymphocytes.

In general, clonal B-cell populations derived from patients with Burkitt's lymphoma, B-cell precursor acute lymphocytic leukemia, or B-cell chronic lymphocytic leukemia retained T_β genes in the germline configuration. However, in rare cases (3 of 21), there were rearrangements of T_β genes that did not fit this pattern. The three leukemias with T_β gene rearrangements were confirmed to be B cells in that each manifested clonal rearrangements of both heavy and light chain immunoglobulin genes. The rearrangement of T_β genes in a small subset of B cells may be analogous to the immunoglobulin heavy chain gene rearrangements observed in 10% of the leukemic T-cell populations we have examined. The DNA sequences that provide signals for the enzymes active in recombining D and J segments in T and B cells are distinct but have considerable similarities. It is possible that recombinases normally acting in T cells to rearrange T_β genes may occasionally lead to rearrangements of this T_β gene in cells of the B-cell series. The T_β rearrangements observed with certain B-cell leukemias can hinder efforts to define the lineage of a particular lymphoid malignancy in an individual patient. A pattern of gene rearrangements that may allow a more definitive assignment of lineage has been defined. Recently, an additional gene complex now termed T_γ was shown to rearrange in T cells and to be expressed in cells of this series (17, 18). In preliminary studies performed in collaboration with K. Muire and J.G. Seidman, we have shown that clonal T cells rearrange their T_γ genes, whereas the clonal B cells examined did not show rearrangements of this gene complex. Thus, rearrangement of both T_β and T_γ genes appears to occur in cells of the T-cell lineage, providing a molecular arrangement that may be specific for T lymphocytes.

There are few techniques available to define clonality in T-cell populations. In a number of disorders there is controversy as to whether an expansion of T-lymphocyte populations reflects a clonal expansion of T cells or a polyclonal expansion of immunoregulatory cells. For example, there is controversy con-

cerning the clonality of the T8-cell populations in the syndrome characterized
by lymphocytosis of large granular lymphocytes expressing the T3-positive,
T8-positive phenotype that is associated with granulocytopenia and
anemia (19-21): specifically, whether this disorder represents an indolent
chronic lymphocytic leukemia of T cells or merely an expansion of an immunoregulatory polyclonal population. In conjunction with E. Winton we
have demonstrated that peripheral blood mononuclear cells of five of seven
such patients studied with T8 lymphocytosis associated with granulocytopenia
had a clonal pattern of T_β gene rearrangement. Thus, the T8 lymphocytosis
associated with granulocytopenia frequently represents a clonal expansion of
this subset of T lymphocytes.

Thus, in summary the analysis of T-cell receptor rearrangements, taken in
conjunction with studies of immunoglobulin rearrangements, aids in the definition of the lineage (T-cell versus B-cell) and the clonality of lymphoid populations of all lineages. The application of this molecular genetic approach has
great potential for complementing conventional marker analysis, cytogenetics, and histopathology, thereby broadening the scientific basis for diagnos-
ing, monitoring the therapy, and classifying lymphoid neoplasms.

None of the hereditary immunodeficiency disorders have as yet been shown
to have a deletion or abnormality of the genes encoding the T-cell antigen
receptor. However, it is of interest that T-cell lines and leukemias derived
from patients with ataxia telangiectasia manifest breaks and translocations at
the sites of T-cell receptor genes. The sites of translocations and breaks in T
cells observed in patients with ataxia telangiectasia are at chromosome 14 at
band q11, chromosome 7 at band q32-35, and chromosome 7 at band p13-15.
These sites correspond to the chromosomal localization of the T-cell receptor
genes which are present on chromosome 14q11 for the T_α gene, chromosome
7q32 for the T_β gene, and chromosome 7p15 for the T_γ gene. Thus the
translocations and breaks in the T cells of patients with ataxia telangiectasia
are at the bands that bear the T-cell receptor genes (22). It is known that
patients with ataxia telangiectasia are very sensitive to X-irradiation and are
presumed to have a defect in DNA repair. This defect in DNA repair may
underlie many of the defects in this syndrome. Site-specific breaks in the DNA
and then reconstitution of the DNA is involved in the generation of an active
immunoglobulin gene in immunoglobulin class switch and in the generation
of the active T-cell receptor genes. It is known that patients with ataxia
telangiectasia frequently have reduced serum concentrations or absence of
IgA, IgG 2, IgG 4, and IgE, immunoglobulins that are encoded by genes at
the 3' end of the heavy chain gene cluster. The production of such immunoglobulins requires DNA deletion and repair. Similarly, the demonstration that
T cells of such patients have breaks and translocations at the site of the T-cell
receptor genes suggests that here, too, site-specific DNA breaks involved in
the generation of an active T-cell receptor gene are not normally repaired in
the patients with ataxia telangiectasia, an abnormality that may underlie the
defects in specific T-cell-mediated immune responses of such patients.

Interleukin-2 Receptor Gene Expression

T-cell activation is initiated following the interaction of antigen with the complex antigen-specific T-cell receptor discussed above. Two principal events occur at this point which are required for T-cell proliferation and the development of functionally active effector T cells. First, following interaction with antigen and the macrophage-derived interleukin-1, T cells synthesize and secrete the lymphokine interleukin-2 (23, 24). In order to exert its biological effects, interleukin-2 must interact with high-affinity-specific membrane receptors (25). Resting T cells do not express interleukin-2 receptors, but receptors are rapidly expressed on T cells following activation with antigen or mitogen. Thus, both the growth factor interleukin-2 and its receptor are absent in resting T cells, but following activation the genes for both proteins become expressed. Thus, both the production of interleukin-2 and the expression of the interleukin-2 receptors are pivotal events in the full expression of the human immune response. While the antigen confers specificity for a given immune response, the interaction of interleukin-2 and interleukin-2 receptors determines its magnitude and duration.

The specific membrane receptor for interleukin-2 on human lymphocytes has been identified using a monoclonal antibody (anti-Tac) directed towards this molecule (26-28).

Utilizing the anti-Tac monoclonal antibody, we have defined a variety of T- and B-lymphocyte functions that require an interaction of interleukin-2 with its inducible receptor on activated lymphocytes (29, 30). The addition of anti-Tac to in vitro culture systems blocked the interleukin-2-induced DNA synthesis of interleukin-2-dependent T-cell lines an inhibited soluble auto-and alloantigen-induced T-cell proliferation. Furthermore, it abrogated the generation of cytotoxic and suppressor effector T cells but did not inhibit their action once generated. The antireceptor antibody also inhibited the proliferation and immunoglobulin synthesis of purified B cells stimulated with staphylococcus Cowan Strain I organisms.

The human interleukin-2 receptors was characterized (28, 31) and cDNAs encoding this receptor have been cloned and expressed. The interleukin-2 receptor was shown to be a 55 Kd glycoprotein composed of a 33 Kd peptide precursor. Mature receptors contain both N-linked and 0-linked sugars and are both sulfated and phosphorylated. cDNAs encoding the human interleukin-2 receptor have been molecularly cloned (31). The deduced amino acid sequence of the interleukin-2 receptor indicates that this peptide is composed of 272 amino acids including a 21 amino acid signal peptide. The receptor contains two potential N-linked glycosylation sites as well as multiple possible 0-lined carbohydrate sites. Furthermore, there is a single hydrophobic transmembrane region and a vary short (13 amino acid) cytoplasmic domain. The cytoplasmic domain of interleukin-2 receptor appears to be too small for enzymatic function. Thus, this receptor differs from other known growth factor receptors that are tyrosine kinases. Potential phosphate acceptor sites (serine and threonine, but not tyrosine) are present within the intracytoplasmic domain.

In the present study the anti-Tac monoclonal antibody was used to characterize interleukin-2 receptor expression in HTLV-I-associated adult T-cell leukemia. We have analyzed the interleukin-2 receptor expression on three forms of T-cell leukemia: acute T-cell leukemia, the Sézary leukemia, and adult T-cell leukemia (32). The acute T-cell leukemic populations and lines derived from such cells we examined did not express the interleukin-2 receptor. Furthermore, 9 of the 10 populations of Sézary leukemic T cells not associated with HTLV-I examined were Tac antigen negative (32). In contrast, all of the populations of leukemic cells from patients with the adult T-cell leukemia, associated with HTLV-I, expressed the Tac antigen. Thus, the demonstration of interleukin-2 receptors on leukemic T cells may aid in differentiating leukemias caused by HTLV-I which are Tac antigen positive from other forms of T-cell leukemia which are, in general, Tac antigen negative.

The interleukin-2 receptor expression on adult T-cell leukemic cells differed from that on normal T cells. First, unlike normal T cells, adult T-cell leukemic cells did not require prior activation to express the interleukin-2 receptors. Furthermore, using the ^{3}H-anti-Tac receptor assay, HTLV-I-infected leukemic T-cell lines characteristically expressed five- to tenfold more receptors per cell (270,000 to 640,000) than did maximally PHA-stimulated T lymphoblasts (30,000 to 60,000) (33). In addition, whereas normal human T lymphocytes maintained in long-term culture with interleukin-2 demonstrated a rapid decline in receptor number, adult T-cell leukemia lines did not show a similar decline. Furthermore, we have noted that some but not all HTLV-I-infected cell lines display aberrantly sized interleukin-2 receptors (34).

Finally, in studies by Uchiyama and coworkers (35), interleukin-2 receptors on adult T-cell leukemic cells, unlike normal activated T cells, were not modulated (down regulated) by anti-Tac and interleukin-2 receptors on adult T-cell leukemia cell lines were spontaneously (interleukin-2 independently) phosphorylated, whereas the phosphorylation of receptors on PHA-stimulated T cells required the addition of interleukin-2. It is conceivable that the constant presence of high numbers of interleukin-2 receptors on the adult T-cell leukemic cells and/or the aberrancy of these receptors may play a major role in the pathogenesis of uncontrolled growth of these malignant T cells.

We have initiated a clinical trial to evaluate the efficacy of intravenously administered anti-Tac monoclonal antibody in the treatment of patients with the adult T-cell leukemia. The scientific basis for these studies is the observation that adult T-cell leukemic cells express the Tac antigen whereas normal resting T cells and their precursors do not (32). Three patients with adult T-cell leukemia were treated with intravenously administered anti-Tac. None of the patients suffered any untoward reactions nor did they produce antibodies reactive with mouse immunoglobulin or the idiotype of the anti-Tac monoclonal. Two patients with a very rapidly developing form of adult T-cell leukemia had a very transient response. However, therapy of the other patient was followed by a 6-month remission as assessed by routine hematological tests, by immunofluorescence analysis of circulating T cells, and by molecular genetic analysis of the arrangement of T-cell β receptor genes. Prior to anti-Tac therapy the patient had 2,200 circulating malignant T cells/mm^3 as assessed by immunofluorescence analysis using the anti-Tac monoclonal antibody. Furthermore, some (1,200/mm^3) but not all of these circulating leukemic lymphocytes reacted with an antibody to the transferrin receptor, a receptor expressed on malignant T cells but not on normal circulating cells. Following anti-Tac therapy there was a decline in the number of circulating T cells bearing the Tac antigen from 2,200 to less than 100/mm^3 and in transferrin-receptor-expressing T cells from 1,200 to less than 100/mm^3. During the 4-week period following the anti-Tac infusions, there were no cells with free interleukin-2 receptors, that is, cells with receptors unblocked by the infused anti-Tac monoclonal. Cells with blocked interleukin-2 receptors were identified as cells that were not reactive with FITC-conjugated anti-Tac but were reactive with FITC-conjugated anti-mouse IgG and with the 7G7 monoclonal antibody, an antibody that identifies an epitope of the interleukin-2 receptor peptide other than that identified by anti-Tac. The remission of the T-cell leukemia in this patient was confirmed utilizing molecular genetic analysis of the arrangement of the gene encoding the β chain of the antigen-specific T-cell receptor. Prior to therapy Southern analysis of the arrangement of the T-cell β receptor gene, utilizing a radiolabeled probe to the constant region of the T_β chain, revealed a new band not present with germline tissues, the hallmark of a clonal expansion of T lymphocytes. This band, reflecting the clonally rearranged T-cell receptor gene, was not demonstrable on specimens obtained following anti-Tac therapy when the patient was in remission. Approximately 6 months following the initial remission, the leukemia recurred with a reappearance of circulating leukemic cells identified by immunofluorescence and molecular genetic analysis. The patient also developed large (5 x 7 x 1 cm) malignant skin lesion. A new course of intravenous infusions of anti-Tac was followed by the virtual disappearance of the skin lesions and an over 90% reduction in the number of circulating leukemic cells. Three months later leukemic cells again were demonstrable in the circulation. At this time the leukemia was no longer responsive to infusions of anti-Tac and the patient required chemotherapy.

These therapeutic studies have been extended in vitro by examining the efficacy of toxins coupled to anti-Tac in selectively inhibiting protein synthesis and viability of Tac-positive adult T-cell leukemic cell lines. The addition of anti-Tac antibody coupled to the A chain of the toxin ricin effectively inhibited protein synthesis by the HTLV-I-associated, Tac-positive adult T-cell leukemia line HUT 102-B2. In contrast, conjugates of ricin A with a control monoclonal of the same isotype did not inhibit protein synthesis when used in the same concentration (36). The inhibitory action of anti-Tac conjugated with ricin A could be abolished by the addition of excess unlabeled anti-Tac or interleukin-2. In parallel studies performed in collaboration with David FitzGerald, Mark Willingham, and Ira Pastan (37) pseudomonas exotoxin conjugates of anti-Tac inhibited the protein synthesis by HUT 102-B2 cells but not that of the Tac-negative acute T-cell line Molt-4 that does not express the Tac antigen. Again, the toxicity of the anti-Tac toxin conjugates could be inhibited by adding excess unlabeled anti-Tac. Thus, the development of toxin conjugates of the monoclonal anti-Tac that are directed toward the interleukin-2 receptor expressed on adult T-cell leukemic cells may permit the development of a rational approach for the treatment of this almost uniformly fatal form of leukemia.

SUMMARY

Immunoglobulin and T-cell antigen receptor genes in their germline form are separated DNA segments that are joined by recombinations during lymphocyte development. The analysis of immunoglobulin and T-cell receptor gene arrangements has been of value in the study of lymphoid neoplasms. The identification of T-cell receptor gene rearrangements taken in conjunction with studies of immunoglobulin gene rearrangments aids in the elucidation of the lineage (T-cell or B-cell) and the clonality of lymphoid populations of all series. The application of this molecular genetic approach has great potential for complementing conventional marker analysis, cytogenetics, aand histopathology, thus broadening the scientific basis for the classification, diagnosis, and monitoring of the therapy of lymphoid neoplasia.

Interleukin-2 is a lymphokine synthesized by some T cells following activation. Resting T cells do not express interleukin-2 receptors, but receptors are rapidly expressed on T cells following the interaction of antigens, mitogens, or monoclonal antibodies with the antigen-specific T-cell receptor complex. Normal resting T cells and most leukemic T-cell populations do not express interleukin-2 receptors; however, the leukemic cells of all patients with HTLV-I-associated adult T-cell leukemia examined expressed the Tac antigen. The constant display of large numbers of interleukin-2 receptors which may be aberrant may play a role in the uncontrolled growth of these leukemic T cells. Patients with the Tac-positive adult T-cell leukemia are being treated with the anti-Tac monoclonal antibody directed toward this growth factor receptor.

REFERENCES

1. Leder, P. (1982). The genetics of antibody diversity. *Sci. Amer.* 246: 102-15.
2. Tonegawa, S. (1983). Somatic generation of antibody diversity. *Nature* 302:575-81.
3. Hedrick, S.M., Cohen, D.I., Nielsen, E.A. and Davis, M.M. (1984). Isolation of cDNA clones encoding T-cell specific membrane-associated proteins. *Nature* 308:149-53.
4. Hedrick, S.M., Nielsen, E.A., Kavaler, J., Cohen, D.I. and Davis, M.M. (1984). Sequence relationships between putative T-cell receptor polypeptides and immunoglobulins. *Nature* 308:153-8.

5. Yanagi, Y., Yoshikai, Y., Leggett, R., Clark, S.P., Aleksander, I. and Mak, T.W. (1984). A human T-cell specific cDNA clone encodes a protein having extensive homology to immunoglobulin chains. *Nature* 308:145-9.

6. Chien, Y.H., Becker, D.M., Lindsten, T., Okamuras, M., Cohen, D.I. and Davis, M.M. (1984). A third type of murine T-cell receptor gene. *Nature* 312:31-5.

7. Saito, H., Kranz, D.M., Takagki, Y., Hayday, A.C., Eisen, H.N. and Tonegawa, S. (1984). A third rearranged and expressed gene in a clone of cytotoxic T lymphocytes. *Nature* 312:771-5.

8. Sim, G.K., Yague, J., Nelson, J. et al. (1984). Primary structure of human T-cell receptor α-chain. *Nature* 312:771-5.

9. Korsmeyer, S.J., Arnold, A., Bakhshi, A., et al. (1983). Immunoglobulin gene rearrangement and cell surface antigen expression in acute lymphocytic leukemias of T-cell and B-cell precursor origins. *J. Clin. Invest.* 71:301-13.

10. Arnold, A., Cossman, J., Bakhshi, A., Jaffe, E.S., Waldmann, T.A. and Korsmeyer, S.J. (1983). Immunoglobulin gene rearrangements as unique clonal markers in human lymphoid neoplasms. *N. Eng. J. Med.* 309:1593-9.

11. Bakhshi, A., Minowada, J., Arnold, A. et al. (1983). Lymphoid blast crisis of chronic myelogenous leukemia represents stages in the development of B-cell precursors. *N. Eng. J. Med.* 309:826-31.

12. Cleary, M.I., Warnke, R. and Sklar, J. (1984). Monoclonality of lymphoproliferative lesions in cardiac transplant recipients. *N. Eng. J. Med.* 310:477-82.

13. Sklar, J., Cleary, M.L., Thielman, K., Gralow, J., Warnke, R. and Levy, R. (1984). Biclonal B-cell lymphoma. *N. Eng. J. Med.* 311:20-7.

14. Allison, J.P., McIntyre,, B.W. and Bloch, D. (1982). Tumor-specific antigen of murine T-lymphoma defined with monoclonal antibody. *J. Immunol.* 129:2293-300.

15. Haskins, K., Kubo, R., White, J., Pigeon, M., Kappler, J. and Marrack, P. (1983). The major histocompatibility complex-restricted antigen receptor on T cells. Isolation with a monoclonal antibody. *J. Exp. Med.* 157: 1149-69.

16. Meuer, S.C., Fitzgerald, K.A., Hussey, R.E., Hodgdon, J.C., Schlossman, S.F. and Reinherz, E.L. (1983). Clonotypic structures involved in antigen-specific human T-cell function. *J. Exp. Med.* 157:705-19.

17. Saito, H., Kranz, D.M., Takagaki, Y., Hayday, A.C., Eisen, H.N. and Tonegawa, S. (1984). Complete primary structure of a heterodimeric T-cell receptor deduced from cDNA sequences. *Nature* 309:757-62.

18. Hayday, A.C., Saito, H., Gillis, S.D. et. al. (1985). Structure, organization, and somatic rearrangement of T-cell gamma genes. *Cell* 40:259-81.

19. Aisenberg, A., Wilkes, B., Harris, N., Ault, K., and Carey, R. (1981) Chronic T-cell lymphocytosis with neutropenia: report of case studied with monoclonal antibody. *Blood* 58:818-22.

20. Chan, W., Check, I., Schick, C., Brynes, R., Kateley, J. and Winton, E. (1984). A morphologic and immunologic study of the large granular lymphocyte in neutropenia with T lymphocytosis. *Blood* 63:1133-40.

21. Reynolds, C. and Foon, K. (1984). T$_\gamma$-lymphoproliferative disease and related disorders in humans and experimental animals: a review of the clinical, cellular, and functional characteristics. *Blood* 64:1146-58.

22. Murre, C., Waldmann, R.A., Morton, C.C., et al. (1985). Human γ-chain genes are rearranged in leukaemic T cells and map to the short arm of chromosome 7. *Nature* 316:549-52.

23. Smith, K.A. (1980). T-cell growth factor. *Immunol. Rev.* 51:337-57.

24. Morgan, D.A., Ruscetti, F.W. and Gallo, R.C. (1976). Selective in vitro growth of T lymphocytes from normal human bone marrows. *Science (Wash. D.C.)* 193:1007-8.

25. Robb, R.J., Munck, A. and Smith, K.A. (1981). T-cell growth factor receptors. *J. Exp. Med.* 154:1455-74.

26. Uchiyama, T., Broder, S. and Waldmann, T.A. (1981). A monoclonal antibody (anti-Tac) reactive with activated and functionally mature human T cells. I Production of anti-Tac monoclonal antibody and distribution of Tac (+) cells. *J. Immunol.* 126:1393-97.

27. Leonard, W.J., Depper, J.M., Uchiyama, T., Smith, K.A, Waldmann, T.A. and Greene, W.C. (1982). A monoclonal antibody that appears to recognize the receptor for human T-cell growth factor; partial characterization of the receptor. *Nature (Lond.)* 300:267-9.

28. Leonard, W.J., Depper, J.M., Robb, R.J., Waldmann, T.A. and Greene, W.C. (1983). Characterization of the human receptor for T cell growth factor. *Proc. Natl. Acad. Sci. U.S.A.* 80:6957-61.

29. Uchiyama, T., Nelson, D.L., Fleisher, T.A. and Waldmann, T.A. (1981). A monoclonal antibdy (anti-Tac) reactive with activated and functionlly mature human T cells. II. Expression of Tac antigen on activated cytotoxic killer T cells, suppressor cells, and on one of two types of helper T cells. *J. Immunol.* 126:1398-403.
30. Depper, J.M., Leonard, W.J., Waldmann, T.A. and Greene, W.C. (1983). Blockade of the interleukin-2 receptor by anti-Tac antibody:inhibition of human lymphocyte activation. *J. Immunol.* 131:690-6.
31. Leonard, W.J., Depper, J.M., Crabtree, G.R., et al. (1984). Molecular cloning and expression of cDNAs for the human interleukin 2 receptor. *Nature* 311-626-31.
32. Waldmann, T.A., Greene, W.C., Sarin, P.S., et al. (1984). Functional and phenotypic comparison of human T-cell leukemia/lymphoma virus negative Sézary leukemia and their distinction using anti-Tac, monoclonal antibody identifying the human receptor for T-cell growth factor. *J. Clin. Invest.* 73:1711-18.
33. Depper, J.M., Leonard, W.J., Krönke, M., Waldmann, T.A. and Greene, W.C. (1984). Augmentation of T-cell growth factor expression in HTLV-I-infected human leukemic T cells. *J. Immunol.* 133:1691-5.
34. Leonard, W.J., Depper, J.M., Roth, J.S., Rudikoff, S., Waldmann, T.A. and Greene, W.C. (1983). Aberrant T-cell growth factor (TCGF) receptors on human T-cell leukemia virus (HTLV) infected leukemic cells. *Clin. Res.* 31:348a.
35. Uchiyama, T., Wano, Y., Tsudo, M. et al. (1985). Abnormal expression of Tac antigen (IL-2 receptor) in adult T-cell leukemia. *In* Miwa, M., ed. Retroviruses in Human Lymphoma/ Leukemia: The Fifteenth International Symposium of the Princess Talaùatsi Cancer Research Fund. *Japan Sci. Soc. Press (in press).*
36. Krönke, M., Depper, J.M., Leonard, W.J., Vitetta, E.S., Waldmann, T.A. and Greene, W.C. (1985). Anti-Tac-ricin A conjugates selectively inhibit protein synthesis in human T-cell leukemia/lymphoma virus infected leukemic cells. *Blood* 65:1416-21.
37. FitzGerald, D.J.P., Waldmann, T.A., Willingham, M.C. and Pastan, I. (1984). Pseudomonas exotoxin-anti-Tac: cell-specific immunotoxin active against cells expressing the human T-cell growth factor receptor. *J. Clin. Invest.* 74:966-71.

Modulation of T Cell Activation by Lymphokines and other Biologically Active Compounds

Alain L. de Weck, Beda M. Stadler, Christine Mazingue,
Christoph Walker, Florence Bettens

*Institute of Clinical Immunology, Inserspital,
University of Bern, Bern, Switzerland*

Lymphocyte proliferation and differentiation represent basic functions of the immune system, since they are required for acquisition of immunological memory, for clonal expansion of specific lymphocyte populations and for production of specific antibodies. In recent years, the combination of techniques such as separation of various lymphocyte subsets on the basis of membrane markers, analysis of the cell cycle by flow cytometry, measurement of H^3-thymidine uptake, detection of membrane receptors and markers by immunofluorescence or ligand binding and quantitative assessment of various lymphokines produced by lymphoid cells have yielded an integrated picture of the events associated with the proliferation and differentiation of T lymphocytes. The identification of «cascades» of events in lymphokine-lymphocyte interactions at the levels of the cell membrane only starts, however, to give definite clues about the corresponding intracellular events, in particular about the biochemical mechanisms leading to selective gene expression within the cell, following activation.

The aim of this paper is: a) to briefly review the current state of knowledge about the role of lymphokines in T cell activation and proliferation; b) to emphasize the interest of flow cytometric cell cycle analysis in identifying biological compounds modulating lymphocyte activation and in evaluating their mode of action.

Cell cycle analysis of activated T lymphocytes

Techniques enabling to stain lymphoid cells simultaneously for cellular RNA and for various membrane markers have permitted to follow lymphoid cells undergoing activation and proliferation through various phases of the cell cycle (8,20) by flow cytometry. A dynamic follow up during the first 48 hours of culture, i.e. while most of the cells have only completed their first proliferative cycle, reveals that several signals and concomitant events are required for the cell to process from a resting G_0 phase through an early activation phase (G_{Ia}), a late activation phase (G_{Ib}), a DNA synthesis phase (S), a premitotic phase (G_2) and mitosis (M) (16).

It is by now well recognized that most substances formerly designated as T cell «mitogens», such as lectins (e.g. PHA, ConA) are only providing a first activating signal enabling the cell to initiate RNA synthesis and to proceed from the resting G_0 to an early G_{Ia} phase (12). This signal presumably is provided by the T3-T receptorcomplex, since it can also be provided by specific antigen or by anti-T3 antibodies. A second concomitant signal, provided experimentally by phorbol myristic acetate and more physiologically by interleukin 1, seems required for initiating the chain of intracellular events (in particular Ca^{++} mobilization and protein kinase C activation) leading to the expression of lymphokine genes, as revealed by the production of interleukin 2 (IL-2) or of interferon gamma. Having within 6-10 hours of initial activation reached the G_{Ia} phase, the majority of T cells appear to require, in order to proceed further, an additional signal provided by interaction of IL-2 with its specific receptor. The main but possibly not the only effect of that lymphokine seems to be the promotion of further RNA synthesis, manifested by the passage of cells from the G_{Ia} into the G_{Ib} phase (12,21). The postulate that the G_1 phase can be subdivided not only quantitatively but possibly also qualitatively into separate subphases has first been met with some skepticism. However, this has been confirmed by direct measurements of RNA synthesis (J.F. Gauchat, F. Bettens, unpublished experiments). In addition, some manipulations in cell culture, such as the addition of dexamethasone, which prevents IL-1 (10) and IL-2 production (1, 10) stops the cell during the G_1 phase and RNA synthesis. Since IL-2 receptor expression is not impaired by this manipulation, addition of exogenous IL-2 triggers a new RNA synthesis, as can be assessed by flow cytometry (1) and biochemically.

Most activated T lymphocytes appear to be dependent for their continued proliferation upon the interaction of IL-2 produced either in an autocrine fashion (2) or by some other T cell subset with specific IL-2 membrane receptors, formed during the early G_1 phase (11). The formation of such IL-2 receptors has been studied kinetically by direct binding of labelled IL-2 (17) and by flow cytometry (1) using a monoclonal antibody (anti-Tac) (23). The appearance of IL-2 receptors follows closely the increase in RNA synthesis characterizing the G_{Ia} phase, they become detectable approximately 2-4 hours after stimulation. The number of T lymphocytes carrying IL-2 receptors and the density of such receptors per cell increase then progressively for the next 18-24 hours. At all phases, the density of IL-2 receptors appears to remain very heterogeneous in the stimulated cell population. Production of IL-2 is apparently the function of some subsets of activated T cells (11). As judged from kinetic analysis, IL-2 becomes detectable in the supernatant of activated lymphocyte cultures about 10-12 hours after the activating signal induced by a lectin. As stated above, the production of IL-2 is dependent in lectin- or antigen activated lymphokines upon a second signal provided by IL-1, which can be the product of activated monocytes or macrophages (19). IL-1 itself becomes detectable in supernatants of activated mononuclear cell populations about 2-4 hours after activation.

Following successful interaction of IL-2 with the IL-2 receptor, the cells proceed to a new burst of RNA synthesis (G_{1b} phase) and start DNA synthesis some 6 hours later. The passage of the G_{1b} to the S phase was thought first to require no additional signal, since there is a close correlation between the number of cells reaching the G_{1b} stage and the incorporation of H^3 thymidine. However, it has been shown (15) that the interaction of transferrin with its activation-induced transferrin receptor is also essential for initiation of the S phase (DNA synthesis). Monoclonal antibodies directed against the transferrin receptor block the proliferative burst induced by IL-2/IL-2 receptor interaction (22) and the appearance of the transferrin receptor follows the appearance of the IL-2 receptor with a lag phase of about 2 hours. It is therefore presumed that the two events are linked. Since there are a number of other early activation antigens, which have been detected with monoclonal antibodies on activated T and B cells (7), it may well be that further elements in the cascade of lymphokine or signal molecules interacting with their receptors during the G_1 phase will be uncovered.

The early events occurring during the G_1 phase seem to be most decisive for the fate of proliferating T lymphocytes, once activated and furnished with the appropriate signals, they will continue on their committed path throughout the cell cycle. However, further events and signals possibly required at later stages, such as completion of the S phase, duration of the G_2 phase and initiation of the M phase have not yet been analyzed for human peripheral blood lymphocytes proliferating in vitro as throughly as for lymphoid cell lines (16).

Following mitosis, T cells either return to a resting G_0 stage or directly enter a new proliferation cycle, provided the required activation and proliferation inducing signals (e.g. IL-2) are continuously present. PHA activated T cells may steadily proliferate in the presence of exogeneous IL-2, while deprival of IL-2 replaces the cells in the G_0 phase, where they remain susceptible to renewed activation (2). Stimulated T cells which have been deprived of IL-2 before entering the S phase and have returned to G_0 show an accelerated expression of IL-2 receptors upon restimulation (11): such cells might be considered as T memory cells.

Modulation of T cell proliferation by various biologically active compounds

As discussed above, a variety of molecules produced by lymphoid cells and thereby qualified as lymphokines, promote T cell activation and proliferation. Since transferrin also appears to be produced by activated T cells, it may also belong to the same category. The fact that various serum batches may have very different effects on lymphocyte proliferation suggests that besides the well characterized IL-1, IL-2 and transferrin, other factors may modulate T lymphocytes during the G_1 phase.

Indeed, a number of biologically active modulating agents have been described in recent years. We will review here those agents which have been reported to interfere with T cell proliferation and which have been analyzed in terms of mechanism and location of interference, by the flow cytometric approach described above. These flow cytometric techniques provide a potent tool for screening of immunopharmacological properties of compounds interfering with the proliferation of the one or the other lymphoid subset.

The effect of various compounds on the production of lymphokines, such as IL-1, IL-2 and IL-3, the expression of activation receptors, such as the IL-2 and the transferrin receptors, and the corresponding effect on the G_1 phase of the cell cycle are summarized in Table 1. Histamine (26), prostaglandin

TABLE 1.   *Effect of various compounds on cell cycle events*

	Inhibit. of Lymphokine Production			Inhibit. of Receptor Expression		Block in Cell Cycle Step		
	IL 1	IL 2	IL 3	IL 2 (Tac)	TF (T9)	G_0-G_1	G_{Ia}-G_{Ib}	G_{Ib}-S
Dexamethasone	+ +	+ +	+ +	$-$*	$-$	$-$	+ +	$-$
Prostaglandin E2		+ +		$-$		$-$	+ +	$-$
Histamine		+		$-$		$-$	+ +	$-$
Cyclosporin A	+	+ +		$\pm$	$-$	$-$	+ +	$-$
Serotonin		$-$		+ +		$-$	+ +	$-$
Schistosome SDIF		$-$		$-$		$-$	$- -$	+ +
C3 Fragment (C3 FP)		$-$		$-$	$-$	$-$	+ +	$-$
Hydroxyurea		$-$		$-$		$-$	$-$	+ +

*Only in vitro.

E2 (24), corticosteroids (1, 10) and cyclosporin A (3, 6), have a marked inhibitory effect on the production of IL-2. These substances, however, with the exception of cyclosporin A (3), do not seem to markedly impair the expression of IL-2 receptors in activated T cells. Indeed, addition of exogenous IL-2 completely restores proliferation and G_{Ia} to G_{Ib} transition. While histamine, prostaglandin E2 and corticosteroids may exert similar inhibiting effects on activation phenomena in various cell types, others such as cyclosporin A are apparently more specific in terms of their cell targets. Although there are reports indicating that cyclosporin A may also affect B lymphocytes or even blood basophils, the current consensus is that this drug, at the pharmacological levels used in vivo, shows a marked T cell specificity (3, 11) and preferentially interferes with T4 helper cells (3). It is recently claimed that cyclosporin A does not interfere with the expression of IL-2 receptors, alternatively, that the slight impairment in IL-2 receptors expression detected is merely a consequence of the impairment in IL-2 production, which modulates the expression of its own receptor. In recent experiments, we definitely observed a difference between the effects of dexamethasone and cyclosporin A in vitro: while exogenous IL-2 fully reconstitutes dexamethasone-treated cells, at least in vitro (1), this is not the case for cyclosporin A-treated T cells (3). Since cyclosporin A does not affect the expression of some early activation antigens (e.g. eF2) (3), it is obvious that its effect is a rather restricted one during the G_{1a} phase.

These experiments have provided clear cut evidence that the production of IL-2 and the expression of IL-2 receptors, although both dependent upon RNA synthesis following activation (25), represent two independent processes. A further inverse example of this dissociation is provided by serotonin, which does not affect IL-2 production but impairs IL-2 receptor expression (19) and thereby inhibits T cell proliferation.

Recently, our interest has been captivated by two compounds which also appear to have a definite T cell selectivity as a targets of action and which prevent T cell proliferation by acting at a later time in the G_1 phase than cyclosporin A, corticosteroids or prostaglandin E2.

The first of these compounds is a 6-8 KD fragment of guinea pig C3, provided to us by Dr. Bitter-Suermann (Mainz). This fragment, produced during the splitting of the C3 molecule by the cobra venom-factor C3 convertase is not yet fully characterized but might be similar to the C3e or to a fragment of the C3d-K split products of C3, which have been described earlier as inhibiting lectin-induced T cell proliferation (14). The interest of this fragment, provisionally denominated C3 FP (C3 fragment peptide) is due to the following observations:

a) C3 FP is a potent inhibitor of IL-2 dependent human T cell proliferation (90% inhibition at doses of 1-4 ng/ml (10^{-9} to 10^{-10} M). It does not affect the proliferation of T cells independent of exogenous IL-2, of B cells, or of other human lymphoid cell lines tested so far.

b) C3 FP does not impair IL-2 production

c) C3 FP does not impair IL-2 receptor expression

d) C3 FP does not prevent binding of IL-2 to the IL-2 receptor

e) Nevertheless, C3 FP prevents the passage of G_{1a} into G_{1b} cells, presumably after IL-2/IL-2 receptor interaction.

Therefore, as indicated also by its kinetics of action (addition at 24 hours after activation still inhibits T cell proliferation), C3 FP interferes rather late in the G_1 phase and represents a hitherto unique inhibitor of human T cell proliferation.

Another interesting inhibitor of T cell proliferation, described in recent years by the group of Capron (9) and which we have had the opportunity of investigating in collaboration (13) is the Schistosome Derived Inhibitory Factor (SDIF). This is a very small molecule (500 daltons), not yet fully characterized, which is released by Schistosome worms. As previously shown, this molecule also affects T cell mediated immunity in vivo (4) and suppresses natural defenses against parasites. In our hands, it had the following properties:

a) SDIF is a very potent inhibitor of T cell proliferation

b) SDIF has no effect on IL-2 production

c) SDIF has no effect on IL-2 receptor expression

d) SDIF has an inhibiting effect exclusively on cell lines of T cell lineage, including those independent of exogenous IL-2. In this it apparently differs from the C3FP.

e) SDIF exerts its inhibiting effect on the G_{1b} - S transition, at a stage independent of IL-2 - IL-2 receptor interaction.

In *summary*, the current conceptions about the factors required for T cell activation and the cascade of lymphokine-receptor interactions promoting activated cells through the G_1 and S phase of the cell cycle, although revealing the existence of various successive steps which may not always be directly correlated, is probably much too simple. Further studies at the molecular biological level, analysing the various specific mRNAs formed will be required for better understanding.

However, the analytical flow cytometric approach described here already permits a powerful screening of immunomodulating agents, since it permits to analyse in a single step the kinetics of modulation of activation antigens, the effects on RNA and DNA synthesis, as well as the target cell specificity, in terms of set or subset of lymphoid cell affected. Ideal immunomodulating agents should be those showing selectivity, both in mechanism and target of action.

REFERENCES

1. Bettens, F., Kristensen, F., Walker, C., Schwulera, U., Bonnard, G.D., de Weck, A.L. (1984): Lymphokine regulation of activated (G_1) lymphocytes. II. Glucorticoid and anti-Tac induced inhibition of human T lymhocyte proliferation. *J. Immunol.*, 132:161.
2. Bettens, F., Kristensen, F., Walker, C., Bonnard, G.D., de Weck, A.L. (1984): Lymphokine regulation of human lymphocyte proliferation. Formation of resting (G_0) cells by removal of interleukin 2 in cultures of proliferating T lymphocytes. *Cell Immunol.*, 86:337-346.
3. Bettens, F., Walker, C., Gauchat, J.-F., Bonnard, G.D., Weil, R., de Weck, A.L.: Effect of CS-A on the early activation of human T helper lymphocytes. Inhibition of RNA-synthesis and modification of the expression of activation antigens. submitted.
4. Camus, D., Nosseir, A., Mazingue, C., Capron, A. (1981): Immunoregulation by schistosoma mansoni. *Immunopharmacology* 3:193.
5. Cantrell, D.A., Smith, K.A. (1983): Transient expression of interleukin 2 receptors. *J. Exp. Med.*, 158:1895.
6. Carpenter, C.B., Strom, T.B. (1984): Immunosuppressive therapy for renal transplantation. *Springer Seminar Immunopathol.* 7:43-57.
7. Cortner, T., Williams, J.M., Christenson, L., Shapiro, H.M., Strom, T.B., Strominger, J. (1983): Simultaneous flow cytometric analysis of human T cell activation. Antigen expression and DNA content. *J. Exp. Med.* 157:461.
8. Darzunkiewiez, Z., Traganos, F., Sharpless, T., Melamed, M.R. (1976): Lymphocyte stimulation: a rapid multiparameter analusis. *Proc. Natl. Acad. Sci. USA* 73:2881.
9. Dessaint, J.P., Camus, D., Fischer, E., Capron, A. (1977): Inhibition of lymphocyte proliferation by factor(s) produced by Schistosoma mansoni. *Eur. J. Immunol.*, 7:624.

10. Gillis, S., Crabtree, G.R., Smith, K.A. (1979): Glucocorticoid-induced inhibition of T cell growth factor production. I. The effect of mitogen-induced lymphocyte proliferation. *J. Immunol.*, 123:1624.
11. Kasahara, T., Hooks, J.J., Dougherty, S.F., Oppenheim, J.J. (1983): Interleukin-2 mediated immune interferon production by human T cells and T cell subsets. *J. Immunol.*, 130:1784.
12. Kristensen, F., Walker, C., Bettens, F., Jouncourt, F., de Weck, A.L. (1982): Assessment of IL 1 and IL 2 effects on cycling and noncycling murine thymocytes. *Cell Immunol.* 74:140.
13. Mazingue, C., Dessaint, J.P., Schmitt-Verhulst, A.M., Cerottini, J.C., Capron, A. (1983): Inhibition of cytotoxic T lymphocytes by a Schistosoma-derived inhibitory factor is independent of an inhibition of the production of interleukin 2. *Int. Archs. Allergy Appl. Immunol.* 72:22.
14. Morgan, E.L., Thoman, M.L., Hoeprich, P.D., Hugli, T.E. (1985): Bioactive complement fragments in immunoregulation. *Immunology Letters* 9:207.
15. Neckers, L.M., Cossman, J. (1983): Transferrin receptor induction in mitogen-stimulated humant T lymphocytes is required for DNA synthesis and cell division and is regulated by interleukin 2. *Proc. Natl. Acad. Sci. USA* 80:3494.
16. Pardee, A.B., Dubrow, R., Hamlin, H.L., Kletzren, R.F. (1978): Animal cell cycle. *Annu. Rev. Biochem.* 47:715.
17. Robb, R.J., Munck, A., Smith, K.A. (1981): T cell growth factor receptors. Quantitation, specificity and biological relevance. *J. Exp. Med.* 154:1455.
18. Slauson, D.O., Walker, C., Kristensen, F., Wang, Y., de Weck, A.L. (1983): Mechanisms of serotonin-induced lymphocyte proliferation inhibition. *Clin. Exp. Immunol.* 54:501.
19. Smith, K.A., Lachman, L.B., Oppenheim, J.J., Favata, M.F. (1980): The functional relationship of the interleukins, *J. Exp. Med.* 151:1551.
20. Stadler, B.M., Kristensen, F., de Weck, A.L. (1980): Thymocyte activation by cytokines: direct assessment of G_0-G_1 transition by flow cytometry. *Cell. Immunol.* 55:436.
21. Stadler, B.M., Dougherty, S., Farrar, J.J., Oppenheim, J.J. (1981): Relationship of cell cycle to recovery of IL-2 activity from human mononuclear cells, human and mouse T cell lines. *J. Immunol.*, 127:1936.
22. Trowbridge, I.S., Lopez, F. (1982): Monoclonal antibody to transferrin receptor blocks transferrin binding and exhibits human tumor cell growth in vitro. *Prox. Natl. Acad. Sci. USA* 79:1175.
23. Uchiyama, T., Nelson, D.L., Fleisher, T.A., Waldmann, T.A. (1981): A monoclonal antibody (anti-Tac) reactive with activated and functionally mature human T cells. II. Expression of Tac antigen on activated cytotoxic killer T cells, suppressor cells and on one of the two types of helper T cells. *J. Immunol.*, 126:1398.
24. Walker, C., Kristensen, F., Bettens, F., de Weck, A.L. (1983): Lymphokine regulation of activated (G_1) cells. I. Prostaglandin E2 induced inhibition of interleukin 2 production. *J. Immunol.*, 130:1770.
25. Wang, Y., Walker, C., Stadler, B.M., de Weck, A.L. (1984): Transcription and translation dependent induction of interleukin 2 (IL-2) and IL-2 receptors. *Immunology Letters* 8:227-231.
26. Yu, H., Tadokoro, K., Stadler, B.M., de Weck, A.L.: Inhibitory effect of histamine on interleukin-2 production. Submitted.

Peripheral Immunodeficiency Associated with Experimental Arthritic Disease in Rats

Steven C. Gilman, PH. D.

*Deparment of Experimental Therapeutics Wyeth Laboratories, Inc.
Philadelphia, PA, USA*

Rheumatoid arthritis is a chronic, debilitating autoimmune disorder, the most severe pathological consequences of which are manifested within the joint capsule itself and consist of a progressive deterioration of articular integrity with eventual loss of joint function (16). These articular events are believed to occur as a result of an abnormal immune response occurring within the joint against an as yet unidentified autoantigen (12). More recently, however, abnormalities in peripheral lymphoid function have been reported in arthritic patients (13, 14), although the precise relationship between peripheral immune function and articular destruction has not been established.

Several animal models of arthritic disease have been described which have significantly contributed to our current understanding of arthritogenesis and the immunopathology of arthritic disease (2). In an attempt to more clearly delineate the immunological consequences of arthritis, we have examined peripheral lymphoid function in a model system in which arthritis is induced in rats by injection of *Mycobacterium butyricum*. In this paper, we present data which demonstrates that a severe immunodeficiency sundrome accompanies the development of arthritic disease in this model and will discuss the role of lymphokine synthesis and responsiveness in mediating this hyporesponsive state.

MATERIAL AND METHODS

Animals and induction of arthritis

Groups of 2-4 Lewis rats (Charles River, Wilmington, MA) were injected in the right hind footpad with 0.5 mg *Mycobacterium butyricum* suspended in 0.1 ml light mineral oil. Spleens were removed from these animals 16-22 days following *M. butyricum* injection, at the peak of the edematous arthritic response as measured by mercury plethysmography of the uninjected hind paw.

Cell cultures

Spleens were aseptically removed and single cell suspensions were prepared by passage through wire mesh screens. After treatment with NH_4Cl to lyse erythrocytes, the cells were washed and resuspended in RPMI 1640 medium containing 10% bovine calf serum, 20 mM glutamine, 50 μg/ml streptomycin, 50 U/ml penicillin and 50 μM 2-mercaptoethanol. For use in some experiments, spleen cells were fractionated into T cell-enriched (nylon wool nonadherent) or macrophage-enriched (plastic adherent) populations. T cell populations contained $\geq 95\%$ W3/13$^+$ T cells, 1-3% B cells and $\leq 2\%$ macrophages while the splenic adherent cells were >85% macrophages based on morphologic and phagocytic criteria.

To assess proliferative responsiveness, spleen cells were cultured for 4 days at 37°C (5% CO_2 in air atmosphere) with 0.1 μg/ml concanavalin A (Con A, Miles Laboratories, Elkhart, IN) or 0.1 μg/ml pokeweed mitogen (PWM, Sigma Chemical Co., St. Louis, MO) in triplicate in 96 well microtiter plates (2 x 10^5 cells/0.2 ml/well). One μCi of [^{3}H] thymidine was added to each well 7 hours prior to harvesting the cells onto glass fiber filters for scintillation counting.

The ability of splenic adherent macrophages to produce IL-1 was determined by culturing 5 x 10^6 plastic adherent spleen cells in 1 ml of medium containing 10 μg/ml *E. coli* lipopolysaccharide (LPS, Sigma Chemical Co., St. Louis, MO) for 24-48 h. Supernatant fluids from these cultures were then assayed for IL-1 activity in a thymocyte costimulator assay in which 1.5 x 10^6 C3H/HEJ mouse thymocytes/0.2 ml medium were cultured for 3 days with 20 μg/ml phytohemagglutinin (PHA, Burroughs-Wellcome, Research Triangle Park, NC) plus varying dilutions of test supernatant (8). The cells were pulsed with [^{3}H] thymidine as described above, and IL-1 activity was calculated by subtracting the disintegrations per minute (dpm) of thymocytes alone from the dpm of thymocytes cultured with PHA plus test supernatant (Δ dpm).

The ability of spleen cells to produce IL-2 was assessed by culturing spleen cells (10^6/ml) with 0.1 μg/ml con A. Twenty-four hours later, the supernatant fluids from these cultures were assayed for IL-2 levels by their ability to support the growth of an IL-2-dependent mouse cytotoxic T cell line, CTLL-2 (7).

In some experiments, Con A-stimulated spleen cell cultures were supplemented with an exogenous source of IL-1 or IL-2. The IL-1 used in these experiments was purchased from Genzyme (Boston, MA) and is a purified human IL-1 isolated from *Staphylococcus albus*-stimulated normal human monocytes. This preparation had no detectable endotoxin, interferon or IL-2. The IL-2 source used was purified recombinant human IL-2 (Genzyme) which had no detectable amounts of IL-1, interferon, colony stimulating factor, macrophage activating factor, endotoxin or phorbol ester. In addition, similar results to those shown here have been observed using purified mouse IL-1 (a generous gift from Dr. S. Mizel, Penn State University) and partially purified preparations of rat IL-1 and IL-2 prepared in our own laboratory.

RESULTS

Splenic immune function in arthritic rats

Figure 1 shows that a marked splenic hyporesponsiveness to *in vitro* stimulation with con A develops in arthritic rats and illustrated the temporal relationship between the diminished spleen cell function and the edematous

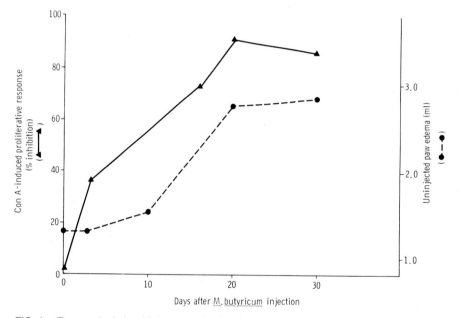

FIG. 1. Temporal relationship between the development of an arthritic response (paw edema) and splenic immunodeficiency in rats. To induce arthritis, rats were injected on day 0 with a homogenized suspension of *M. butyricum* in the right hind paw. At intervals thereafter, paw edema in the uninjected paw (●—●) was measured by mercury plethysmography and 2 animals were sacrificed and the ability of their spleen cells to proliferate *in vitro* to 0.1 μg/ml Con A was assessed (▲—▲). Results of proliferative assays are expressed as a percentage inhibition in [³H] thymidine uptake of spleen cells from arthritic rats compared to [³H] thymidine uptake of normal spleen cells assayed on the same day.

arthritic response. Splenic hyporesponsiveness to mitogenic stimulation developed in parallel with detectable arthritis as measured by paw edema. The splenic immunodeficiency was apparent by day 4 after *M. butyricum* injection and by day 16-22 the Con A responsiveness of "arthritic" cells was reduced by 80-90%. *In vitro* proliferative responses to other mitogens such as PHA and PWM are also reduced and spleen cells from ovalbumin-immune arthritic rats responded poorly when stimulated *in vitro* with ovalbumin (data not shown).

The immunodeficiency observed in arthritic rats was dependent upon the development of arthritis and was not simply a consequence of exposure of the animals to *M. butyricum* as spleen cell proliferative responses was normal in *M. butyricum*-injected animals which did not develop arthritis (10).

The reduced proliferative responsiveness of arthritic cells was not due to down-regulation of proliferative by prostaglandins. Thus, treatment of "arthritic" spleen cells with 1 μM indomethacin inhibited >90% of prostaglandin synthesis but did not restore to normal the ability of these cells to proliferate in response to Con A or PHA (10).

Lymphokine regulation of T cell responsiveness

Since IL-1 and IL-2 are important soluble mediators of T cell activation, we addressed the possibility that the reduced proliferative response of "arthritic" spleen cells could be due to abnormal production of and/or response to IL-1 and IL-2 by "arthritic" cells. LPS-stimulated IL-1 synthesis by macrophages from the spleens of arthritic rats was equal to or greater than IL-1 synthesis by normal macrophages, while IL-2 synthesis by "arthritic" spleen cells was reduced (Table 1). Moreover, the Con A-induced proliferative response of "arthritic" cells was lower than normal even if the cultures were supplemented

TABLE 1.   *Synthesis of IL-1 and IL-1 and IL-2 by Spleen Cells from Normal and Arthritic Rats*

	IL-1 Synthesis by LPS-Stimulated Splenic Macrophages[a]			IL-2 Synthesis by Con A-Stimulated Spleen Cells[b]		
		IL-1 activity (Δdpm x 10^{-3})			IL-2 activity (dpm x 10^{-3})	
Supernatant Dilution	Normal	Arthritic	Supernatant Dilution	Normal	Arthritic
1/16	632	615	1/4	225	228
1/64	522	643	1/16	236	172*
1/256	352	433	1/64	177	58*
1/512	69	70	1/256	85	15*

[a] For IL-1 production, plastic adherent spleen cells (>85% macrophages) from normal and arthritic rats (16 days after *M. butyricum* injection) were cultured (5 x 10^6/ml) for 24 h. with 10 μg/ml LPS. Supernatant fluids were collected and assayed for IL-1 levels using a thymocyte costimulator assay (C3H/HEJ thymocytes). The numbers are the mean dpm [^{3}H] thymidine uptake for triplicate cultures (x 10^{-3}) with the dpm of thymocytes plus PHA alone (11,425) subtracted (i.e., Δdpm).

[b] For IL-2 production, spleen cells from normal and arthritic rats were cultured with 0.1 μg/ml Con A for 24 h and supernatant fluids were collected and assayed for IL-2 levels using an IL-2 dependent T cell line, CTLL-2. Numbers indicate the mean dpm [^{3}H] thymidine uptake (x 10^{-3}) for triplicate cultures.

* $P \leq 0.05$ compared to the same dilution of supernatant fluid from normal spleen cells (Dunnett's t-test).

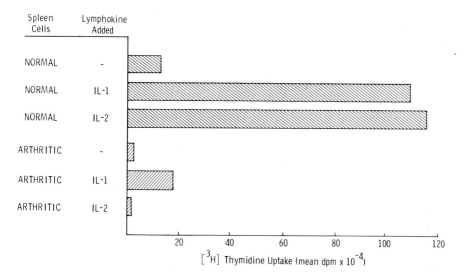

FIG. 2.   Effects of exogenous IL-1 and IL-2 on the proliferative response of spleen cells from normal and arthritic rats to Con A. Spleen cells from normal or arthritic rats (16 days after *M. butyricum* injection) were cultured *in vitro* with 1 μg/ml Con A plus either 0.5 units/ml purified human IL-1 or 10 units/ml recombinant human IL-2 and [³H] uptake was assessed on day 4.

with exogenous purified human IL-1, partially purified rat IL-2 or recombinant human IL-2 (Figure 2). In addition, Con A-activated spleen cells from arthritic rats did not utilize IL-2 in culture or bind and absorb this T cell growth factor as did normal cells (10). These results suggest that the deficient spleen cell proliferative response of arthritic cells results primarily from a reduced ability of T cells from the animals to recognize and respond to IL-1 and IL-2.

Role of suppressor cells

Whether the reduced mitogen and lymphokine responsiveness of "arthritic" spleen cells was an intrinsic T cell defect or the result of an active suppressive mechanism was assessed by cell subset analysis and cell fractionation studies. Fluorescent antibody studies using monoclonal antibodies to rat T helper (W3/25) or T suppressor/cytotoxic (OX8) cells did not reveal any dramatic alteration in the percentage of total T cells (50-55%) or W3/25⁺/OX8⁺ ratio (2:1) in "arthritic" spleen cells which could explain the functional changes observed. However, nylon wool purified T cells from the spleens of arthritic rats becam IL-2 responsive and actively proliferated to Con A stimulation when supplied with normal splenic macrophage accessory cells (Figure 3) and splenic macrophages from arthritic rats suppressed the *in vitro* Con A-induced proliferative response of normal spleen cells to a greater degree than did equivalent numbers of normal macrophages (Table 2). Finally, macrophages isolated from the spleen of arthritic rats elaborated in culture a soluble factor

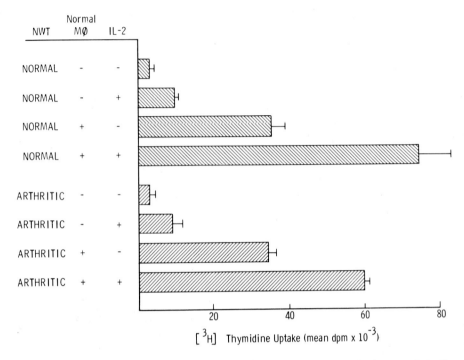

FIG. 3.   Ability of T cells form arthritic rats to proliferate and respond to IL-2 when supplied with normal macrophage accessory cells. T cells were purified by nylon wool filtration from the spleens of normal and arthritic rats (16 days after *M. butyricum* injection) and cultured *in vitro* (2 x 10⁵/well) with 0.1 μg/ml Con A. T cell cultures were supplemented with 10⁴ normal splenic macrophages and/or 5 U/ml rat IL-2. Proliferation (mean [³H] thymidine uptake of triplicate cultures was assessed on day 4.

TABLE 2.   *Effects of Macrophages from Normal and Arthritic Rats on the Proliferative Response of Normal Spleen Cells[a]*

| | Source of Added Macrophages | | | |
| | Normal | | Arthritic | |
Macrophages Added	[³H] Thymidine Uptake	% Change	[³H] Thymidine Uptake	% Change
± 18[b]	—	212 ± 18[b]	—	
1%	190 ± 19	↓10	183 ± 15	↓14*
5%	177 ± 12	↓17	134 ± 6	↓37*
10%	160 ± 12	↓25	118 ± 10	↓44*

[a] Splenic macrophages (>85% purity) were isolated from the spleens of normal and arthritic rats (16 days after *M. butyricum* injection). Varying numbers of these cells were cultured with 2 x 10⁵ unfractionated normal spleen cells in the presence of 1 μ/ml Con A and proliferation ([³H] thymidine uptake) assessed on day 4.
[b] Numbers indicate the mean dpm [³H] thymidine uptake (x 10⁻³) ± S.D. for triplicate cultures.
* P ≤ 0.05 compared to cultures containing the same percentage of normal macrophages (Dunnett's t-test).

TABLE 3. *Effects of Macrophages Culture Supernatants on the Mitogen-Induced Proliferative Response of Normal Spleen Cells*[a]

Macrophages Supernatant Added	Proliferative Response			
	Con A (1 µg/ml)		PWM (0.1 µg/ml)	
	[³H] Thymidine Uptake	% Change	[³H] Thymidine Uptake	% Change
—	240 ± 44[b]	—	419 ± 44[b]	—
Normal	267 ± 40	↑11	425 ± 13	↑2
Arthritic	7 ± 8	↓99*	4 ± 3	↓99*

[a] Macrophages were isolated from the spleens of normal and arthritic rats (16 days after *M. butyricum* injection) and cultured for 4 days at 37°C (10^7 cells/ml). Supernatant fluids from these cultures were dialysed against phosphate-buffered saline and assessed for their ability to inhibit the Con A or PWM response of normal spleen cells at a final supernatant concentration of 10%.
[b] Numbers indicate the mean dpm [³H] thymidine uptake ($\times 10^{-3}$) $\pm$ S.D. of triplicate cultures.
* $P \leq 0.05$ compared to cultures without macrophage supernatant (Dunnett's t-test).

which suppressed the mitogen-induced proliferative response of normal spleen cells (Table 3). This monokine activity was non-dialysable (3500 MW exclusion) and trypsin sensitive but resistant to heating at 75°C for 10 minutes.

DISCUSSION

We have characterized an immunodeficiency syndrome associated with experimental arthritic disease in rats in which *in vitro* spleen cell proliferative responsiveness is markedly impaired (3, 10). This syndrome is particularly interesting in view of the close resemblance between the lymhoid hyporesponsiveness observed in this animal model and that described in patients with rheumatoid arthritis (13, 14).

It has become increasingly clear that a variety of cytokines regulate T cell activation processes. In particular, interleukins 1 and 2 are critically important for optimal T cell activation to occur (5, 15). We and others have proposed that altered production of and/or responsiveness to mediators such as IL-1 and IL-2 could explain at least some of the abnormalities in lymphoid cell function observed in autoimmune and immunodeficiency disorders (6, 9). The data presented here provide additional support for this hypothesis as lymphokine abnormalities appear to contribute to the immunoregulatory imbalance observed in rats with experimentally-induced arthritic disease.

We focused our efforts on the roles of IL-1 and IL-2 in the reduced proliferate responsiveness of spleen cells from arthritic rats. No evidence was found that this proliferative defect is due to a lack of available IL-1. While the synthesis of IL-1 by "arthritic" cells appears normal, T cells from arthritic rats do not respond as well as normal T cell to IL-1. Thus, the relative increase in [³H] thymidine uptake induced by exogenous IL-1 is lower in cultures of "arthritic" spleen cells than in similar cultures of normal cells and the absolute amount of [^{3}H] thymidine uptake is lower in "arthritic" cells cultured with or without exogenous IL-1.

Spleen cells from arthritic rats produce lower than normal amounts of IL-2, but this does not appear to be physiologically meaningful as addition of exogenous IL-2 to cultures of "arthritic" cells does not restore their proliferative activity. In fact, "arthritic" cells are virtually unresponse to exogenous IL-2. Cell fractionation experiments suggest that the reduced proliferative capacity and lymphokine responsiveness of arthritic cells results from the action of a plastic adherent suppressor cell (e.g., macrophage). Thus macrophage-enriched spleen cells from arthritic rats actively suppress the Con A response of normal spleen cells and purified "arthritic" T cells produce and respond to IL-2 and proliferate normally when cultured with normal macrophages. Moreover, recent studies indicate that arthritic macrophages elaborate a soluble, trypsin-sensitive monokine which mediates their suppressive activity, but the importance of this mediator and its biochemical characteristics are not well defined at present.

We conclude from these observations that in the arthritic spleen suppressor macrophages interact with T cells in such a way as to reduce their ability to respond to IL-1 and IL-2 and that the failure of these cells to recognize and utilize IL-1 and IL-2-mediated growth signals limits their proliferative capacity. Whether the reduced lymphokine responsiveness occurs at a membrane receptor level or at some post-receptor event is unknown, although the finding that "arthritic" T cells bind less IL-2 than normal supports the former possibility (10).

The relationship between abnormal peripheral immune function and those articular events leading to joint destruction are not known at present, nor is it known whether restoring these peripheral manifestations to normal levels would result in clinical beneficial effects. These questions become particularly relevant in light of the recent data suggesting that IL-1 may be an important inflammatory mediator within the rheumatoid joint (5) and that many antirheumatic drugs have dramatic effects on immune responsiveness (11). However, aberrant cytokine regulation of T cell activation is not unique to arthritic disease as similar functional defects have been reported in systemic lupus erythematosus, acquired immune deficiency syndrome, and aged animals and humans (1, 4, 9). Further studies are required to determine the precise relevance of such immune defects to clinical expression of these important human diseases.

Acknowledgements

The collaborative efforts and helpful discussions by Drs. Richard Carlson and Alan Lewis and technical assistance by Louis Datko, John Daniels and Robert Wilson are gratefully acknowledged.

REFERENCES

1. Alcocer-Varela, J. and Alarcon-Segovia, D. (1982). Decreased production of and response to interleukin 2 by cultured lymphocytes from patients with systemic lupus erythematosus. *J. Clin. Invest.* 69:1388-1392.
2. Billingham, M.E.J. (1983). Models of arthrits and the search for antiarthritic drugs. *Pharmacol. Ther.* 21:389-428.
3. Binderup, L., Bram, E. and Arrigoni-Martelli, E. (1983). The effect of some antirheumatic drugs *in vivo* on the response of spleen cells to concanavalin A in rats with chronic inflammation. *Int. J. Immunopharmac.* 4:57-66.
4. Dauphinee, M.J., Kepper, S.B., Wofsy, D. and Talal, N. (1981). Interleukin 2 deficiency is a common feature of autoimmune mice. *J. Immunol.* 127:2483-2487.
5. Dinarello, C.A. (1984). Interleukin 1. *Rev. Infect. Dis.* 6:51-95.
6. Dosch, H.-M. and Shore, A. (1982). Hypothesis: the role of interleukins in lymphopoesis - important in autoimmune disease *J. Rheumatol.* 9:353-358.
7. Gilman, S.C., Rosenberg, J.S. and Feldman, J.D. (1982). T lymphocyte of young and aged rats. II. Functional deficits and the role of intelukin 2. *J. Immunol.* 128:644-650.
8. Gilman, S.C., Rosenberg, J.S. and Feldman, J.D. (1983). Inhibition of interleukin synthesis and T cell proliferation by a monoclonal anti-Ia antibody, *J. Immunol.* 130:1236-1240.
9. Gilman, S.C. (1984). Lymphokines in immunological aging. *Lymphokine Res.* 3:119-123.
10. Gilman, S.C., Daniels, J.F., Wilson, R.E., Carlson, R.P. and Lewis, A.J. (1984). Lymphoid abnormalities in rats with adjuvant induced arthritis. I. Mitogen responsiveness and lymphokine synthesis. *Ann. Rheum. Dis.* 43:847-855.
11. Gilman, S.C. and A.J. Lewis, (1985). Immunomodulatory drugs in the treatment of rheumatoid arthritis. In: *Antiinflammatory and Antirheumatic Drugs*, edited by Rainsford, K.D., CRC Press, Boca Raton, FL (in press).
12. Harris, E.D. (1984). Pathogenesis of rheumatoid arthritis. *Clin. Orthoped. Rel. Res.*, 182:14-23.
13. Miyasaka, N., Nakamura, T., Russell, I.J. and Talal, N. (1984). Interleukin 2 deficiencies in rheumatoid arthritis and systemic lupus erythematosus. *Clin. Immunol. Immunopathol*, 31:109-117.
14. Seitz, M., Diemann, W., Gram, N., Hunstein, W.D. and Gemsa, D. (1982). Characterization of blood mononuclear cells of arthritis patients. 1. Depressed lymphocyte proliferation and enhanced prostanoid release from monocytes. *Clin. Immunol. Immunopathol.*, 25:405-416.
15. Smith, K.A. (1980). T cell growth factor. *Immunol. Rev.* 51:337-357.
16. Zvaifler, N.J. (1973). The immunopathology of joint inflammation in rheumatoid arthritis. *Adv. Immunol.*, 16:265-336.

Immunoregulatory Activity of Thymosin alpha - 1

Gino Doria, Luciano Ardorini, Camillo Mancini,
and Daniela Frasca

Laboratory of Pathology, ENEA C.R.E. Casaccia
C.P. 2400, 00100 Rome, A.D., Italy

The calf thymus extract Fraction 5 (12) contains several immunoregulatory peptides including thymosin α_1 which has been purified to homogeneity and sequenced (17). This peptide consists of 28 amino acid residues (m.w. 3,108) and has been synthesized chemically (26) and by recombinant DNA technology (27). The role of thymosin α_1 in promoting and maintaining T cell maturation to effector cells has important immunoregulatory effects in several experimental animal models and clinical trials, as recently reviewed (28, 22).

Following thymus involution, the decline in circulating thymosin α_1 concentration (19) may be correlated with reduction in rate of T lymphocyte maturation and decrease in cell-mediated and antibody responses observed in aged mice (13). Hence, profound functional defects in helper T cell activity (16, 1, 5) as well as in IL-2 production (24) and expression of IL-2 receptors (2) have been described in aged mice.

Injection of immunodeficient old mice with synthetic thymosin α_1 has been previously described to be effective in restoring defects in helper activity of whole spleen cells (10) and of T cell subpopulations (6). In the present study aging mice have been used as an experimental model of secondary immunodeficiency to investigate the *in vivo* effects of synthetic thymosin α_1 or its fragments on helper T cell activity and IL-2 production. Data presented in this paper demonstrate that the N-terminal half of thymosin α_1 is as effective as the entire α_1 molecule to enhance helper activity, IL-2 production, and expression of IL-2 receptors in old mice, whereas the C-terminal half has no enhancing effects. Part of these results have been presented elsewhere (4, 9).

MATERIALS AND METHODS

Animals. Male (C57BL/10xDBA/2) F1 mice, bred and maintained in our animal facilities, were used at the age of 3-24 months.

Antigens. Horse red blood cells (HRBC) and sheep red blood cells (SRBC) were obtained from Sclavo (Siena, Italy). Two,4,6-Trinitrobenzene sulfonic acid (TNBS) purchased from Eastman Organic Chemicals (Rochester, NY) was further purified by recrystallization from 1 N HCl. Two,4,6-trinitrophenyl (TNP)-HRBC was prepared by heavy conjugation of TNBS to HRBC (14) and used *in vitro* as immunogen. TNP-SRBC, prepared by light conjugation of TNBS to SRBC (21) was used as test antigen in the Cunningham and Szenberg assay (3) to detect anti-TNP plaque forming cells (PFC).

Cell culture. Spleen cell suspensions were cultured in microtissue culture plates (Falcon 3040) according to Mishell and Dutton (20). Complete culture medium contained: RPMI 1640 (Gibco, NY) supplemented with 10% fetal calf serum (FCS) (Flow Laboratories, UK), 2 mM L-glutamine (Gibco) and 10 μg/ml gentamicin (Shering, Kenilworth, NY). Only for IL-2 production and titration, complete medium was supplemented with 5×10^{-5} M 2-mercaptoethanol (2-ME). CTLL cells (from K.A. Smith) were cultured in 2-ME-containing medium supplemented with 5% MLA 144 cell culture supernatant as IL-2 source. Ig-non producing mouse myeloma cells, P3X63 Ag8.563 (from M.D. Scharff) were cultured in 2-ME-containing medium.

Titration of helper cell activity. Mice were carrier-primed by intravenous injection of 2×10^5 HRBC in 0.2 ml phosphate-buffered saline (PBS) to induce helper activity 4 days before sacrifice. Helper activity of spleen cells from carrier-primed mice was titrated by a modification of the method originally described by Kettman and Dutton (15). Briefly, in each experiment triplicate culture wells received 0.1 ml medium containing 2×10^5 TNP-HRBC and 1×10^6 nucleated spleen cells from a pool of 8-10 uninjected 3 month old mice. Culture wells of one group received no further cells and were used as background control, while wells of other groups received graded numbers ($5\text{-}25\times10^4$) of nucleated spleen cells pooled from 4-6 carrier-primed mice of a given age. Previous experiments demonstrated that under these conditions helper activity of carrier-primed spleen cells is limited by T cells and is not influenced by B cells or macrophages (5). The anti-TNP antibody response of cells pooled from triplicate wells was evaluated at day 4 and 5 of culture and expressed as PFC/culture. The PFC response of 1×10^6 nucleated spleen cells from the unprimed 3 month old mice was subtracted from the PFC responses exhibited by the same spleen cells co-cultured with $5\text{-}25\times10^4$ spleen cells from carrier-primed mice. Helper activity was evaluated from the anti-TNP PFC versus primed cells/culture regression coefficient ± Se (standard error) of a straight line forced through the origin by the least squares method (23).

Thymosin treatment. Six-24 month old mice were injected intraperitoneally with 0.2 ml saline containing 10 μg synthetic thymosin α_1, 3 days before carrier-priming or 7 days before sacrifice. Alternatively, mice received one intraperitoneal injection of 0.2 ml saline containing 5 μg N_{14} (N-terminal amino acid residues 1-14) or C_{14} (C-terminal amino acid residues 15-28) synthetic fragment of the α_1 molecule. Thymosin α_1 and its fragments were kindly provided by A.L. Goldstein.

IL-2 treatment. Twenty-four month old mice were injected with 0.1 ml medium containing 1 U of IL-2 from EL-4, or AOFS (from J. Kappler), or Concanavalin A (Con A)-stimulated spleen cells. Each IL-2 preparation was injected subcutaneously immediately before carrier-priming.

IL-2 production. Gibbon IL-2 was produced by culturing MLA 144 cell line ($4x10^5$ cells/ml) in tissue culture dishes (Falcon 3003) at 37° C in a 5% CO_2 humidified incubator. Culture supernatant was collected by centrifugation 3 days later, when the initial cell density reached $1-2x10^6$/ml. The IL-2 containing supernatant was filtered through 0.2 μ Millex Filter (Millipore, France) and stored at –20°C. MLA 144 culture supernatant was routinely used to maintain IL-2 dependent CTLL cells and as standard preparation in the IL-2 titration assay.

Murine IL-2 production was induced by stimulating spleen cells ($1x10^7$/ml) in culture (Falcon 3008) with 2 μg/ml Con A (Miles-Yeda Laboratories, Rehowoth, Israel) and 10 ng/ml Phorbol Myristic Acetate (PMA) (Sigma, St. Louis, MO). After 48 hrs under the same culture conditions supernatants were collected, filtered and stored until use, as described above. Con A and PMA concentrations were optimal for maximum IL-2 production.

IL-2 titration. The assay was based on the method of Gillis et al. (11) but involved statistical validation of titration data according to the principles of the biological assay by parallel lines as applied to probit analysis of quantitative responses (8). Briefly, supernatants were two-fold serially diluted in medium from 1:2 to 1:256, and 100 μl samples of each dilution were added to triplicate microwells (Falcon 3040) containing 100 μl of IL-2 dependent CTLL cell suspension ($1x10^4$/well). Triplicate cell control wells received 100 μl medium instead of dilution samples. After 20 hrs incubation at 37° C all cultures received 0.5 μCi of ^{3}HTdR in 20 μl (specific activity 2 μCi/mole, The Radiochemical Centre, Amersham, U.K.). Four hrs later, cells were harvested by an automated cell harvester (Skatron). Filter disks were transferred to vials containing liquid scintillation fluid (Filtercount, Packard) and radioactivity was measured as counts per minute (cpm) in a Tri-Carb 460 CD scintillation counter (Packard, Downers Grove, IL). The mean cpm from triplicate control wells containing cells cultured in medium without IL-2 was subtracted from cpm in each well. Net cpm were then referred, as percent, to the maximum cpm observed in the assay. Sigmoid curves fitting percent of the maximum response as a function of the reciprocal of supernatant $\log_2$ final dilutions were transformed in straight lines by substituting percentage with probit value for each well. In each titration assay, probit transformation was applied to standard dilutions of MLA 144 culture supernatant (arbitrarily defined to contain 10 U gibbon IL-2/ml) and to experimental dilutions of spleen cell culture supernatants. Parallelism between the standard regression and each experimental regression as well as linearity of the two combined regressions were verified by analysis of variance. The potency of an experimental supernatant relative to that of the standard supernatant was calculated as the antilog of the orizontal distance between the experimental and standard lines. Then, the relative potency was multiplied by 10 to estimate the IL-2 titer of the experimental supernatant in terms of U/ml. A factor by which the titer should be multiplied or divided to obtain the variation due to one standard error was also calculated.

Radioimmuno assay. IL-2 receptors on mitogen-activated spleen cells from mice of different ages have been detected by radioimmuno assay (RIA) carried out at room temperature. Flexible microtiter plates (Flacon 3912) were treated (100 μl/well) with a solution of poly-L-lysine hydrobromide (approximate m.w. 300,000, Sigma P-1524) in distilled water (25 μg/ml). After 45 min the solution was flicked off, plates were washed twice with balanced salt solution (BSS), and each well received 50 μl of a cell suspension in BSS ($4x10^6$/ml). The cells used in each assay were mitogen-activated mouse spleen cells (see *IL-2 production*), P3X63 Ag8.653 Ig-non producing mouse myeloma cells (negative control) and CTLL cells (positive control). Each cell suspension was washed in BSS and distributed in a series of triplicate wells. After 1 hr, plates were washaed with BSS, incubated for 5 min with 0.1% glutaraldehyde in 0.1 M phosphate buffer pH 7.4, washed twice with BSS and then incubated for 5 min with 0.1 M glycine buffer pH 7.0. After two washings with BSS each well received 200 μl of 1% bovine serum albumin (Sigma) and 0.02% NaN_3 in BSS. Plates were covered with plastic sealers and stored at 4° C up to 3 months. Before use, cell-coated wells were washed three times with 2% FCS in PBS (RIA Buffer, RIAB). Rat IgM monoclonal antibory 7D4 (from E.M. Shevach) specific for the mouse IL-2 receptor (18) was two-fold serially diluted in RIAB from 1:200 to 1:12,800 and 100 μl samples of each dilution were added to cell-coated triplicate wells. For each cell population additional triplicate wells received 100 μl of RIAB instead of monoclonal antibody. After 1 hr incubation unbound antibody was flicked off and plates were washed three times with RIAB. All cell-coated wells received 100 μl of rabbit antibodies anti-rat Ig (RARIg) diluted 1:1000 in RIAB. After 1 hr incubation unbound RARIg was removed by repeated washings of the plates with RIAB. Finally, all wells received 100 μl RIAB containing ^{125}I-Protein A ($1x10^5$ cpm) from *Staphilococcus aureus* and after 45 min unbound radioactivity was removed by washing the plates four times with RIAB. Wells were cut and radioactivity was measured as cpm in a gamma counter (Kontron). Results are expressed as net cpm: mean cpm from triplicate wells with 7D4 - mean cpm from triplicate wells without 7D4.

RESULTS

Results in Table 1 illustrate that helper T cell activity is impaired by aging but is restored to a large extent by injection of 10 μg thymosin α_1. Moreover,

TABLE 1. *Effect of thymosin α_1 peptide, N_{14} or C_{14} fragment injection on helper T cell activity in aging mice*

Exp. No.	Age (mos.)	Material injected	Anti-TNP PFC vs. primed cells/culture regression coefficient $\pm$ SE
1	3	none	141 $\pm$ 4
	6	none	81 $\pm$ 1
	6	α_1 (10 µg)	104 $\pm$ 6
	6	N_{14} (5 µg)	147 $\pm$ 3
	6	C_{14} (5 µg)	83 $\pm$ 5
2	3	none	241 $\pm$ 19
	18	none	104 $\pm$ 4
	18	α_1 (10 µg)	179 $\pm$ 12
	18	N_{14} (5 µg)	208 $\pm$ 9
	18	C_{14} (5 µg)	112 $\pm$ 6

Helper activity of spleen cells pooled from 4 mice, HRBC-primed at the age of 3-18 months, was titrated by adding graded numbers ($5-25 \times 10^4$) of these primed cells to cultures containing 1×10^6 normal spleen cells from 3 month old mice and 2×10^5 TNP-HRBC. Helper activity was evaluated from the anti-TNP PFC versus primed cells/culture regression coefficient of a straight line forced through the origin. Thymosin α_1 peptide, N_{14} or C_{14} fragment was injected intraperitoneally 3 days before HRBC-priming.

injection of an equimolar amount of the N_{14} fragment is at least as effective as the entire α_1 molecule in restoring helper T cell activity in 6 and 18 month old mice, whereas injection of the C_{14} fragment has no effect.

Results in Table 2 indicate that helper T cell activity in 24 month old mice is increased, up to the same level as in young mice, by injecting 1 unit of IL-2 from any of the three different sources.

TABLE 2. *Effect of IL-2 injection on helper T cell activity in aging mice*

Age (mos.)	Material injected	Anti-TNP PFC vs. primed cells/culture regression coefficient $\pm$ SE
3	none	231 $\pm$ 9
24	none	87 $\pm$ 9
24	EL-4 IL-2 (1 U)	205 $\pm$ 24
24	AOFS IL-2 (1 U)	298 $\pm$ 31
24	Con A sup. IL-2 (1 U)	203 $\pm$ 19

Helper activity of spleen cells pooled from 4 mice, HRBC-primed at the age of 3 or 24 months, was titrated as described in table 1. Each IL-2 preparation (0.1 ml) was injected subcutaneously immediately before HRBC-priming.

The results reported in Table 1 and 2 suggest the possibility that thymosin α_1 and the N_{14} fragment act on helper T cells via the induction of IL-2 production. This possibility is supported by the results in Table 3 showing that aging negatively affects IL-2 production while the injection of either thymosin

TABLE 3.   *Effect of thymosin α_1 peptide, N_{14} or C_{14} fragment injection on IL-2 production by spleen cells from aging mice*

Age (mos.)	Material injected	IL-2 U/ml $\pm$ SE
3	none	6.59 (1.16)[a]
12	none	0.93 $\pm$ 0.07
12	α_1 (10 μg)	5.57 $\pm$ 0.44
12	N_{14} (5 μg)	6.94 $\pm$ 0.49
12	C_{14} (5 μg)	0.90 $\pm$ 0.11

IL-2 units refer either to a single value from a pool of 4 mice (3 mos.) or to mean values from 8 individual mice (12 mos.). Thymosin α_1 peptide, N_{14} or C_{14} fragment was injected intraperitoneally 7 days before sacrifice.
[a] Figure in parentheses is the factor by which the IL-2 units should be multiplied or divided to obtain the variation due to one standard error.

α_1 or its N_{14} fragment in 12 month old mice enhances IL-2 production up to the level of uninjected 3 month old mice. Again, injection of the C_{14} fragment was devoid of any effect.

Enhancement of IL-2 production as induced by injecting 12 month old mice with thymosin α_1 or its N_{14} fragment could favour the expression of IL-2 receptors. Results in Table 4 indeed demonstrate that thymosin α_1 or its N_{14} fragment, unlike the C_{14} fragment, induces the expression of IL-2 receptors on mitogen-activated spleen cells from old mice. This effect in turn could increase cell sensitivity to the IL-2 signal.

TABLE 4.   *Effect of thymosin α_1 peptide, N_{14} or C_{14} fragment injection on the expression of IL-2 receptors on mitogen-activated spleen cells from aging mice*

Age (mos.)	Material injected	^{125}I-Protein A bound (net cpm $\pm$ SE)
3	none	1,609 $\pm$ 156
12	none	280 $\pm$ 48
12	α (10 μg)	1,035 $\pm$ 134
12	N_{14} (5 μg)	1,194 $\pm$ 103
12	C_{14} (5 μg)	391 $\pm$ 45

Mitogen-activated spleen cells pooled from 4 mice, young (3 mos.) or old (12 mos.), were incubated stepwise with rat monoclonal antibody 7D4 (dilution 1:200), rabbit antibodies anti-rat Ig, and ^{125}I-Protein A. Net cpm represent the difference between mean cpm from triplicate wells containing 7D4 and mean cpm from triplicate wells in which 7D4 has been replaced by RIAB. Old mice were uninjected or injected intraperitoneally with thymosin α_1 peptide or its N_{14} or C_{14} fragment 7 days before sacrifice. Net cpm $\pm$ SE in controls: P3X63 Ag8.653 cells, 28 $\pm$ 18; CTLL cells, 2,263 $\pm$ 195.

DISCUSSION

The present findings demonstrate that the age-related decline of helper T cell activity, IL-2 production, and expression of IL-2 receptors can be counteracted by injecting old mice with synthetic thymosin α_1. This enhancing activity of thymosin α_1 is restricted to the first 14 amino acid residues from the N-terminal end of the α_1 molecule, whereas the other half of the thymosin molecule is devoid of any demonstrable activity. A similar effect on helper T cell activity can also be induced by injecting 24 month old mice with IL-2 from different sources. This result is in line with the observation that although IL-2 synthesis is decreased in aged mice the ability to respond to IL-2 is unimpaired, as their immune responses can be reconstituted by injecting exogenous IL-2 (25).

It is apparent from the present study that thymosin α_1-induced enhancement of helper T cell activity in old mice may be mediated by increase in IL-2 production and expression of IL-2 receptors. Thus, the major activity of thymosin α_1 in maintaining and regulating T cell functions is likely to involve an increase in the cell precursor frequency of IL-2 producing T cells. Since IL-2 is a necessary signal not only for the expansion of helper T cells but also for the production of other lymphokines required for the generation of effector cells (7), modulation of IL-2 production by thymosin α_1 provides a rational basis for therapeutic intervention in several immunodeficiency syndromes.

Acknowledgements

Work supported by ENEA-EURATOM Contract and by Istituto Pasteur - Fondazione Cenci Bolognetti. Publication No. 00 of the EURATOM Biology Division.

REFERENCES

1. Callard, R.E., and Basten, A. (1978): Immune functions in aged mice. IV. Loss of T cell and B cell functions in thymus-dependent antibody responses. *Eur. J. Immunol.*, 8:552-558.
2. Chang, M.P., Makinodan, T., Peterson, W.J., and Strehler, B.L. (1982): Role of T cells and adherent cells in age-related decline in murine interleukin 2 production. *J. Immunol.*, 129:2426-2430.
3. Cunningham, A.J., and Szenberg, A. (1968): Further improvements in the plaque technique for detecting single antibody-forming cells. *Immunology*, 14:599-606.
4. Doria, G., Adorini, L., and Frasca, D. (1984): Recovery of T cell functions in aged mice by injection of immunoregulatory molecules. In: *Lymphoid Cell Functions in Aging*, edited by A.L. De Weck, pp. 59-68. EURAGE.
5. Doria, G., D'Agostaro, G., and Garavini, M. (1980): Age-dependent changes of B-cell reactivity and T cell-T cell interaction in the in vitro antibody response. *Cell. Immunol.*, 53:195-206.
6. Doria, G., Frasca, D., and Adorini, L. (1984): Immunoregulation of antibody response in aging. In: *Progress in Immunology V*, edited by T. Tada, and M. Yamamura, pp. 1549-1562. Academic Press, Tokyo.
7. Farrar, J.J., Benjamin, W.R., Hilfiker, M.L., Howard, M., Farrar, W.L., and Fuller-Farrar, J. (1982): The biochemistry, biology, and role of interleukin 2 in the induction of cytotoxic T cell and antibody-forming B cell responses. *Immunol. Rev.*, 63:129-166.
8. Finney, D.J. (1964): *Statistical Method in Biological Assay*, Charles Griffin, and Co., London.
9. Frasca, D., Adorini, L., and Doria, G. (1984): Production of and response to interleukin 2 in aging mice. Modulation by thymosin α_1. In: *Lymphoid Cell Functions in Aging*, edited by A.L. De Weck, pp. 155-160. EURAGE.

10. Frasca, D., Garavini, M., and Doria, G. (1982): Recovery of T-cell functions in aged mice injected with synthetic thymosin α_1. *Cell. Immunol.*, 72:384-391.
11. Gillis, S., Ferm, M.M., Ou, V., and Smith, K.A. (1978): T cell growth factor parameters of production and a quantitative microassay for activity. *J. Immunol.*, 120:2027-2032.
12. Hooper, J.A., McDaniel, M.C., Thurman, G.B., Cohen, G.H., Schulof, R.S., and Goldstein, A.L. (1975): The purification and properties of bovine thymosin. *Ann. N.Y. Acad. Sci. USA*, 249:125-144.
13. Kay, M.M.B. (1978): Effect of age on T cell differentiation. *Fed. Proc.*, 37:1241-1244.
14. Kettman, J., and Dutton, R.W. (1970): An in vitro primary immune response to 2,4,6,trinitrophenyl substituted erythrocytes: response against carrier and hapten. *J. Immunol.*, 104:1558-1561.
15. Kettman, J., and Dutton, R.W. (1971): Radioresistance of the enhancing effect of cells from carrier-immunized mice in an in vitro primary immune response. *Proc. Natl. Acad. Sci. USA*, 68:699-703.
16. Krogsrud, R.L., and Perkins, E.H. (1977): Age-related changes in T-cell function. *J. Immunol.*, 118:1607-1617.
17. Low, T.L.K., and Goldstein, A.L. (1979): The chemistry and biology of thymosin. II. Amino acid sequence analysis of thymosin α_1 and polypeptide β_1. *J. Biol. Chem.*, 254:987-995.
18. Malek, T.R., Robb, R.J., and Shevach, E.M. (1983): Identification and initial characterization of a rat monoclonal antibody reactive with the murine interleukin 2 receptor-ligand complex. *Proc. Natl. Acad. Sci. USA*, 80:5694-5698.
19. McClure, J.E., Lameris, N., Wara, D.W., and Goldstein, A.L. (1982): Immunochemical studies on thymosin: radioimmunoassay for thymosin α_1. *J. Immunol.*, 128:368-375.
20. Mischell, R.J., and Dutton, R.W. (1967): Immunization of dissociated spleen cells from cultures of normal mice. *J. Exp. Med.*, 126:423-442.
21. Rittenberg, M.B., and Pratt, K.L. (1969): Antitrinitrophenyl (TNP) plaque assay. Primary response of Balb/c mice to soluble and particulate immunogens. *Proc. Soc. Exp. Biol. Med.*, 132:575-581.
22. Sculof, R.S., and Goldstein, A.L. (1983): Clinical applications of thymosin and other thymic hormones. In: *Recent Advances in Clinical Immunology*, edited by R.A. Thompson, and N.R. Rose, pp. 243-286. Churchill Livingstone, London.
23. Steel, R.G.D., and Torrie, J.H. (1960): *Principles and procedures of statistics*. McGraw-Hill Book Company, New York.
24. Thoman, M.L., and Weigle, W.O. (1981): Lymphokines and aging: interleukin-2 production and activity in aged animals. *J. Immunol.*, 127:2102-2106.
25. Thoman, M.L., and Weigle, W.O. (1985): Reconstitution of in vivo cell-mediated lympholysis. Responses in aged mice with interleukin 2. *J. Immunol.*, 134:949-952.
26. Wang, S.S., Douvan Kulesha, I., and Winter, D.P. (1979): Synthesis of Thymosin α_1. *J. Am. Chem. Soc.*, 101:253-254.
27. Wetzel, R., Heyneker, H.L., Goeddel, D.V., Jhurani, P., Shapiro, J., Crea, R., Low, T.L.K., McClure, J.E., Thurman, G.B., and Goldstein A.L. (1980): Production of biologically active N^{α}-desacetylthymosin α_1 in E. Coli through expression of a chemically synthesized gene. *Biochemistry*, 19:6096-6104.
28. Zatz, M.M., Low, T.L.K., and Goldstein, A.L. (1982): Role of thymosin and other thymic hormones in T-cell differentiation. In: *Biological Responses in Cancer*, edited by E. Mihich, pp. 219-247. Plenum Publishing Co., New York.

The Role of Thymic Hormones in Regulating T Cell Activity and Lymphokine Production

Jacob Shoham

Department of Life Sciences, Bar Ilan University
Ramat Gan 52100, Israel

INTRODUCTION

The evidence linking the thymus with proper development and maturation of the immune system belong already to the sphere of classical immunology. It was also established beyond any doubt that the thymus exerts its maturational and regulatory effects on T cells by both microenvironmental, direct influence on immature T cells migrating into it (5) and by soluble factors secreted from its epithelial-endocrine cell compartment (1, 37). Several groups of investigators have been involved in the isolation and characterization of thymic soluble factors (1, 10, 26, 37) and it is widely recognized today that more than one, the exact number is still unknown, of such soluble factors are involved in performing the humoral function of the thymus (2).

Numerous studies demonstrated thymic humoral effect on almost all aspects of T cell activity (for reviews see 1, 35, 37). The aim of the present communication is not to catalogue documented effects of various thymic factors on T cell functions, but rather to suggest some general principles of thymus hormonal activity. By doing so I hope to contribute to the emerging trend of transition from the phenomenological and descriptive era of research on thymus factors to the stage in which the mechanism of the effects of these factors is better understood, leading to a more sensible clinical use of these factors, in conditions associated with immunodeficiencies or other diseases. I will use mostly studies performed in my laboratory (14-16; 26-34) in order to illustrate the proposed general principles. These studies were done primarily with one thymus preparation called thymostimulin (TS or TP-1). TP-1 is a partially purified extract of calf thymus prepared by Istituto Farmacologico Serono, Rome and initially characterized by Falchetti et al. (8). Proliferative T cell response (PR) in mixed lymphocyte tumor cell (MLTC) cultures (30, 31) and induction of cell mediated cytotoxicity (CMC) in vitro (29) as analysed with human peripheral blood mononuclear cells (PBMC), will serve as the two main examples for the present discussion.

THYMIC HORMONAL EFFECT ON PROLIFERATIVE RESPONSE AND CELL MEDIATED CYTOTOXICITY

The experimental system

Human PBMC isolated by Ficoll-Hypaque centrifugation (3), were incubated with TP-1 in the dose range 1 ng - 100 µg/ml (usually 1 µg/ml) for 1-18 hr at 37°C in serum free medium. Spleen and/or heart extracts, prepared similarly to TP-1 served as controls. After preincubation the PBMC were allowed to interact in culture with mitomicyn C treated human tumor cell lines (Raji lymphoma cells or IgR3 malignant melanoma cells). The outcome of this interaction was measured: (1) by proliferative response (PR) as judged by 3 H-thymidine incorporation (30, 31); (2) by cytotoxic activity CMC as measured by ^{51}Cr release from target cells (29); (3) by titrating the level of a lymphokine, immune interferon (IFNγ) secreted into the medium of these culture (34).

Main features of monitored effects

The observation made with this experimental system can be summarized as following:

a) TP-1 had a strong effect on PR and on induction of CMC, with a significant mean enhancement of their expression (Fig. 1). Such strong effects were demonstrated also with other thymic factors (1, 37).

b) The scatter of individual effects was however very wide, spanning from strong enhancement to strong suppression. Fig. 2 represents the scatter of effects of TP-1 on PR. Similar wide scatter with CMC (29). These results cannot be attributed to the nature of thymic factor under study, since such a wide scatter of effects was demonstated not only with the partially purified extract TP-1 but also with the synthetic serum thymic factor (FTS) (12), and it thus seems to be a general phenomenon.

c) The effect of TP-1 is negatively correlated with the level of PR in control: enhancement (or suppression) of PR by TP-1 became progressively greater as control PR became progressively lower (Fig. 2).

d) The mean effect (Fig. 1) and its scatter (Fig. 2) were similar in healthy subjects and cancer patients.

e) The maximal effect of TP-1 was obtained with suboptimal number of stimulating cells (Fig. 3). No effect was obtained under optimal stimulations conditions with both PR and CMC (29, 30).

f) The dose-effect relationships of TP-1 are in the form of a bell shape curve., i.e. doses higher and lower than the optimum one are without effect (Fig. 4). Such relationships were observed also in vivo for TP-1 (15) and for thymopoietin (17), and, in fact, may be regarded as a general characteristic of immunomodulating agents (28).

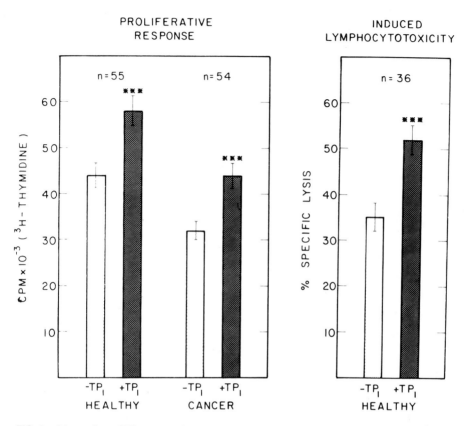

FIG. 1. Mean effect of TP-1 on proliferative response and induced lymphocytotoxicity of human PBMC using Raji lymphoma cells as stimulators. The PBMC were incubated with TP-1 (1 mg/ml, 1 hr, 37 c) and then cultured in MLTC for 4 days.

g) Target selectivity (specificity) of CMC, when present, was not masked by TP-1 induced enhancement, and in some case even become more pronounced (Fig. 5). However non-selective reactions may also be enhanced (29).

Implications as to some principles governing thymic hormonal activity on effector T cell functions

1. It was suggested that the effects of thymic factors on the immune system can be described as "normalizing" or "restorative" (9, 24). This general concept (11) was interpreted as suggesting higher ones in mixed lymphocyte culture and that thymosin corrects deficient and cancer patients (observation d, above) attest against this notion. The cancer patients did not respond better than the healthy subjects in spite of their documented immunodeficiency and

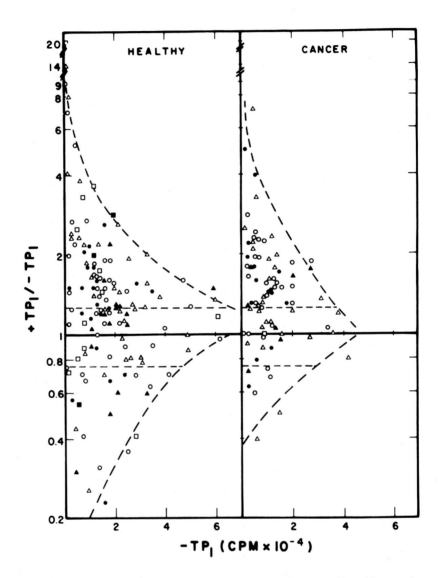

FIG. 2. Distribution of response to TP-1 treatment of PBMC from healthy subjects and cancer patients tested in MLTC assay with IgR3 melanoma cells after 4 ($\triangle$, $\blacktriangle$), 5 ($\bigcirc$, $\bullet$) or 6 ($\square$, $\blacksquare$) days in culture. Open symbols -2×10^4 IgR$_3$ cells; solid symbols -1×10^4 cells. Correlation between PR in control ($-TP_1$) and the ratio $+TP_1/TP_1$ was tested by Spearman rank correlation test, for each culture time separately. See text and ref. 31 for more details.

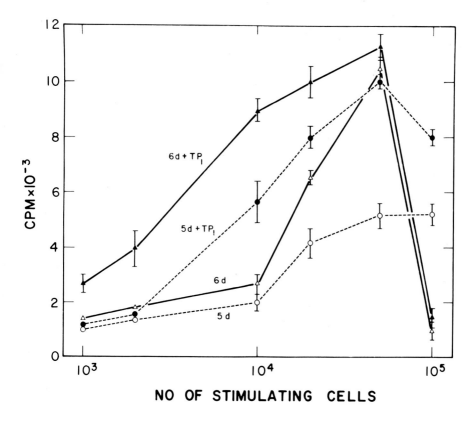

FIG. 3. TP-1 effect on PR as a function of number of stimulating cells. IgR$_3$-MLTC. Conditions as in Figs. 1-2.

lower control PR. Moreover, the distribution of results in the 2 groups (Fig. 2, observation c, above) is not compatibile with "normalization" which implies enhancement of low PRs and suppression of high ones. Instead, both enhancing and suppressive effects were more pronounced with lower control PRs. Apparently, when the allogeneic stimulation is weaker, it is more liable to be modified by thymic factors. Indeed, suboptimal stimulation conditions were found to reflect better TP-1 effects, on the one hand (observation e), and cell mediated immunoregulatory activities, on the other hand (7). The possibility that thymic factors may regulate *normal* immune functions, not only restore deficient functions to normal, may have interesting clinical implications.

2. The results (mainly observation b) are best explained if we assume that the effect of thymic factors on lymphocyte function is primarily an *indirect* one, probably via modulation of the production of certain lymphokines (see below) which comprise a "second wave" of immunoregulatory functions elicited in culture. Such complex interactions amplify subtle differences among

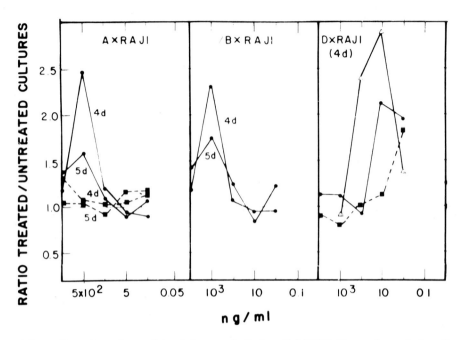

FIG. 4.   Dose dependency of thymic hormonal effect on Raji-MLTC. Responding cells from 3 individuals (A, B and D) were incubated for 1 hr with the indicated concentrations of TP-1 (O——O); thymopoietin pentapeptide (TP5) (△—△); spleen extract (■——■) on heart extract (□----□).

individuals, causing the wide scatter of end point measurements of TP-1 effect on PR an CMC. In contrast, in an immediate and direct assay for surface markers (e.g. active T-rosettes) which does not involve stay in culture, TP-1 effect was only enhancing and not so widely scattered (33). There are additional evidence that thymic hormonal effect on T cell effector functions is an indirect one (12, 18, 19). This notion is schematically represented in Fig. 6.

3. Thymic factors are active not only as inducers of T cell differentation but also as homeostatic regulators of the function of mature T cells. The fact that TP-1 effect was manifested only under suboptimal stimulation conditions, (observation e) can be taken as a presumptive evidence that TP-1 regulates the activity of a mature responding cell pool. If, instead, TP-1 would cause recruitment of non-responding, less mature T cells to the responding pool, this should occur with all stimulatory cell numbers. There are additional evidence for this notion, including the fact that the functional activity of apparently mature lymph node cells is strongly affected by thymic factors (40).

THYMIC HORMONAL EFFECT ON LYMPHOKINE PRODUCTION

The data presented above suggested to us that T cell functions like PR or CMC are not directly regulated by thymic hormones and that certain inter-

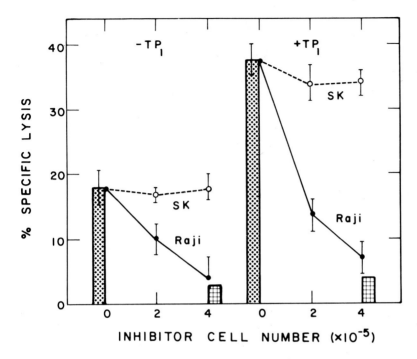

FIG. 5. Cytotoxicity inhibition assay. PBMC from a healthy donor were cultured with Raji cells □ or in medium only □ for 4 days, after 1 hr preincubation with TP-1 or medium control. Cytotoxicity was assayed on 51^{Cr} labelled Raji cells (1×10^4 cells/tube) in the presence of the indicated amounts of unlabelled Raji or SK-mel cells used as inhibitor cells (cold competition).

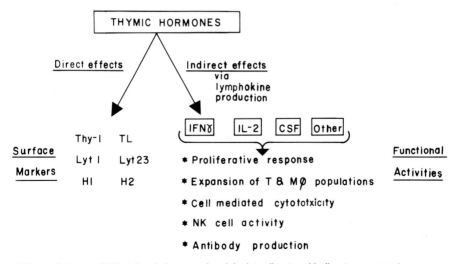

FIG. 6. Scheme dividing thymic hormonal activity into direct and indirect components.

mediary events take place in culture. Lymphokines, the non-antibody products of activated lymphocytes, some of them have effector functions, some regulate the expansion of lymphocyte populations and the expression of their differentiative functions.

The regulation of lymphokine production is based on an interplay between positive and negative signals. The strongest positive signal is an antigenic or a mitogenic stimulus. The activation stimulus initiates the production of a large array of effector and regulatory lymphokines. A certain balance of negative and positive regulatory signals is achieved as part of the activation of inducer and suppressor cells in the regulatory circuit (4). However, there is evidence that different stimulatory events cause the production of sets of lymphokines which are different quantitatively or qualitatively (6, 20) resulting in different levels of regulatory balance.

Thymic hormones have a central role in the maturation of T-lymphocytes, as well as in the regulation of their functional activity (1, 26). Accordingly, it is concievable that their regulatory function will be reflected also in the control of lymphokine production. However, this prediction was only recently started to be tested as more quantitative assays for lymphokines were developed. The first regulatory lymphokine to be evaluated in this connection was immune interferon (IFNγ) (34). Subsequently, colony stimulating factor (CSF) (16) and interleukin-2 (IL-2) (22 and Shoham, Sharabi and Eshel, manuscript in preparation) were also studied.

Enhancement of the production of IFNγ by Thymic factors.

In the experimental system described above, TP-1 had a significant enhancing effect on production of IFNγ by Con A (but not by PHA) stimulated human PBMC (Fig. 7). Enhancement by TP-1 was generally stronger in cultures with lower production of IFNγ (34). It was observed using PBMC of healthy subjects. Interestingly, the dissociation between Con A and PHA induction in regard to IFNγ production was observed in other experimental systems (13, 38). The experiment presented in Figure 7 demonstrates that TP-1 can enhance both IFNγ production and PR as time dependent phenomena. Yet, cell replication was not needed for IFNγ production and enhancement of the latter was apparent before cell replication took place. Effect of thymosin on IFNγ production in vitro was subsequently demonstrated (36).

In a subsequent study we were able to show that TP-1 increases also serum levels of interferon when injected to virus (Mengo virus or MP-virus) infected mice (Fig. 8). This effect is associated with increase NK cell activity, and, most importantly, with significant impact on the survival rate of Mengo virus infected mice (14).

These results make a very strong point for the role of thymic factors in the regulation of interferon production both *in vitro* and *in vivo* and suggest the application of such factors with demonstrable effect on interferon production

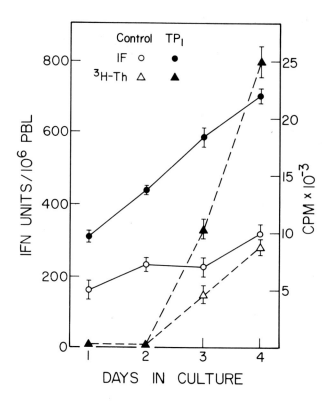

FIG. 7. Time dependency of TP-1 effect on IFN production and PR in Con A activated culture of PBMC. IFN production with (●——●) or without (○——○) pretreatment by TP-1. PR, measured by ^{3}H thymidine incorporation with ▲----▲ or without △----△ pretreatment by TP-1.

for the treatment of viral diseases, not only in the immunocompromised hosts but also in subjects without known immunodeficiency prior to their viral infection.

Production of CSF

We compared CSF production by spleen cells of normal versus tumor bearing mice (C57BL/6 mice inoculated with Lewis Lung Carcinoma) treated with TP-1 (4mg/kg, ip, 4 times/wk) or with phosphate buffered saline control. Animals were sacrificed after different time intervals (3-17 days) and their spleen cells cultured for 4 days without mitogenic stimulation. The medium conditioned in these cultures was tested for its colony stimulating activity on Balb/c bone marrow cells using the bilayer agar method (23). Granulocyte macrophage colonies were counted after 7 culture days. Our previous experience with this method indicated a linear corelation between concentration of GM-CSF and number of colonies.

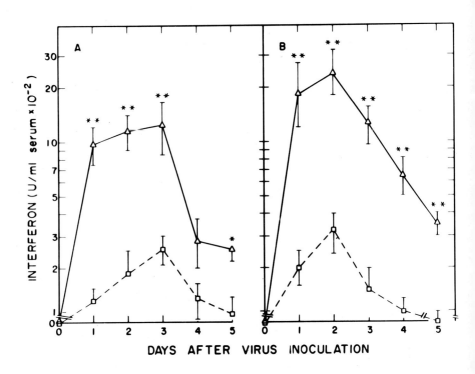

FIG. 8. IFN levels in the serum of C57B1/6(A) or ICR(B) mice inoculated with Mengo virus and treated (△——△) or untreated (□----□) with TP-1. Plaque reduction assay. Each point = results with 5 animals determined separately. Bars ± 1SD.
* .p< 0.05; ** .p< 0.01 (student's t test)

The results (Fig. 9) indicate that the presence of tumor cells causes a significant (p < 0.01, student's t-test) increase in CSF production by spleen cells 3 days after inoculation but not later. TP-1 treatment of the tumor-bearing mice further increased CSF production on the 3rd day and the increase was still significant (p < 0.01) on the 10th day. TP-1 treatment of uninoculated mice resulted in a small (statistically insignificant) decrease in CSF production. Similar experiments done with the virus inoculated mice failed to show any effect of TP-1 on CSF production. Thus, the effect of TP-1 on lymphokine production is not an indiscriminate general process, but is rather selective, according to the antigenic stimulus eliciting the response — in tumur bearing mice TP-1 enhances CSF but not IFN production, whereas in virus infected mice IFN but not CSF production is enhanced.

Production of IL-2

IL-2, a product of activated helper T cells, has a central regulatory position in the immune system. It influences T-cell maturation and proliferation and

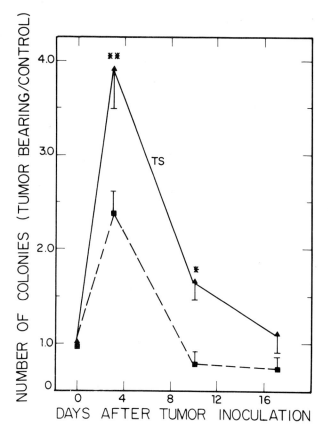

FIG. 9. CSF activity in supernatants of spleen cells taken from mice inoculated with 3LL cells and treated with TP-1 (△—△) or diluent (PBS) control (□----□). Bars and p values as in Fig. 8.

regulates T-cell activities such as the production of other lymphokines (i.e. IFNγ). Accordingly, the chain of arguments that linked thymic factors and lymphokines, in general, was particularly strong for IL-2. Several research groups (21, 22, 40) including ours, investigated the modulatory action of thymic factor on IL-2 production. We tested TP-1 effect on IL-2 production in 2 experimental systems of immature T cells which were basically similar to those used by Palacios (21, 22): (a) Mixed lymphocyte cultures of thymocytes using allogeneic combinations (C57Bl/6 mouse thymocytes as responders and mitomycin C treated C3H thymocytes as stimulators). (b) Splenocytes of athymic mice (nu/nu of Balb/c background) stimulated by Con A. In the 2 experimental systems, the responder cells were incubated with various doses of TP-1 or FTS (kindly donated by Dr. Bach) for 2-5 days, before stimulation by allogeneic cells (a), or Con A (b). Supernatant was collected from stimulated cultures and tested for IL-2 activity on an IL-2 dependent line (CTL-L).

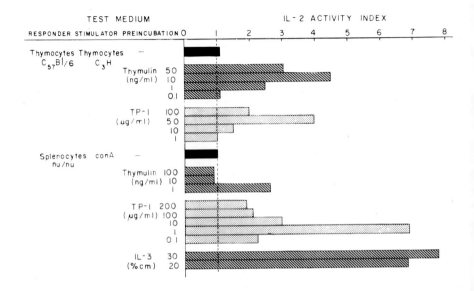

FIG. 10. IL-2 activity in supernatants of 5 days mixed lymphocyte reactions (C57B1/6 mouse thymocytes as responders and mitomycin c treated C₃H mouse thymocytes as stimulators) or 2 days Con A stimulated nude mouse splenocytes. Responder cells were inoculated for 4 days in medium containing the indicated doses of FTS (thymulin), TP-1, or WEHI-3 cells conditioned medium (% cm, WEHI-3 cells are a known source of IL-3), or left in medium only, before initiation of MLC or Con A stimulated culture. IL-2 activity was assayed on the IL-2 dependent CTL-L cell line.

Fig. 10 demonstrates results obtained with the 2 experimental systems. Both factors had a strong effect on IL-2 production with some difference in their relative potency in the 2 systems, suggesting the possibility that they represent 2 different active molecules (i.e. the activity of TP-1 in this connection is probably not because of its possible FTS contents). The effect is dose-dependent with a bell shape dose-effect relationships.

Other Lymphokines

The production of some other lymphokines is also regulated by thymic factors — including migration inhibition factors for macrophages and leucocytes (37) and additional regulatory molecules of helper or suppressor cells (12, 18, 19, 39).

Concluding Comments

Converging lines of evidence, only few of them cited here, suggest that a large part of the effects of thymic factors on the immune system is imparted via effects on the production of lymphokines, as schematically shown in Fig. 6.

The study of the regulation of lymphokine production by thymic factors is still in an early stage of development and our knowledge of this field is, at best, fragmentary. However, the available data allow us to draw some general conclusions as to the relationships between thymic factors and lymphokines.

a) Thymic factors have a significant effect on lymphokine production. In general, and only with a few exceptions, thymic factors modulate the production induced by an antigenic or mitogenic stimulus and no direct independent effect of thymic factors could be observed on quiescent lymphocytes.

b) The modulatory effect of thymic factors on production was observed with several lymphokines. However, this is not a total, indiscriminate effect expressed to the same degree on all lymphokines in any given situation. The effect is selective and is dependent on the nature of the experimental model, the activation agent (antigen) and probably the type of the thymic factor used, as shown in the comparison of TP-1 effect on the production of IFN and CSF in virus-infected or tumor inoculated mice (see above).

c) Generally, the modulatory effect *in vitro* correlates with a similar effect *in vivo*.

d) The dose of the thymic factor used, the duration of exposure to it and the temporal relationships between this exposure and antigenic stimulation are of utmost importance in determining the direction and intensity of the modulatory effect.

Acknowledgements

The autor's research described in this review was supported in part by a grant from Istituto Farmacologico Serono, Rome. The skillful assistance of Yedidah Sharabi, Ph.D., Miriam Cohen, M. Sc., and Ilana Eshel, M. Sc., is gratefully acknowledged.

REFERENCES

1. Bach, J.F. and Carnaud, O. (1976): Thymic Factors. *Prog. Allergy.* 21:342-398.
2. Bach, J.F. and Goldstein, G. (1980): Newer concepts of thymic hormones. *Thymus* 2:1-4.
3. Boyum, A. (1968): Isolation of leucocytes from human blood. *Scand. J. Clin. Lab. Invest. Suppl.* 97:31-35.
4. Cantor, H. and Gershon, R.K. (1980): T cell sets: the role of their genetic programme in immunoregulation. In: *The Immune System: Functions and Therapy of Dysfunction.* Edited by: G. Doria and A. Eshkol, pp. 13-25. Academic Press, London.
5. Clark, S.L. (1973): The intrathymic environment. *Contemp Topics Immunobiol.* 2:72-98.
6. Dianzani, F., Monaham, T.M., Scupham, A. and Zucca, M. (1979): Enzymatic induction of interferon production by galactose oxidase treatment of human lymphoid cells. *Infect. Immunity,* 26:879-885.
7. Dwyer, J.M., Jonson, C. and Desaules, M. (1929): Behaviour of human immunoregulatory cells in culture. I. Variables requiring consideration for clinical studies. *Clin. Exp. Immunol.* 38:499-513.
8. Falchetti, R., Bergesi, G., Eshkol, A., Cafiero, C., Adorini, L. and Caprino, L. (1977). Pharmacological and biological properties of a calf thymus extract (TP-1). *Drugs Exptl. Clin. Res.* 3:39-47.
9. Goldstein, A.L., Cohen, G.H., Rossio, J.L., Thurman, G.B., Brown, C.N. and Ulrich, J.T. (1976). Use of thymosin in the treatment of primary immunodeficiency diseases and cancer. *Med. Clinics N. Am.* 60:591-615.

10. Goldstein, A.L., Low, T.L., Zata, M.M., Hall, N.R. and Naylor, P.H. (1983). Thymosins. *Clinics Immunol.* 3:119-132.
11. Hadden, J.W. (1977): Mechanisms of immunopotentiation. In: *Comprehensive Immunology*, edited by R.A. Good and S.B. Day, vol. 3 pp. 279-314. Plenum Comp., New York.
12. Kaufman, D.C. (1980): Maturational effects of thymic hormones on human helper and suppressor T cells: Effects of FTS (Facteur Thymique Serique) and thymosin. *Clin. Exp. Immunol.* 39:722-727.
13. Kirchner, H., Fenkl, H., Zawatzky, R., Engles, H. and Becker, H. (1980): Dissociation between interferon production induced by phytohemagglutinin and concanavalin A in spleen cell cultures of nude mice. *Eur. J. Immunol.* 10:224-227.
14. Klein, A.S., Fixler, R. and Shoham, J. (1984): Antiviral activity of a thymic factor in experimental viral infections. I. Thymic hormonal effect on survival, interferon production and NK cell activity in Mengo virus infected mice. *J. Immunol.* 132:3159-3163.
15. Klein, A.S. and Shoham, J. (1981): The effect on the thymic estract TP-1 (thymostimulin) on the survival rate of tumor bearing mice. *Cancer Res.* 41:3217-3221.
16. Klein, A.S. and Shoham (1984): Regulation of the production of interferon and other lymphokines by thymic factors. In *Thymic Factor Therapy*. Edited by N.A. Byrom, and J.R. Hobbs. pp. 83-94. Raven Press. New York.
17. Lau, C.Y. and Goldstein, G. (1980): Functional effects of thymopoietin 32-36 (TP5) on cytotoxic lymphocyte precursor units (CLP-U). Enhancement of splenic CLP-U *in vitro* and *in vivo* after suboptimal antigenic stimulation. *J. Immunol.* 124:1861-1865.
18. Marshall, G.D., Thurman, G.B. and Goldstein, A.L. (1980): Regulation of *In vitro* generation of cell mediated cytotoxicity. I. *In vitro* induction of suppressor T-cells by thymosin. *J. Reticuloendothel. Soc.* 28:141-149.
19. Marshall, G.D., Thurman, G.B. and Goldstein, A.L. (1980): Regulation of *In vitro* generation of cell mediated cytotoxicity. II. Characterization of thymosin induced suppressor T-cells *Immunopharmacology* 2:301-312.
20. Monaham, T.M. and Abell, C.W. (1978): The requirement for cell surface galactosyl residues during oxidative activation of normal and chronic lymphocytic leukemia lymphocytes. *Exp. Cell Res.* 116:47-58.
21. Palacios, R. (1983): Role of serum thymic factor (FTS) in the development of interleukin-2 producer lymphocytes. *Clinics Immunol.* 3:83-94.
22. Palacios, R., Fernandez, C. and Sideras, P. (1982): Development and continuous growth in culture of interleukin 2 producer lymphocytes from athymic nu/nu mice. *Eur. J. Immunol.* 12:777-782.
23. Pluznik, D.H. and Sachs, L. (1965). The cloning of normal "mast" cells in tissue culture. *J. Cell. Comp. Physiol.* 66:319-327.
24. Rotter, V., Fink, A. and Trainin, N. (1978) *In vitro* allogenic response of human lymphocytes dependent upon dialyzable plasma components and a thymic hormone, THF. *Cell. Immunol.* 36:242-250.
25. Schafer, L.A., Goldstein, A.L., Gutterman, J.U. and Hersch, E.M. (1976) *In vitro* and *in vivo* studies with thymosin in cancer patients. *Ann. N.Y. Acad. Sci.* 277:609-614.
26. Shoham, J. (1980): The thymus extract TP-1 and human immune reactivity. In: *Thymus, Thymic Hromones and T-Lymphocytes*. Edited by F. Aiuti and H. Wigzell, pp. 273-293. Academic Press, London.
27. Shoham, J. (1982): Definition of the activity of peptides isolated from the thymic extract thymostimulin. In: *Current Chemotherapy and Immunotherapy*. Edited by P. Periti and G.G. Grassi, Vol. 2, pp. 1185-1187. The American Society for Microbiology, Washington, D.C.
28. Shoham, J. (1983): Clinical assessment of the safety of immunostimulating drugs - past experience and guidelines for the future. In: *Current Problems in Drug Toxicology*, edited by G. Zbinden, J.Y. Detaille and G. Mazue, pp. 264-282. J. Libbey Eurotext, Paris.
29. Shoham, J. and Cohen, M. (1983): Thymic hormonal activity on human peripheral blood lymphocytes, in vitro. V. Effect on induction of lymphocytotoxicity. *Int. J. Immunopharmacol.* 5:523-532.
30. Shoham, J. and Eshel, I. (1980): Thymic hormonal effect on human pheripheral blood lymphocytes in vitro. III. Conditions for mixed lymphocyte tumor culture assay. *J. Immunol. Methods.* 37:261-273.
31. Shoham, J. and Eshel, I. (1983): Thymic hormonal activity on human peripheral blood lymphocytes in vitro. IV. Proliferative response to allogeneic tumor cells in healthy adults and cancer patients. *Int. J. Immunopharcol.* 5:515-522.
32. Shoham, J., Ben-David, E., and Sandbank, U. (1982): Feedback inhibition of thymic secretory activity in mice treated by the thymic extract thymostimulin. *Immunology* 45:31-39.

33. Shoham, J., Cohen, M., Chandali, Y. and Avni, A. (1980): Thymic hormonal activity on human peripheral blood lymphocytes, *in vitro*. I. Reciprocal effect on T and B rosette formation. *Immunology* 41:353-359.
34. Shoham, J., Eshel, I., Aboud, M. and Salzberg, S. (1980): Thymic hormonal activity on human peripheral blood lymphocytes *in vitro*. II. Enhancement of the production of immune interferon by activated cells. *J. Immunol.* 125:54-58.
35. Stutman, O. (1983): Role of thymic hormones in T-cell differentiation. *Clinics Immunol.* 3:9-82.
36. Svedersky, L.P., Nui, A., May, L., McKay, P. and Stebbing, N. (1982): Induction and augmentation of mitogen-induced immune interferon production in human peripheral blood lymphocytes by Nµ-desacetylthymosin. *Eur J. Immunol.* 12:244-249.
37. Trainin, N., Pecht, M. and Handzel, Z.T. (1983): Thymic hormones: inducers and regulators of the T-cell system. *Immunol. Today* 4:16-20.
38. Weitzerbin, J., Stefanos, S., Falcoff, R., Lucevo, M., Catinot, L. and Fakoff, E. (1978): Immune interferon induced by phytohemagglutinin in nude mouse spleen cells, *Infect. Immun.* 21:966-970.
39. Wolf., R.E. (1979): Thymosin induced suppression of proliferative response of human lymphocytes to mitogens. *J. Clin. Invest.* 63:677-683.
40. Zatz, M.M. and Goldstein, A.L. (1985): Mechanism of action of thymosin. I. Thymosin fraction 5 increases lymphokine production by mature murine T-cells responding in a mixed lymphocyte reaction. *J. Immunol.* 134:1032-1038.

SECTION III
MEMBRANE DEFECTS

Characterization of Phagocytic and Cytotoxic Abnormalities in Patients who have an Inherited Deficiency of Neutrophil Complement Receptor Type Three (CR_3) and the Related Membrane Antigens LFA-1 and pl50,95

Gordon D. Ross, Ph. D.

Professor of Medicine and of Microbiology and Immunology
Division of Rheumatology and Immunology, Department of Medicine
University of N. Carolina, Chapel Hill, NC, USA

INTRODUCTION

This report summarizes the clinical and laboratory findings about a group of patients from several families who have a genetic deficiency in three related leukocyte membrane surface antigens known as CR3, LFA-1, and pl50,95. Each surface antigen has an identical β-chain linked non-covalently to one of three distinct α-chain types. Patients who are similar or identical to this group of patients have now been identified by several investigators (1-3, 5, 8, 9, 11, 13, 21, 26, 28, 30), and in accompanying report, Springer and Anderson describe some other characteristics of patients with this deficiency. The patients have an increased susceptibility to bacterial infections that is similar to patients who have other types of neutrophil functional deficiencies or neutropenia. Laboratory tests have indicated that isolated neutrophils from these patients have two major types of functional deficiencies that probably contribute to their reduced ability to overcome bacterial infections. First, neutrophils exhibit a reduced ability to adhere to substrates, and this may explain the reduced chemotactic activity of neutrophils noted in some (2, 8, 28), but not all of the patients (3, 30). Second, isolated neutrophils from the patients have a reduced phagocytic and respiratory burst response to both opsonized and unopsonized bacteria and yeast. At this time it is unclear which of these two types of neutrophil functional defects are primarily responsible for the diminished host defense syndrome exhibited by these patients. This report focuses exclusively on the phagocytic and cytotoxic abnormalities of neutrophils from these patients.

CLINICAL CHARACTERISTICS

Patients with this disorder have either a total or partial deficiency of the CR_3/LFA-1/pl50,95 antigen family. In most cases, the patients with total deficiency have had more serious problems with infections than the patients with partial deficiency. The histories of two patients with total deficiency and two patients with partial deficiency will be summarized.

Patient #1, a Caucasian female, was first reported in 1981 (1), and later in 1984 was shown to be totally deficient in CR_3/LFA-1/pl50,95 (2). Delayed separation of the umbilical cord was noted at 3 weeks of age. At 5 weeks of age she presented with peritonitis. *Klebsiella, Proteus*, and enterococcus were isolated from ascites fluid. At 4 months of age she was hospitalized for a perianal abscess from which the same types of bacteria were isolated. During the next 8 months she had 3 bouts of otitis media, conjunctivitis, candidal diaper rash, and vaginitis. During the second year of life she had recurrent problems with inflammation of the gingiva, sinusitis, and facial cellulitis. *Staphylococcus aureus* was isolated from the facial cellulitis. Her parents were unrelated and had no other children (1).

Patient #2, a Caucasian male, was shown to be totally deficient in a neutrophil membrane surface glycoprotein of 180,000 daltons (180K M_r) that was subsequently shown to be the α-chain of CR_3 (8). Omphalitis had developed at 5 days of age, and umbilical cord separation was delayed until 3 weeks of age. Cultures were positive for *Staphylococcus aureus, E. coli*, and β-hemolytic streptococcus. Cellulitis without pus formation was noted. A subumbilical cyst that was unresponsive to antibiotic therapy required excision at 3 months of age. At 1 year he had a penile ulcer from which *Klebsiella* and *Pseudomonas aeruginosa* were grown. At 2 years he presented with a perianal and rectal ulcer and *Pseudomonas aeruginosa* septicemia. He also had frequent bouts of otitis media and recurrent skin infections (*S. aureus*) without pus formation, and recurrent pneumonia. Periodontitis appeared with eruption of primary teeth, and anaerobic cultures of periodontal pockets consistently grew capnocytophaga. At 6 years of age he developed appendicits requiring appendectomy. An abdominal wall cellulitis then developed that was treated successfully with normal white cell infusions after being unresponsive to intravenous gentamicin and clindamycin. One month later he developed spreading gas gangrene of the left leg that required amputation above the knee. He was the only child in a family with no history of bacterial infections or periodontitis (8).

Patients #3, a Caucasian female who is now 12 years old, was shown to express ~10% of the normal amount of CR_3/LFA-1/pl50,95 (21, 26, 30). She presented with a groin abscess at 3 weeks of age and there was delay in separation of the umbilical cord, which finally detached at 7 weeks. At 18 months of age she was hospitalized with a *Pseudomonas pyocynaeus* septicemia. She developed a number of further chronic skin ulcers over the succeding years. Frequently, superficial skin infections developed into subcutaneous abscesses which broke down to give ulcers with sharply demarcated edges and marked eschar formation, often requiring surgical debridement. On healing these left characteristics paper thin scars. She also had persistent gingivitis and dental sepsis, and multiple dental extractions. From 8 years old until the present, the frequency of infections has appeared to diminish, except for occasional skin infections and persistent gingivitis. She was one of three children from unrelated parents who had no history of infections. An older brother was fit, but a younger brother had a similar clinical history and partial deficiency of CR_3/LFA-1/pl50,95. At 6 years of age, the affected brother was severely ill with peritonitis that followed perforation of a necrotic ileal ulcer.

Patient #4, a Caucasian female who is presently 15 year old, was recently shown to have ~10% of the normal amount of each of the CR_3/LFA-1/pl50,95 antigen family members. She is unlike most of the other patients in that her umbilical cord separation was apparently normal and she has never suffered from a systemic bacterial infection. Between the ages of 5-10 years old, she had 21 reported episodes of pyoderma, including documented β-streptococcus. However, these did not always require antibiotic treatment for resolution. Furthermore, the incidence of skin infections diminished after the age of 10 years, and between the ages of 11 to 15 years she had only 3 reported skin infections. Her major problem with infection has been persistent gingivitis since the age of 4 years. This has frequently been accompanied by oral ulcers, and has resulted in significant bone loss around her teeth. The parents were unrelated and had no history of infections. She has two half-sisters and one half-brother, all of whom are healthy (B. L. Myones and G.D. Ross, unpublished observation).

Over the last three years, ~20 patients have been identified with this disorder worldwide. Almost all of the patients have had problems with skin infections and persistent gingivitis. However, at least one patient with partial deficiency had primarily skin infections and did not suffer from gingivitis.

LABORATORY FINDINGS AND DIAGNOSIS

The majority of standard tests of neutrophil function fail to detect this abnormality. In contrast to chronic granulomatous disease, tests for the respiratory burst response to phorbol myristate acetate (PMA) are normal. Phagocytosis of opsonized bacteria and sheep erythrocytes coated with IgG (EAIgG) are also occasionally normal, although a lower rate of ingestion may be detected with certain strains uf unopsonized bacteria (*E. coli, S. epidermidis, S. aureus*) (1, 26) or with EAIgG bearing small amounts of IgG (3, 4, 24, 30). Patients with total deficiency or CR_3/LFA-1/pl50,95 have all been reported to exhibit abnormal adherence and chemotaxis. However, abnormal adherence and chemotaxis has only been observed in some of the patients with partial deficiency. A consistent finding in all of the patients so tested is the greatly reduced phagocytic and respiratory burst response to unopsonized zymosan (26, 30). Responses to serum-opsonized zymosan are also frequently <50% of normal (1, 3, 11, 30).

The definitive finding is absence of reaction with monoclonal antibodies directed to CR_3/LFA-1/pl50,95 antigens. Three antibodies to the α-chain of CR_3 are available commercially: anti-Mac-1 (Hybritech Inc., San Diego, CA, and Boehringer Mannheim, Indianapolis, IN), OKM1 (Ortho Pharmaceuticals, Raritan, NJ), and anti-Leu-15 (Becton-Dickinson Co., Sunyvale, CA). In addition, anti-Leu-M5 sold by Becton-Dickinson Co., has recently been shown to be specific for the α-chain of pl50,95 (18). Antibodies to the α-chain of LFA-1 and to the common β-chain shared by all three antigen family members are not as yet commercially available. Indirect immunofluorescence assay may be used, but care must be taken to avoid false-positive Fc-receptor-dependent staining of cells that are actually deficient in CR_3/LFA-1/pl50,95 antigens (31). Aggregates should be removed from monoclonal antibodies by high-speed centrifugation, and the fluorescence-labeled second antibody reagent should be a F(ab')$_2$ fragment. Fluorochrome labeled F(ab')$_2$ fragments of anti-mouse IgG (and anti-rat IgG for use with anti-Mac-1) are available from Cappel Worthington Biochemicals, Malvern, PA. Analysis by flow cytometry is required to distinguish patients with partial deficiency form patients with total deficiency (29).

Analysis of the parents and siblings of patients has frequently shown approximately half-normal amounts of CR_3/LFA-1/pl50,95 antigens, suggesting a codominant inheritance pattern. In some families heterozygotes expressing half-normal amounts of antigens were more easily identified with chemotactic factor stimulated neutrophils than with unstimulated neutrophils (29). In other families however, both parents had normal amounts of CR_3/LFA-1/pl50,95 antigens (26) or only one of the parents had half-normal amounts of antigen (5). These findings and the existence of patients who are either totally or partially deficient in all of the antigens suggest the existence of more than one type of genetic lesion among the different pedigrees.

STRUCTURE AND FUNCTION OF CR₃/LFA-1/pl50,95 DETERMINED FROM IN VITRO TESTS

Structure of CR₃/LFA-1/pl50,95.

All three surface antigen types are made up of two non-covalently linked glycoprotein chains (27). The smaller of the two chains is the 95K M_r β-chain which is structurally identical in all three antigen types (17). The larger α-chain of the three antigen types share no antigens detected by polyclonal or monoclonal antibodies (17). Furthermore, no similarities in the α-chain from CR_3 and LFA-1 were apparent in tryptic mapping studies (17). The approximate molecular weights of the α-chains of CR_3/LFA-1/pl50,95 are 165K, 175K, and

150K respectively. These have been determined by sodium dodecyl sulfate polyacrylamide gel electrophoresis (SDS-PAGE), and different values have been reported that are dependent upon both the SDS-PAGE conditions and the molecular weight markers used. Neutrophils contain far more CR_3 than the other two antigen types, and the α-chain of CR_3 may be visualized on SDS-PAGE gels of solubilized normal neutrophils. In early studies, comparison on SDS-PAGE gels of normal versus CR_3/LFA-1/pl50,95-deficient neutrophils revealed the missing CR_3 α-chain. However, it was not initially appreciated that the several patients described by different laboratories might all be missing the same glycoprotein because molecular weights ranging from 110-229K were reported. Later, monoclonal antibody fluorescence staining demonstrated that each patient was deficient in the same CR_3/LFA-1/pl50,95 antigens, and immunoblotting analysis indicated that the α-chain of CR_3 was the missing protein visualized in SDS-PAGE gels of normal neutrophils (25).

Biosynthetic studies of CR_3 and LFA-1 have revealed that α and β chains were synthesized separately, glycosylated, and then joined together prior to membrane insertion (15). Examination of LFA-1 synthesis in a B cell line stablished from one of the patients revealed an apparently normal LFA-1 α-chain precursor, whereas no β-chain precursor was seen. It was hypothesized that the molecular basis of the deficiency might be the absent ability to synthesize the normal β-chain precursor required for processing of the α-chain precursor into a complete surface molecule. Unfortunately, attempts to visualize the β-chain precursor in a normal B cell line were also unsuccessful (29). This was unexpected as α and β chain precursors had been demonstrated previously in studies of a myeloid cell line (15).

Expression of CR₃/LFA-1/pl50,95 on different leukocyte types

LFA-1 is found on all leukocyte types (27), whereas CR_3 and pl50,95 are found only on phagocytic cells, a proportion of T cells, and natural killer (NK) cells (6, 18). Monocytes express nearly equal amounts of CR_3 and LFA-1, whereas neutrophils express far more CR_3 than LFA-1 (27). Quantitation by radioimmune assay and flow cytometry indicates that individual neutrophils bear approximately 65,000 molecules of CR_3, 9000 molecules of LFA-1, and 7000 molecules of pl50,95. With neutrophils and monocytes, vast stores of CR_3 are maintained in specific granules near the membrane surface, and stimulation of cells by either chemotactic factors, PMA, or even cell isolation conditions triggers an immediate 10-20 fold increase in the number of CR_3 expressed on the membrane surface (19). Neutrophils isolated and maintained strictly at 4°C express only 4000 CR_3 per cell, whereas neutrophils isolated at room temperature and exposed to PMA express <100,000 CR_3 per cell. Similar findings have been made with monocyte CR_3 and the pl50,95 of neutrophils (18). However, the amount of LFA-1 on phagocytic cell does not change with the stimuli that cause increased surface expression of CR_3 and pl50,95 (5). Only the LFA-1 of lymphocytes exhibits increased surface expression following cell stimulation; either mitogens or mixed lymphocyte culture reactions stimulate increased LFA-1 expression (5).

Functions of CR₃/LFA-1/pl50,95

CR₃ functions as a major opsonin receptor on phagocytic cells that has the ability to trigger phagocytosis, a respiratory burst, degranulation, and the release of leukotrienes (7, 23, 24). In addition, CR₃ may also play a role in the adherence of neutrophils required for chemotaxis (T.A. Springer and D.C. Anderson, accompanying article in this volume). The function of CR₃ on T cells and NK cells has not been defined. LFA-1 (lymphocyte function-associated antigen 1) has been shown to have a role in the cytotoxic functions of both T cells and NK cells, and is believed to be responsible for mediating firm adherence to target cells prior to cell-mediated killing (16). LFA-1 may also play a role in the required adherence functions of B and T cells in the immune response (14). Although little is known of the function of LFA-1 on phagocytic cells, preliminary studies have suggested that the LFA-1 of neutrophils may be involved in the phagocytosis of bacteria (26). There is as yet no definitive data on the function of pl50,95.

Since the patients with deficiency of CR₃/LFA-1/pl50,95 have what appears to be a neutrophil functional deficiency and have no apparent abnormalities of their immune system, studies have been focused on the functions of these antigens on neutrophils. Furthermore, it appears likely that most of the functional defects of the patients' neutrophils result primarily form their deficiency of CR₃, as similar functional defects can be induced in normal neutrophils by treatment with monoclonal antibodies to CR₃, but not with monoclonal antibodies to LFA-1 or pl50,95 (4, 24).

CR₃ has a binding site for the fixed iC3b present on opsonized bacteria (22, 23), and recent tests of phagocytic cells treated with antibodies to CR₃ and CR₁ (the C3b-receptor) have suggested that CR₃ may be more important than CR₁ as a phagocyte receptor for C3 (10, 24). This is because serum-opsonized bacteria may have more fixed iC3b available for CR₃ than they have fixed C3b available for CR₁, and because CR₃ has a greater range of cytotoxic functions that it may trigger. Even though both CR₁ and CR₃ of activated neutrophils may trigger ingestion (20), only CR₃ can trigger degranulation and a respiratory burst (24). Furthermore, in addition to its C3-binding site, CR₃ also contains a second distinct binding site for yeast and bacteria (24, 26). These two binding sites of CR₃ can be blocked selectively with different monoclonal antibodies to the α-chain of CR₃. Anti-Leu 15 blocks the iC3b-binding site of CR₃, whereas OKM1 selectively blocks the yeast binding site of CR₃ demonstrated that it was lectin-like because it bound to zymosan (a yeast cell wall fraction from which all proteins had been removed), and because the binding of CR₃ to yeast was blocked by the sugar N-acetyl-D-glucosamine (22, 24). Subsequently, it was shown that yeast binding to monocytes was inhibited by the β-glucan component of yeast (12), and that particulate β-glucan binding and ingestion by neutrophils was inhibited by monoclonal anti-CR_3 (G.D. Ross, unpublished observation). Thus, the yeast binding site of CR_3 is a lectin with specificity for β-glucan.

Only the yeast (β-glucan) binding site of CR_3 is able to trigger functions with neutrophils prior to activation of CR_3. However, ligation of the yeast binding site in CR_3 with either yeast cells walls (zymosan) or β-glucan particles activates CR_3 so that particles attached to CR_3 by way of the iC3b-binding site are ingested (26). Yeast activation of CR_3 for particle ingestion requires only 1 min, and preliminary studies have indicated that it may involve phosphorylation of the β-chain of CR_3 and linkage of the receptor to microfilaments and microtubules. CR_3 can also be activated for particle ingestion by sequential stimulation of neutrophils with chemotactic mediators such as C5a or FMLP followed by fibronectin (20). The rapid ingestion of iC3b-opsonized bacteria suggests that bacteria may trigger the glucan-binding site of CR_3 in a similar manner as yeast. The absence of this natural bacteria recognition system on neutrophils may be one reason for the increased susceptibility of patients with deficiency of CR_3/LFA-1/pl50,95. It remains to be demonstrated if LFA-1 and pl50,95 may be lectin, similar to CR_3 with specificity for different bacterial polysaccharides.

REFERENCES

1. Abramson, J.S., Mills, E.L., Sawyer, M.K., Regelmann, W.R., Nelson, J.D., and Quie, P.G. (1981): Recurrent infections and delayed separation of the umbilical cord in an infant with abnormal phagocytosis. *J. Pediatr.*, 99:887-894.
2. Anderson, C.D., Schmalstieg, F.C., Arnaout, M.A., Kohl, S., Tosi, M.F., Dana, N., Buffone, G.J., Hughes,B.J., Brinkley, B.R., Dickey, W.D., Abramson, J.S., Springer, T., Boxer, L.A., Hollers, J.M., and Smith, C.. (1984): Abnormalities of polymorphonuclear leukocyte function associated with heritable deficiency of high molecular weight surface glycoproteins (GP138): common relationship to diminished cell adherence. *J. Clin. Invest.* 74:536-551.
3. Arnaout, M.A., Pitt, J., Cohen, H.J., Melamed, J., Rosen, F.S., and Colten H.R. (1982): Deficiency of a granulocyte-membrane glycoprotein (gp150) in a boy with recurrent bacterial infections. *N. Engl. J. Med.*, 306:693-699.
4. Arnaout, M.A., Todd III, R.F., Dana, N., Melamed,J., Schlossman, S.F., and Colten, H.R. (1983): Inhibition of phagocytosis of complement C3- or immunoglobulin G-coated particles and of C3bi binding by monoclonal antibodies to a monocyte-granulocyte membrane glycoprotein (Mo1). *J. Clin. Invest.* 72:171-179.
5. Arnaout, M.A., Spits, H., Terhorst, C., Pitt, J., and Todd III, R.F. (1984): Deficiency of a leukocyte surface glycoprotein (LFA-1) in two patients with Mo1 deficiency. Effects of cell activation on Mo1/LFA-1 surface expression in normal and deficient leukocytes. *J. Clin. Invest.*, 74:1291-1300.
6. Ault, K.A., and Springer, T.A. (1981): Cross-reaction of a rat-anti-mouse phagocyte-specific monoclonal antibody (anti-Mac-1) with human monocytes and natural killer cells. *J. Immunol.*, 126:359-364.
7. Austen, K.F., and Czop, J.K. (1985): Release of leukotrienes by human monocytes on stimulation of their phagocytic receptor for β-glucan and other particulate activators of complement. *Fed. Proc.*, 44:736.
8. Bowen, T.J., Ochs, H.D., Altman, L.C., Price, T.H., Van Epps, D.E., Brautigan, D.L., Rosin, R.E., Perkins, W.D., Babior, B.M., Klebanoff, S.J., and Wedgwood, R.J. (1982):

Severe recurrent bacterial infections associated with defective adherence and chemotaxis in two patients with neutrophils deficient in a cell-associated glycoprotein. *J. Pediatr.*, 101:932-940.

9. Buchanan, M.R., Crowley, C.A., Rosin, R.E., Gimbrone, M.A., Jr., and Babior, B.M. (1982): Studies on the interaction between GP-180-deficient neutrophils and vascular endothelium. *Blood*, 60:160-165.

10. Cain, J.A., Newman, S.L., and Ross, G.D., (1985): Role of fixed C3 fragments versus yeast (Y) cell wall components in the superoxide (0_2) burst response of human neutrophils (PMN). *Fed. Proc.*, 46:1877.

11 Crowley, C A , Curnutte, J T , Rosin, R E , Andre-Schwartz, J , Gallin, J I , Klempner, M., Snyderman, R., Southwick, F.S., Stossel, T.P., and Babior, B.M. (1980): An inherited abnormality of neutrophil adhesion. Its genetic transmission and its association with a missing protein. *N. Engl. J. Med.*, 302:1163-1168.

12. Czop, J.K., and Austen, K.F. (1985): A β-glucan inhibitable receptor on human monocytes: its identity with the phagocytic receptor for particulate activators of the alternative complement pathway. *J. Immunol.*, 134:2588-2593.

13. Dana, N., Todd III, R.F., Pitt, J., Springer, T.A., and Arnaout, M.A. (1984): Deficiency of a surface membrane glucoprotein (Mo1) in man. *J. Clin. Invest.*, 73:153-159.

14. Davignon, D., Martz, E., Reynolds, T., Kurzinger, K., and Springer, T.A. (1981): Monoclonal antibody to a novel lymphocyte function-associated antigen (LFA-1): mechanism of blockade of T lymphocyte-meditated killling and effects on other T and B lymphocyte functions. *J. Immunol.*, 127:590-595.

15. Ho, M.-K., and Springer, T.A. (1983): Biosynthesis and assembly of the α and β subunits of Mac-1, a macrophage glycoprotein associated with complement receptor function. *J. Biol. Chem.*, 258:2766-2769.

16. Krensky, A.M., Sanchez-Madrid, F., Robbins, E., Nagy, J.A., Springer, T.A., and Burakoff, S.J. (1983): The functional significance, distribution, and structure of LFA-1, LFA-2, and LFA-3: cell surface antigens associated with CTL-target interactions. *J. Immunol*

21. Ross, G.D., Thompson, R.A., Ward, R.H.R., Walport, M.J., Harrison, R.A., and Lachmann, P.J. (1983): Identification of a genetic deficiency of leukocyte membrane complement receptor type three (CR₃). In: *Proceedings of the Workshop on Clinical Aspects of Complement-Mediated Diseases*, Bellagio, Italy, page 15.

22. Ross, G.D., Newman, S.L., Lambris, J.D., Devery-Pocius, J.E., Cain, J.A., and Lachmann, P.J. (1983): Generation of three different fragments of bound C3 with purified factor I or serum. II. Location of binding sites in the C3 fragments for factors B and H, complement receptors, and bovine conglutinin. *J. Exp. Med.*, 158:334-352.

23. Ross, G.D., and Medof, M.E. (1985): Membrane complement receptors specific for bound fragments of C3. *Adv. Immunol.*, 37:217-267.

24. Ross, G.D., Cain, J.A., and Lachmann, P.J. (1985): Membrane complement receptor type three (CR₃) has lectin-like properties analogous to bovine conglutinin and functions as a receptor for zymosan and rabbit erythrocytes as well as a receptor for iC3b. *J. Immunol.*, in press.

25. Ross, G.D., Cain, J.A., Davies, C.J., and Lachmann, P.J. (1985): Selective activation of neutrophil complement receptor type three (CR₃) by zymosan. *Fed. Proc.*, 44:1861.

26. Ross, G.D., Thompson, R.A., Walport, M.J., Springer, T.A., Watson, J.V., Ward, R.H.R., Lida, J., Nexman, S.L., Harrison, R.A., and Lachmann, P.J. (1985): Characterization of patients with an increased susceptibility to bacterial infections and a genetic deficiency of leukocyte membrane complement receptor type three (CR₃) and the related membrane antigen LFA-1, submitted for pubblication.

27. Sanchez-Madriz, F., Nagy, J.A., Robbins, E., Simon, P., and Springer, T.A. (1983): A human leukocyte differentiation antigen family with distinct α-subunits and a common β-subunit: The lymphocyte function-associated antigen (LFA-1), the C3bi complement receptor (OKM1/Mac-1), and the p150,95 molecule. *J. Exp. Med.*, 158:1785-1803.

28. Seger, R., Fischer, A., Dupandy, A., Bohler, M.C., Virelizier, J.L., Katatchkine, M., Descamps, B., Trung, P.H., Grospierre, B., and Griscelli, C. (1985): Adhesive protein deficiency resulting in abnormal phagocytic cell functions and impaired cytotoxicities. In: *Third Meeting of the European Group on Germ Line Deficiencies*, edited by C. Griscelli, in press. North Holland Publishing Company, Amsterdam.

29. Springer, T.A., Thompson, W.S., Miller, L.J., Schmalstieg, F.C., and Anderson, D.C. (1984): Inherited deficiency of the Mac-1, LFA-1, p150,95 glycoprotein family and its molecular basis. *J. Exp. Med.*, 160:1901-1918.

30. Thompson, R.A., Candy, D.C.A., and McNeish, A.S. (1984): Familial defect of polymorph neutrophil phagocytosis associated with absence of a surface glycoprotein antigen (OKM1). *Clin. Exp. Immunol.*, 58:229-236.
31. Winchester, R.J., and Ross, G.D. (1985): Methods for enumerating cell population by surface markers using conventional microscopy. In: *Manual of Clinical Immunology*, 3rd Edition, edited by N.L. Rose, and H. Friedman, in press. American Society for Microbiology, Wash. D.C.

The Importance of the Mac-1, LFA-1 Glycoprotein Family in Monocyte and Granulocyte Adherence, Chemotaxis, and Migration into Inflammatory Sites: Insights from an Experiment of Nature[1]

Timothy A. Springer[2] and Donald C. Anderson[3]

[1]This is reprinted from Ciba Foundation Symposium #118, 'Biochemistry of Macrophages'.
[2]Dana-Farber Cancer Institute Harward Medical School
[3]Baylor College of Medicine and Texas Children's Hospital Houston, Texas, USA

Cell surface adherence reactions are of central importance in a wide spectrum of granulocyte, monocyte, and lymphocyte functions wich contribute to host defense against infection. Granulocyte and monocyte translocation *in vitro* and mobilization *in vivo* is influenced by the nature of cell-substrate adherence interactions. Studies emploiyng time lapse photography have shown that granulocytes adhere preferentially to vascular endothelium adjacent to a site of inflammation prior to their diapedesis into tissues (3). This "directed" adherence is facilitated by products of inflammation such as C5a and N-formyl-methionyl peptides which bind to specific receptors on granulocytes and monocytes and initiate a sequence of events that enhance cellular adherence (reviewed in 15, 22). Considerable evidence exists that physical properties of endothelial cells or experimental substrates (glass, plastic, albumin, fibrinogen, fibronectin) influence adherence and secondarily the extent and direction of cell migration (23). Migration toward gradients of chemotactic factor's *in vitro* appears to require intermittent adhesion which is sufficiently strong to allow attachment to a substrate but sufficiently localized temporally to allow selective detachment (23).

Adhesive interactions are fundamental to other granulocyte and monocyte functions. Specific recognition of opsonized microorganisms is facilitated by membrane receptors for IgG and for the third component of complement (C3), which mediate adhesion to opsonized microorganisms prior to the triggering of cytoskeletal events leading to endocytosis. Adhesion mediated by

IgG (Fc) receptors can also trigger antibody-dependent killing of target cells, independently of endocytosis. In the absence of opsonins, some microorganisms may adhere to granulocytes and monocytes without undergoing ingestion or may be phagocytosed inefficiently, depending on the physical properties of the microorganism (9).

Many different cell surface proteins are important in these events. Among these, and of ubiquitous importance in the aforementioned granulocyte and monocyte adhesion reactions, and additionally in lymphoid adhesive interactions, are the Mac-1, LFA-1 family of glycoproteins (Table 1). These

TABLE 1.   The Mac-1, LFA-1 Family[a]

	Mac-1 (OKM1, Mo1)	LFA-1	pI50,95
Subunits ($M_r \times 10^{-3}$)	$\alpha M \beta$ (170, 95)	$\alpha L \beta$ (180, 95)	$\alpha X \beta$ (150, 95)
Cell Distribution	Monocytes Macrophages Granulocytes Large Gran. Lymph.	Lymphocytes Monocytes Granulocytes Large Gran. Lymph.	Monocytes Granulocytes
Stimulation Increases Surface Expression	+	−	+
Functions Inhibited by Monoclonal Antibodies	Complement Receptor Type Three. Granulocyte Adherence, Stimulated Adherence, Spreading, Aggregation, and Chemotaxis	Cytolytic T Lymphocyte Mediated Killing and T Helper Cell Responses Natural Killing. Antibody-Dependent Cellular Cytotoxicity. Phorbol Ester- Stimulated Lymphocyte Aggregation	?

Common Features: The β subunits appear identical. The α subunits αM and αL are 35% homologous in sequence. The α and β subunits are noncovalently associated in $\alpha_1\beta_1$ complexes. Both α and β subunits are glycosylated and exposed on the cell surface. All functions shown require divalent cations.
[a] Reviewed in 16, 13, 18, 19.

molecules appear to synergize with other receptors or act on their own to regulate or mediate a panoply of leukocyte functional interactions. The wide variety of these functions, and their common dependence on cell adhesion, suggests that the Mac-1, LFA-1 glycoproteins are of general importance in leukocyte adhesion reactions. In this sense, they may be analogous to the adhesion molecules of other tissues, such as the nervous system (N-CAM) or liver (L-CAM).

The thesis of this paper is that these glycoproteins regulate monocyte and granulocyte adherence and chemotaxis *in vitro*, and diapedesis and migration into inflammatory sites *in vivo*. Two types of studies are presented. The first utilizes monoclonal antibodies (MAb) to these glycoproteins (13). MAbs have been obtained which are specific for the αM, αL, or αX subunits, and thus react only with Mac-1, LFA-1, or pl50,95, respectively (Table 1). Another type of MAb reacts with the common β subunit, and hence with all three of these glycoproteins. The other type of study described here utilizes cells from patients with a recently discovered heritable deficiency of the entire glycoprotein family. This deficiency is detailed below. Before coming to these studies, we first describe a physiologically important property of the Mac-1, and pl50,95 glycoproteins, their upregulation by inflammatory stimuli.

Upregulation of Mac-1 an pl50,95 on granulocytes and monocytes

N-formyl methionyl peptides such as f-Met-Leu-Phe, which are produced by bacteria, and the C5a anaphylotoxin, a product of complement activation, are chemoattractants for monocytes and granulocytes. These molecules bind with high affinity to specific receptors on these cells (15). They trigger in addition to chemotaxis, increased adherence to surfaces (termed "hyperadherence"), granulocyte aggregation, the respiratory burst, and the secretion of about 20% of the lactoferrin and cobalamin-binding protein stored in granulocytes (23, 10). These proteins are stored in the secondary or "specific" granules of granulocytes. After granulocytes in suspension are stimulated with chemoattractants electron microscope morphometric analysis demonstrates rapid bipolarization of the cell with the formation of lamellipodia at one end, the loss of about 30% of the secondary granules but no loss of primary granules, and an increase of about 25% in surface area. The latter can be accounted for by the fusion of the membrane bilayer surrounding secondary granules with the plasma membrane (12).

Importantly, the chemoattractant f-Met-Leu-Phe stimulates a marked increase in the amount of Mac-1 and pl50,95 expressed on the surface of monocytes (Fig. 1) and granulocytes (17). Quantitation showed a 5-fold increase for Mac-1 and pl50,95 on both granulocytes and monocytes (17, and unpublished). In contrast, the related LFA-1 glycoprotein was not increased. The increases were stimulated by 10^{-8}M f-Met-Leu-Phe, which is within the concentration range for chemotaxis (23). The chemoattractant C5a, and the secretagogues phorbol myristyl acetate (PMA) and calcium ionophore A23187 stimulated similar increases in surface expression (2). Upregulation was maximal after 8 minutes at 37°C, and was not impeded by inhibitors of protein synthesis (D. Anderson, L. Miller, and T. Springer, unpublished).

Thus, Mac-1 and pl50,95 are stored in a latent pool in granulocytes and monocytes, and can be mobilized to the cell surface by chemoattractants (Fig. 2). The 5-fold increase shows that the amount of Mac-1 and pl50,95 is considerably higher than on the unstimulated cell surface. Furthermore, since the 5-fold increase in Mac-1 and pl50,95 is accompanied by only about a 25% increase in granulocyte surface area (12), the density of Mac-1 and pl50,95 in the membrane bilayer of the storage vesicle must be approximately 16-fold higher than on the cell surface. In granulocytes, the intracellular Mac-1 pool

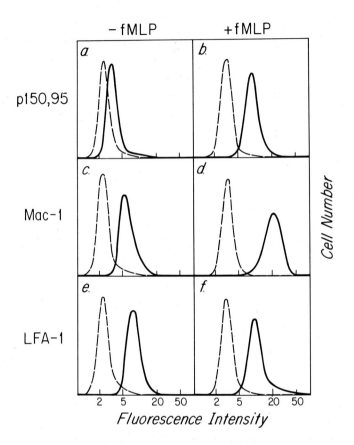

FIG. 1. Chemoattractant stimulates increased expression of p150,95 and Mac-1 but not LFA-1 on monocytes. Mononuclear cells were incubated 1/2 hour at 37°C with 10^{-8}M f-Met-Leu-Phe, or held at 4° as indicated. Cells were stained at 4° with specific (solid curves) or control (dashed curves) MAb, followed by FITC anti-mouse IgG, and subjected to immunofluorescence flow cytometry. Both antibodies were used at saturating concentrations, so that fluorescence is proportional to the number of antigen molecules per cell. Fluorescence of monocytes was determined by gating on 90° and forward angle light scatter to esclude lymphocytes.

cosediments in sucrose gradients with secondary granules (21), but further experiments are needed before it can be definitively established whether Mac-1 and p150,95 are stored in the membrane enclosing secondary granules or some other secretory vesicle. The location of the latent pool in monocytes has not yet been examined.

Mac-1, LFA-1 Deficiency Disease

Recently, a disease has been recognized in which the Mac-1, LFA-1 and p150,95 glycoproteins are deficient (17, 2). Patients have recurrent, life-threatening bacterial infections, a lack of pus formation, and persistent

NEUTROPHIL SECRETORY GRANULE MOBILIZATION

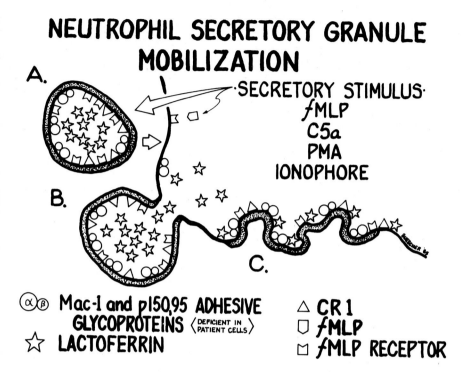

A.

·SECRETORY STIMULUS·
ƒMLP
C5a
PMA
IONOPHORE

B.

C.

ⓐⓑ **Mac-1 and pl50,95 ADHESIVE GLYCOPROTEINS** (DEFICIENT IN PATIENT CELLS)

☆ **LACTOFERRIN**

△ **CR 1**
▢ **ƒMLP**
▱ **ƒMLP RECEPTOR**

FIG. 2. Secretory vesicle mobilization in granulocytes. The components shown are all mobilized to the cell surface or secreted in response to the indicated stimuli. Deficient patient cells lack an intracellular pool of Mac-1 and pl50,95, and thus fail to mobilize them to the cell surface components such as the CR1 and fMLP receptor is otherwise completely normal in patient cells. Mac-1 and pl50,95, the CR1 and fMLP receptor may be in storage sites distinct from one another and from that of lactoferrin in the secondary granule. They are shown in the same secretory vesicle only for ease of representation. (Drawing by Dr. S. Buescher).

granulocytosis (Table 2). The deficiency affects all cell lineages which normally express the Mac-1, LFA-1 glycoprotein family, i.e., monocytes, granulocytes, and lymphocytes, and cell lines established from patients. Deficiency is inherited as an autosomal, recessive mutation. Each of the three α subunits, and the common β subunit, is deficient from the surface of all patients' cells, as shown by immunofluorescent flow cytometry and immunoprecipitation with MAb specific for each subunit (Fig. 3). Two phenotypes have been defined, severe deficiency and moderate deficiency, with surface expression of <0.2% and 5%, respectively, of normal amounts of Mac-1, LFA-1 and pl50,95 (Fig. 3) (2). In both phenotypes, the underlying defect is in the common β subunit (17), as summarized in Fig. 4. In normal cells, α and β subunit precursors (α' and β') are synthesized which become noncovalently associated, probably in the endoplasmic reticulum, and transported to the Golgi, where carbohydrate processing and a slight increase in molecular

TABLE 2. Clinical features of Mac-1, LFA-1 deficiency syndrome Texas Patients[a]

Clinical features	Severe deficiency			Moderate deficiency				
	#1 6Y/O F	#2 16M/O F*	#3 18M/O F*	#4 18Y/O M	#5 15Y/O M	#6 37Y/O M	#7 8Y/O M	#8 12Y/O F
Delayed Umbilical Cord Severance and Infection	+	+	+	–	–	–	–	–
Persistant Granulocytosis (15,000–161,000/mm³)	+++	+++	+++	+	+	+	+	+
Recurrent Soft Tissue Infections:								
— Necrotic/ulcerative cutaneous/subcutaneous abscess or cellulitis	+++	+++	+++	++	+	+++	+	++
— Perirectal abscess/sepsis	+	+	+	–	–	–	–	–
— Mucositis/stomatitis/ pharyngitis/tracheitis	+++	+	++	+++	+++	+	+++	+++
— Gingivitis/periodontitis	+++	+	+	+++	+++	+++	+++	+++
— Pneumonitis	+	+	–	–	–	+	+	–
— Peritonitis/necrotizing Enterocolitis	+	+	+	+	–	++	–	–
Impaired Wound Healing	–	+	+	+	+	±	±	±
Parental Consanguinity	–	–	+	–	–	±	±	±
Ethnic Background	Anglo-Saxon	Hispanic	Iranian	Hispanic	Hispanic	Hispanic	Hispanic	Hispanic

* Deceased
[a] Summarized from Anderson et al. (1985).

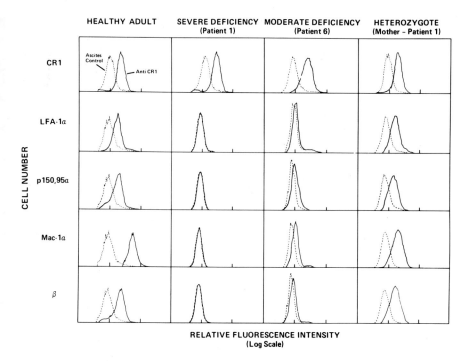

FIG. 3. Immunofluorescence flow cytometry of granulocytes of representative severe and moderate deficiency patients, a heterozygote, and a healthy adult. Unstimulated granulocytes were indirectly stained with antibodies to the CR1 or the indicated α or β subunits (solid lines) or control MAb (dashed lines). Other methods as in Fig. 1 legend. A similar degree of deficiency was found if patient granulocytes were stained after f-Met-Leu-Phe stimulation. From Anderson et al. 1985 with permission.

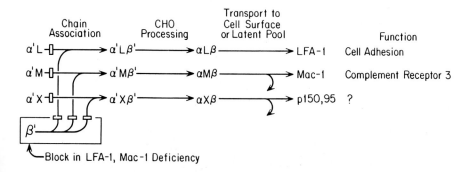

FIG. 4. Biosynthesis of the Mac-1, LFA-1 glycoprotein family (Sanchez-Madrid et al. 1983, Springer et al. 1984). The evidence in patient cells for a primary block in β subunit synthesis, and a secondary block in α subunit processing, is described in the text.

weight occurs. The mature molecules are then transported to the cell surface or to intracellular storage sites. Patient cells, however, appear to lack β subunit synthesis or to make it only in small amounts. Normal α' precursors are made, but do not undergo carbohydrate processing, suggesting biosynthesis is blocked prior to the Golgi. αβ association appears required for processing and transport to the surface. The α chains are not expressed on the surface (severe deficiency) or in amounts which appear stoichiometrically limited by the small quantity of β produced (moderate deficiency). In addition to surface expression, patient granuloytes and monocytes lack the intracellular pool of Mac-1 and pl50,95. After stimulation with f-Met-Leu-Phe or PMA, there is little if any increase in Mac-1 and pl50,95 surface expression (2, 17).

Mac-1, LFA-1 deficiency is a highly specific defect. Patient granulocytes show normal surface expression of the Fc receptor, the complement receptor type 1 (CR1), and many other markers surveyed in an international monoclonal antibody workshop (19). Upregulation of the complement receptor type 1, secretion of granule constituents such as lactoferrin and lysozyme, the respiratory burst, and superoxide production in response to chemoattractants and PMA are completely normal in patient cells. Thus, the granule mobilization response depicted in Fig. 2 and other biochemical changes appear normal in patient cells, with the exception that Mac-1 and pl50,95 are absent from the intracellular compartment that is mobilized to the cell surface. This is in contrast to a distinct disorder involving specific granule deficiency (11).

The Functional Consequences of Deficiency

The effects of this deficiency disease have taught us much about the importance of the Mac-1, LFA-1 glycoprotein family in leukocyte adhesion and migration (1, 2). The first known function of Mac-1 was as the complement receptor type 2, which mediates binding and phagocytosis of particles opsonized with the iC3b ligand (4, 25). Indeed, despite some initial controversy (17), it is clear that patients are deficient in the CR3 (8, 1). However, the functional defects are much broader than this.

The recurrent soft tissue infection in patients (Table 2) appear due to an inability of granulocytes and monocytes to migrate into inflammatory sites (1, 2). There is an absence of pus formation in the common necrotic, ulcerative skin lesions and in other less readily apparent infected sites. This is confirmed by biopsies, which show granulocyte mobilization into infected tissues is profoundly impaired. Patients have severe gingivitis, yet a saline wash of the oral cavity reveals no PMN's, as would be found in other types of gingivitis. Leukocyte mobilization was measured experimentally in patients by the Rebuck skin window test. The skin was abraded, a coverslip placed over the site, and granulocytes and monocytes present in the serous effusions were counted at 2 hour intervals. Healthy controls showed immigrating neutrophils at 2 and 4 hours followed by monocytes at 6 hours. Severely deficient patients showed no mobilization of neutrophils or monocytes to the site even at the 24 hour timepoint, and leukocyte mobilization in moderately deficient patients was strikingly diminished and delayed. Thus, Mac-1, LFA-1 deficiency results in a profound defect in the ability of leukocytes to diapedese, i.e. to leave the circulation by migrating between endothelial cells and through the basement membrane into inflammatory sites.

This dysfunction correlates with *in vitro* defects in chemotaxis and adhesion (1, 2). Chemotaxis to f-Met-Leu-Phe and C5a was markedly depressed (Table 3). Patient granulocytes exhibited normal bipolar shape change in

TABLE 3. *Assessment of adherence dependent granulocyte functions[1]*

FUNCTIONAL ASSAY	SEVERE[2] DEFICIENCY	MODERATE[3] DEFICIENCY	HEALTHY ADULTS
CHEMOTAXIS			
f-Met-Leu-Phe (10^{-8}M)	43 ± 6[4]	66 ± 7	105 ± 4
C5a	42 ± 5	68 ± 14	108 ± 7
ADHERENCE			
Baseline (PBS)	12 ± 2*	16 ± 9	38 ± 6
f-Met-Leu-Phe (10^{-8}M)	12 ± 3	28 ± 12	63 ± 6
PMA (5 μg/ml)	16 ± 4	31 ± 12	67 ± 9
AGGREGATION			
C5a	16 ± 11**	15 ± 12	100 ± 0
f-Met-Leu-Phe (10^{-7}M)	16 ± 4	14 ± 13	40 ± 6
PMA (10 μg/ml)	15 ± 9	22 ± 3	105 ± 7
PHAGOCYTOSIS			
Oil-Red-0-(IgG)	1.4 ± 0.6[5]	1.4 ± 0.5	1.7 ± 0.4
Oil-Red-0-(iC3b)	1.9 ± 1.2[5]	2.4 ± 1.2	7.0 ± 3.1
C3-opsonized Zymosan	4.6 ± 0.7[6]	7.9 ± 3.2	17.4 ± 4.0

[1] Data presented with respect to each functional assay is represented by mean ± 1 SD value for each patient category derived from individual patient mean values of 2-6 separate experiments. Summarized from Anderson et al. 1985.
[2] Includes assessments on severe deficiency Patients 1, 2 and 3.
[3] Includes assessments on moderate deficiency Patients 4, 6, 7 and 8.
[4] Boyden assay values (mean ± 1 SD) for f-Met-Leu-Phe or C5a (10% Zymosan-activated serum) expressed as μm migration/40 min. incubation.
* Percent of granulocytes adhering to serum (6%) coated glass under baseline or stimulated conditions at 21°C.
** Granulocyte aggregation responses to C5a (10% Zymosan activated plasma) f-Met-Leu-Phe or PMA, at 37° C, measured by the increase in light transmittance and expressed as the % of the response to C5a.
[5] Dionylphthalate uptake (μg/10^6 granulocytes in 15 min).
[6] Slope of chemiluminescence evolution (CPM^2 x 10^{-5}).

suspension in response to chemoattractants, but failed to orient to gradients of f-met-Leu-Phe or C5a when attached to surfaces (1). Granulocytes undergoing orientation to f-Met-Leu-Phe in Zigmond chambers were examined by scanning electron microscopy (Fig. 5). Healthy granulocytes oriented normally with lamellipodia at their leading edge facing in the direction of the chemoattractant diffusing from the right (Fig. 5B, C). In contrast, patient granulocytes failed to orient (Fig. 5E, F). Photographs taken in a plane perpendicular to the substrate and parallel to the gradient (Fig. 5C, F) showed

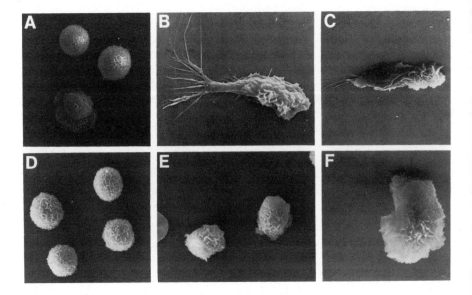

FIG. 5. Orientation of patient or control granulocytes in chemotactic gradients. Scanning electron micrographs show the sequence of cell ruffling and spreading on the substrate (A) and achievment of polarity and orientation by healthy adult PMN (B, C), and parallel experiments on deficient PMNs (D-F). Cells adhere to the coverslip over the bridge in a Zigmond orientation chamber and respond to f-Met-Leu-Phe diffusing from the right. Cells in A, B, D, and E are photographed in plane parallel to the coverslip, and in C and F perpendicular to the coverslip. From Anderson et al. (1984), with permission.

that patient granulocytes were clearly activated since they were bipolar, but in a plane perpendicular to the substrate rather than parallel to it (Fig. 5F). They were unable to initiate lateral or peripheral areas of attachment with the substrate.

The orientation and chemotaxis defects appear secondary to a defect in adherence. The percentage of granulocytes adhering to serum-coated glass under "baseline" conditions was significantly (p < 0.01) diminished compared to healthy controls (Table 3). After stimulation with f-Met-Leu-Phe or PMA, there was no or little increase in adherence by severely deficient PMA and only a modest increase by moderately deficient PMN. In contrast, healthy control PMN demonstrated a normal hyperadherence response. The defect in adherence is also found for glass and plastic coated with other proteins, including fibronectin (1, 6). Patient cells which do adhere to protein-coated glass or to plastic demonstrate a profound defect in their ability to spread. C5a, fMLP, and PMA cause healthy granulocytes to aggregate into clumps, which can be measured in an aggregometer by changes in light transmittance. Deficient patient granulocytes failed to aggregate (Table 3). Although a change in surface charge upon stimulation may contribute to granulocyte aggregation (10), there was no difference in charge between patient and normal granulocytes (1). Phagocytosis was measured of IgG and iC3b-opsonized oil red-0 particles and C3-opsonized zymosan. Phagocytosis of C3-opsonized particles by patient granulocytes was diminished (Table 3), as would be expected from the CR3 defect. Patient granulocytes phagocytosed IgG-opsonized particles normally (Table 3). PMN demonstrate phagocytosis of many microorganisms in the absence of opsonization, although at a slower rate than after opsonization. Under these conditions, patient granulocytes demonstrate diminished phagocytosis of some but not all microorganisms. Defects are found for S. aureus and zymosan (1, 20).

Inhibition of Adherence-Dependent Functions by MAb.

Binding of monoclonal antibodies to normal granulocytes reproduced the defects found in Mac-1, LFA-1 deficient patients. Both baseline and f-Met-Leu-Phe-stimulated adherence were strikingly inhibited (Fig. 6). Spreading,

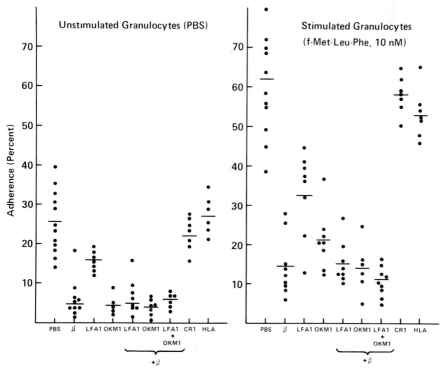

FIG. 6. Effects of MAbs to the Mac-1, LFA-1 glycoprotein family on granulocyte adherence. Granulocytes were preincubated with MAbs, washed and then incorporated into Smith Hollers adherence chambers in which they were allowed to adhere to serum (6%) coated glass substrated under unstimulated (PBS) or stimulated (f-Met-Leu-Phe, 10 nM) conditions at 21°C. MAb preparations used for the studies shown included: the OKM1 MAb to Mac-1 α (5 μg/ml), F(ab')₂ fragments of the TS1/22 MAb to LFA-1 α (5 μg/ml), and F(ab')₂ fragments of the TS1/18 MAb to the common β subunit of Mac-1 and LFA-1 (5 μg/ml). Control MAbs included saturating concentrations of a F(ab')₂ fragment of rabbit IgG directed against the human C3b receptor (anti-CR1) and a MAb to HLA framework antigen (W6/32).

TABLE 4.   *Effects of subunit specific monoclonal antibodies to Mac-1 proteins on adherence-independent granulocyte functions*

Granulocyte function ●	Mac-1 α		LFA-1 α	pl50,95 α	β	HLA-A,B
	OKM1	LM2/1.6	TS1/22 F(ab')$_2$	SHCL-3	TS1/18 F(ab')$_2$	W6/32
Adherence (6% Serum coated glass)	+	+	±	+	+	−
Hyperadherence (6% Serum coated glass-10 nm fMLP)	+	+	±	+	+	−
Spreading - glass	+*	+*	−	±*	+*	−
Aggregation - C5a	+	+	±	+	+	−
Chemotaxis - C5a	+*	+*	−	±*	+*	−
Phagocytosis (iC3b-ORO)	+		−	−	+	−
Shape Change (Suspension)	−	−	−	−	−	−
f-Met-Leu-^{3}H-Phe binding	−	−	−	−	−	−
Superoxide generation (PMA)	−	−	−	−	−	−
Secretion-glucoronidase, Vit B$_{12}$ Transport Protein (PMA)	−	−	−	−	−	−
Phagocytosis (IgG-ORO)	−	−	−	−	−	−

● For most experiments granulocytes were preincubated in saturating concentration of MAbs or their F(ab')$_2$ fragments, washed and then assayed.
+ Consistantly and significantly blocks function
± Incosistant or minimal blockage
− No blockage
* Requires presence of monoclonal antibody during assay for inhibitory effect

chemotaxis, and aggregation were also inhibited (summarized in Table 4). The order of potency was anti-β < anti-Mac-1 α < anti-pl50,95 α < anti-LFA-1. This suggests that all members of the glycoprotein family may contribute to these reactions; the order of potency reflects their relative amounts on the granulocyte surface (19). These effects are quite specific. They are obtained with F(ab')$_2$ fragments (anti-β and anti-LFA-1) and are not given by IgG MAb bound to other surface molecules (the CR1 and HLA-A,B). Functions not deficient in patient cells were not inhibited by these MAb, i.e. shape change in suspension, f-Met-Leu-Phe binding, superoxide generation, secondary granule secretion, and phagocytosis of oil-red-0 (Table 4).

A Dynamic Model of Chemotaxis and Diapedesis

The specific molecular and functional deficits observed in patient cells suggest that in normal cells adherence and chemotaxis are mediated by the Mac-1, LFA-1 glycoprotein family, and that chemoattractant-stimulated hyperadherence and aggregation are mediated by the increase surface expression of Mac-1 an pl50,95. MAb blocking experiments confirm these findings. We believe chemotaxis is profoundly deficient in patients because of the underlying inability to adhere properly to substrates. We propose that *in vivo*, chemoattractants diffusing from sites of inflammation into the circulation induce Mac-1 and pl50,95 upregulation, leading to increased adherence of monocytes and granulocytes to blood vessels in the inflammatory site (Fig. 7).

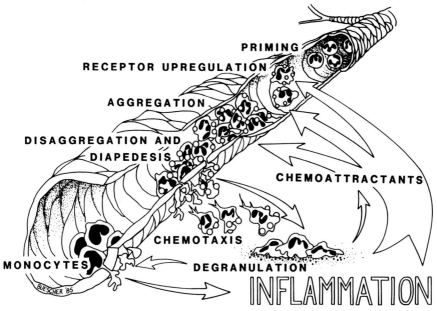

FIG. 7. Chemoattractant-mediated Mac-1 and pl50,95 upregulation, changes in leukocyte adherence, and diapedesis at inflammatory sites. Drawing by Dr. S. Buescher.

We further propose that in analogy to the importance of the Mac-1, LFA-1, and pl50,95 glycoproteins in chemotaxis *in vitro*, these glycoproteins mediate essential adherence functions during diapedesis and migration into the inflammatory site. The most important clinical manifestation of Mac-1, LFA-1 deficiency is the inhability of granulocytes to migrate into inflammatory sites and form pus. We propose that this is due to a lack of upregulation of adhesivess, which is normally regulated by the increased surface expression of Mac-1 and pl50,95.

The molecular mechanisms by which these glycoproteins mediate or regulate adhesivity are not known, and are an interesting area for further research. If adhesion is mediated by binding to specific ligands, the experiments with protein-coated glass and plastic substrates suggest that the ligand would first be secreted by the granulocytes or monocytes, then adhere to the substrate, thus allowing attachment of adhesion proteins. It has been demonstrated that the Mac-1 molecule binds at least one specific ligand, iC3b (25); however, other adhesive interactions mediated by Mac-1 might involve different ligand binding sites or different adhesive mechanisms. It is possible that the Mac-1, LFA-1 glycoproteins each bind several different ligands, or have highly flexibile conformations and act as molecular glues, binding to a wide range of molecules. Alternatively, the Mac-1, LFA-1 glycoproteins might not bind ligands directly, but might regulate adhesion through other surface molecules. It should be pointed out that all of the adhesive interactions in which these molecules participate require metabolic energy and temperatures higher than 4°C, and thus are not dependent on simple receptor-ligand interactions alone. The Mac-1, LFA-1 glycoproteins may regulate active processes, such as energy-dependent modification of the activity of other molecules, or remodeling the topography of the plasma membrane.

Whatever the mechanism, the delivery of adhesive proteins to the cell surface in discrete packages, bu fusion of secretory vesicles with the plasma membrane, allows an interesting speculation about chemotaxis. Cells undergoing chemotaxis orient in the gradient with lamellipodia at their anterior end and the uropod with retraction fibers at their posterior end (Fig. 5). Sensing of the chemoattractant not only stimulates orientation and motility, but release of secondary granules or some other secretory vesicle containing the Mac-1 and pl50,95 glycoproteins. As explained earlier, the concentration of these glycoproteins is much higher in the membrane bilayer of the storage compartment than in the plasma membrane of the unstimulated cell. We propose that during chemotaxis, the secretory vesicles containing Mac-1 and pl50,95 fuse with the plasma membrane at the leading edge of the cell. The site of fusion is hypothesized to be directed by the same chemoattractant-sensing machinery that guides the ruffling lamellipodia toward the chemoattractant.

A focal point of high Mac-1 and pl50,95 concentration would thus be formed in the plasma membrane at the site of fusion. Adhesion would be initiated or strengthened at this focal point. After further cell translocation, this focal point of attachment would near the cell uropod. By this time, diffusion of the adhesion proteins in the plane of the membrane, during moments when they are dissociated from ligand, would have lowered their concentration and the strength of adhesion. Alternatively, other time-dependent processes could regulate dissipation of the adhesive force. Detachment in the area of the uropod and its retraction fibers could thus occur, allowing further translocation. Because each granulocyte contains hundreds of specific granules, this cycle could be repeated many times. This process would allow intermittent adhesion sufficiently strong to allow attachment to a substrate but sufficiently localized temporally to allow selective detachment. This process would be superimposed on endocytic recycling of membrane, with endocytosis over the entire surface of the cell, and readdition at the leading edge of the cell. This allows bulk membrane flow from the leading edge to the uropod, and has been hypothesized to effect cell locomotion (15).

Previous observations are consistent with this model. We found that granulocyte spreading and chemotaxis are inhibited in the continued presence of excess MAb to the Mac-1 α subunit or the common β subunit, but not if cells are pretreated with MAb (Table 4). This is consistent with the idea that these processes require mobilization of Mac-1 from the intracellular latent pool to the cell surface. A role for secondary granule secretion in adherence and chemotaxis has previously been proposed, although it was related to changes in surface charge rather than to Mac-1 and p150,95 upregulation (10). Chemotaxis through micropore filters is accompanied by secondary granule release, and release is greatest from granulocytes that migrate the furthest. Degranulation occurs at the leading edge of the cell, and has been seen to occur from pseudopodia at points of close apposition to the filter matrix. Furthermore, spreading of neutrophils on glass beads or nylon fibers results in secondary but not primary granule release (24). Exudate granulocytes accumulating in sterile heat blister exudates, or in skin chamber, are selectively depleted in secondary granules, and secondary granule constituents are found in the exudate fluid (24). Circulating granulocytes from burn patients are depleted in their stores of secondary granules and deficient in chemotaxis (10). Patients with a granulocyte developmental defect with an absence of secondary granules show a chemotactic defect (10). Exposure of granulocytes to step increases in f-Met-Leu-Phe concentration induces adhesion sites at the lamellipodia, followed by their redistribution to the uropod, as shown by binding of albumin-coated latex beads (14). These observations on chemotaxis, adherence, and secondary granule release may all be related to chemoattractan-stimulated Mac-1 and p150,95 upregulation.

More detailed studies on the intracellular location of Mac-1 and p150,95, the coordination of their upregulation with cell adhesion, orientation, and chemotaxis, the formation and dissipation of the adhesive foci, and the structural basis for the adhesion functions of these proteins, promise to provide important insights into the molecular mechanisms of leukocyte chemotaxis and diapedesis.

REFERENCES

1. Anderson, D.C., Schmalstieg, F.C., Arnaout, M.A., et al. (1984): Abnormalities of polymorphonuclear leukocyte function associated with a heritable deficiency of high molecular weight surface glycoproteins (GP138): Common relationship to diminished cell adherence. *J. Clin. Invest.* 74:536-551.
2. Anderson, D.C., Schmalstieg, F.C., Finegold, M.J., Hughes, B.J., Rothelin, R., Miller, L.J., Kohl, S., Tosi, M.F., Jacobs, R.L., Goldman, A., Sheare, W.T., and Springer, T.A. (1985): The severe and moderate phenotypes of heritable Mac-1, LFA-1, pl50,95 deficiency: Their quantitative definition and relation to leukocyte dysfunction and clinical features. *J. Inf. Dis.*, in press.
3. Atherton, A., Born, G.V.R. (1972): Quantitative investigations of the adhesiveness of circulating polymorphonuclear leucocytes to blood vessel walls. *J. Physiol.* 222:447-474.
4. Beller, D.I., Springer, T.A., and Schreiber, R.D. (1982): Anti-Mac-1 selectively inhibits the mouse and human type three complement receptor. *J. Exp. Med.* 150:1000-1009.
5. Bretscher, M.S. (1984): Entocytosis: Relation to capping and cell locomotion. *Science* 224:681-686.
6. Buchanan, M.R., Crowley, C.A., Rosin, R.E., Gimbrone, M.A., and Babior, B.M. (1982): Studies on the interaction between GP-180-deficient neutrophils and vascular endothelium. *Blood* 60:160-165.
7. Danan N., Todd, R., Pitt, J., Colten, H.R., and Arnaout, M.A. (1983): Evidence tha Mo1 (a surface glycoprotein involved in phagocytosis) is distinct from the C3bi receptor. *Immunobiology* 164:205-206.
8. Dana, N., Todd, R.F., III, Pitt, J., Springer, T.A., and Arnaout, M.A. (1984): Deficiency of a surface membrane glycoprotein (Mo1) in man. *J. Clin. Invest.* 73:153-159.
9. Dawson, P., Mandell, O. (1980): Pagocyte strategy vs. microbial tactics. *Rev. Inf. Dis.* 2:817-836.
10. Gallin, J.I. (1982): Role of neutrophil lysosomal granules in the evolution of the inflammatory response. In Pagocytosis: *Past and Future*, ed. Karnovsky M.L., and Bolis L., pp. 519-541. New York: Academic Press, Inc.
11. Gallin, J.I., Fletcher, M.P., Seligmann, B.E., Hoffstein, S., Cehrs, K., and Mounessa, N. (1982): Human neutrophil-specific granule deficiency: A model to assess the role of neutrophil-specific granules in the evolution of the inflammatory response. *Blood* 59:1317-1329.
12. Hoffstein, S.T., Friedman, R.S., and Weissmann, G. (1982): Degranulation, membrane addition, and shape change during chemotactic factor-induced aggregation of human neutrophils. *J. Cell. Biol.* 95:234-241.
13. Sanchez-Madrid, F., Nagy, J., Robbins, E., Simon, P., and Springer, T.A (1983): A human leukocyte differentiation antigen family with distinct alpha subunits and a common beta subunit: the lymphocyte-function associated antigen (LFA-1), the C3bi complement receptor (OKM1/Mac-1), and the pl50,95 molecule. *J. Exp. Med.* 158:1785-1803.
14. Smith, C.W., and Hollers, J.C. (1980): Motility and adhesiveness in human neutrophils: Redistribution of chemotactic factor-induced adhesion sites. *J. Clin. Invest.* 65:804-812.
15. Snyderman, R., and Pike, M.C. (1984): Chemoattractant receptors on phagocytic cells. In: *Annual Review of Immunology*, Vol. 2, ed. Paul, W.E., Fathman, C.G., and pp. 257-281. Palo Alto, C.A.: Annual Reviews Inc.
16. Springer, T.A., Davignon, D., Ho, M.K., Kürzinger, K., Martz, E., and Sanchez-Madrid, F. (1982): LFA-1 and Lyt-2,3, molecules associated with T lymphocyte-mediated killing; and Mac-1, an LFA-1 homologue associated with complement receptor function. *Immunol. Rev.* 68:111-135.
17. Springer, T.A., Thompson, W.S., Miller, L.J., Schmalstieg, F.C., and Anderson, D.C. (1984): Inherited deficiency of the Mac-1, LFA-1, pl50,95 glycoprotein family and its molecular basis. *J. Exp. Med.* 160:1901-1918.
18. Springer, T.A., Anderson, D.C. (1985): Functional and structural interrelationships among the Mac-1, LFA-1 family of leukocyte adhesion glycoproteins, and their deficiency in a novel, heritable disease. In: *Hybridoma Technology in the Biosciences and Medicine*, ed. Springer, T.A., New York, in press: Plenum.
19. Springer, T.A., Anderson, D.C. (1985): Antibodies specific for the Mac-1, LFA-1, pl50,95 glycoproteins or their family, or for other granulocyte proteins. In: *Second international workshop on human leukocyte differentiation antigens*, ed. Reinherz E. Berlin, in press: Springer Verlag.
20. Thompson, R.A., Candy, D.C.A., and McNeish, A.S. (1984): Familial defect of polymorph

neutrophil phagocytosis associated with absence of a surface glycoprotein antigen (OKM1). *Clin. Exp. Immunol.* 58:229-236.

21. Todd, R.F., III, Arnaout, M.A., Rosin, R.E., Crowley, C.A., Peters, W.A., and Babior, B.M. (1984): Subcellular localization of the large subunit of Mo1 (Mo1 alpha; formerly gp 110), a surface glycoprotein associated with neutrophil adhesion. *J. Clin. Invest.* 74:1280-1290.

22. Tonnesen, M.G., Smedly, L.A., and Henson, P.M. (1984): Neutrophil-endothelial cell interactions: Modulation of neutrophil adhesiveness induced by complement fragments C5a and C5a des arg and Formyl-Methionyl-Leucyl-Phenylalanine in vitro. *J. Clin. Invest.* 74:1581-1592.

23. Wilkinson, Peter C. (1982): Chemotaxis and Inflammation, 2nd Edition. London: Churchill Livinstone.

24. Wright, D.G., and Gallin, J.I. (1979). Secretory responses of human neutrophils: Exocytosis of specific (secondary) granules by human neutrophils during adherence and in vitro and during exudation in vivo. *J. Immunol.* 123:285-294.

25. Wright, S.D., Rao, P.E., Van Voorhis, W.C., Craigmyle, L.S., Iida, K., Talle, M.A., Westberg, E.F., Goldstein, G., and Silverstein, S.C. (1983): Identification of the C3bi receptor of human monocytes and macrophages with monoclonal antibodies. *Proc. Natl. Acad. Sci. USA* 80:5699-5703.

SECTION IV
IMMUNOBIOLOGY
OF IMMUNODEFICIENCIES

Immune Responses to Poliovirus by Lymphocytes from Antibody Deficient Patients

A.R. Hayward, N.A. Halsey and M.J. Levin

Department of Pediatrics and The Barbara Davis Center for Childhood Diabetes
University of Colorado Health Sciences Center
Denver, CO 80262, USA

INTRODUCTION

Paralytic poliomyelitis infections are a rare but well documented complication of immunization with attenuated poliovirus vaccine. The overall incidence is about one in five million doses of vaccine distributed and of 76 cases between 1969 and 1978, 62% were in secondary household contacts, 24% in vaccinees and 11% in children with primary immunodeficiency disorders. The immunodeficiency syndromes reported in the literature include congenital X-linked agammaglobulinemia (2 cases) other hypogammaglobulinemia syndromes (7 cases) IgA deficiency (2 cases) combined immunodeficiency (7 cases) and one with cartilage hair hypoplasia (reviewed, in 10) with subsequent cases described in 1, 2, 3 and 8. The boy we report is the first we are aware of to have had transient hypogammaglobulinemia as an association and the same diagnosis seems likely in a second case. These clinical observations (described below) prompted us to undertake studies on other antibody deficient patients to determine the extent to which they could develop cell mediated immunity to polio-virus.

Case Reports

(1) The boy had no family history of immunodeficiency; he was given his first oral polio vaccine at 68 days' age. Nineteen days later he became febrile (40ºC) and vomited. Three days later he had a right sided 6th and 7th cranial nerve palsy and a flaccid paralysis of the left upper arm. CSF obtained after the cranial nerve palsy developed showed a mononuclear pleocytosis with a slightly raised protein. A stool sample obtained a week later grew out Poliovirus type 2 characterized as vaccine-like at the CDC. Immunologic investigations on the child are summarized in Table 1.

TABLE 1.   *Serum Immunoglobulins of Patient 1*

Age in Months	Serum immunoglobulins (mg%)			Other Tests
	IgG	IgA	IgM	
5	200	8	0	Blood count normal
6	170	4	20	Normal PHA response
				B cells present in blood
				(Ig replacement started)
9	270	18	30	
18	400	16	30	(Ig replacement stopped)
27	380	40	34	Anti-TT titer 1:64
34	430	31	45	Anti-TT titer 1:256
38	524	26	55	
	400 - 1400	30 - 150	50 - 250	Control range

During the 3 years of follow-up the patient developed normally and showed substantial resolution of his paralysis.

(2) This girl was born at 29 weeks' gestation and had multiple complications of prematurity including hyaline membrane disease and a small intraventricular hemorrhage. Hydrocephalus from the hemorrhage was treated with a ventricular-peritoneal shunt. At 4 1/2 months she received her first DPT-OPV. Six days later she was irritable and had a seizure. CSF obtained from the sunt revealed 104 white blood cells, 69% monocytes and 31% lymphocytes, with a protein of 77 mg %. Poliovirus type 2 was cultured from the CSF and characterized as vaccine like at the CDC. Her immunoglobulins (in mg per dl) at 4 months were IgG, 160, IgA 10, IgM 276 and at 8 months were IgG 318, IgA 44, IgM 372. The IgM levels are high but the IgG had risen to the range of healthy controls by 8 months. Follow up revealed some persistent developmental delay but no paralysis.

MATERIALS AND METHODS

Subject and blood processing

Three healthy controls, 2 patients with X-linked agammaglobulinemia and 4 with varied hypogammaglobulinemia syndrome were recruited with informed consent. Ten ml of blood were drawn before and 3 weeks after an im boost with 1 ml of killed poliovirus vaccine (Squibb-Connaught, Inc.). The blood was defibrinated and the serum separated by centrifugation. The mononuclear cells (MNC) were separated by centrifugation of Ficoll-Hypaque.

Poliovirus and antigen preparation

Vaccine-strain poliovirus type 1 was grown to full CPE in the continuous monkey kidney cell line LLC MK2. The poliovirus antigen for in vitro use was prepared by extraction of the infected cells in a glycine buffer according to the method of Zaia, et al (12). A control antigen prepared by an identical extraction process from uninfected cells was included in all experiments. In preliminary studies we determined that the optimal dilution of the antigen for lympho-cyte stimulation was between 1:50 and 1:100, though proliferative responses could be detected at dilutions of up to 1:300.

Catabolism of S labelled poliovirus

A culture of poliovirus was labelled with ^{35}S methionine overnight. The cells were disrupted in 1% deoxycholate. The supernatant was clarified by centrifu-gation and the virus recovered by ultracentrifugation at 28,000 rpm for 2 hours. The trace amounts of unincorporated ^{35}S methionine which remained were removed by dialysis in Hanks balances salt solution +5% human albumin for 4 hours.

Patient and control MNC were incubated in RPMI 1640 + 1% autologous serum for 1 hour on flasks at 37°C to allow attachment of monocytes; non-adherent cell were washed off at this time. Five ml of fresh medium supplemented with 10% fetal calf serum or antibody-containing control serum and containing 0.1 ml of live S labelled vaccine strain poliovirus were added to the cultures. The distribution of label between the cells and supernatant after overnight culture was determined by counting in liquid scintillation fluid. The cellular fraction was recovered by 0.1% SDS lysis of the cells, spinning down the cell debris and running 0.5 ml of the supernatant over a small Sephacryl 200 column with a void volume of 10 ml and a volume for complete elution of 62 ml.

Lymphocyte culture for responder cell frequency analysis

Blood MNC were washed and resuspended in RPMI 1640 medium with 10% human (autologous or healthy donor) serum. Forty-eight replicate Linbro 76-013-05 culture wells were seeded with 60,000; 30,000; 15,000 and 7,500 cells. Polioantigen was added at a final dilution of 1:50 to 24 of the replicates at each cell concentration and 1:50 control antigen to the remaining 24 wells. The plates were cultured for 10 days, then pulsed harvested and counted as before (5).

The data were analysed to determine the percentage of antigen stimulated wells whose counts exceeded the mean +3 SD for control antigen wells and the precursor frequency was established by interpolation at the 37% non-re-sponder well level (6, 9).

RESULTS

In vitro uptake and catabolism of poliovirus

Comparison of ^{35}S counts in the supernatant and cell fractions of adherent cell cultures after overnight incubation indicated that about 0.5% of the label became cell-associated whether or not antibody was added to the culture. The S 200 elution profiles of the cell associated and supernatant label fractions

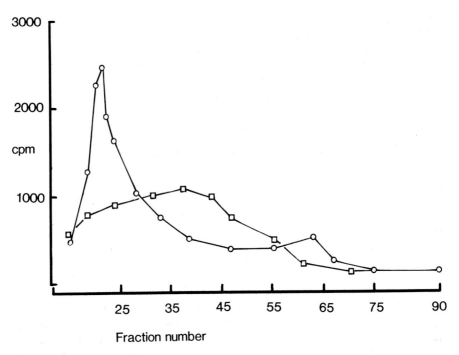

FIG. 1. Elution profile of ^{35}S label from S200 column fractionation of cell associated (–□–) and control supernatant (–O–) fractions.

(Figure 1) show that the sharp peak in the supernatant is replaced by a broad peak in the cells. Identical results were obtained with monocytes from healthy controls, XLA and varied hypogammaglobulinemia patients. These data argue against a failure of antigen uptake by our patients' monocytes.

Responder T cell frequencies before and after immunization

These data are summarized in Table 2. Individuals with a responder cell frequency of 1:30,000 or greater had linear plots of non-responder wells against cell number per well, suggesting that the response was limited by only

TABLE 2. *Immune Responses to Poliovirus Antigen Following Booster Immunization[1]*

Subjects	Responder T Cell Frequency		Serum Antibody
	Before boost	After boost	Increase
X linked agammaglobulinemia	1:30,000	1:12,000	0
Varied hypogammaglobulinemia	1:60,000	1:50,000	0
Controls	1:60,000	1:15,000	4 fold

[1] Responder T cell frequencies measured by limiting dilution. Antibody measurement by ELISA

a single cell population. The responder T cell frequency increased about four fold following the booster immunization with killed polio vaccine in the healthy controls. The congenital X-linked agammaglobulinemia patients had a higher frequency of responder cells before immunization than the controls and this increased after boosting. The unclassified (varied) hypogammaglobulinemia patients' MNC showed a lower response to boosting.

DISCUSSION

Two observations pertinent to the pathogenicity of enteroviruses, and especially poliovirus, are reported here. One is that paralytic polio following oral immunization can occur in transient hypogammaglobulinemia in addition to the other antibody deficiency syndromes previously described. We are unaware of other descriptions of this, perhaps because of the rarity with which transient hypogammaglobulinemia is diagnosed, together with the rarity of paralytic polio in any antibody deficient patients.

A prolonged clinical course and lymphocyte infiltrates of the brain and cord of fatal cases of vaccine polio (reviewed, 11) would be compatible with a cell mediated immune response to the virus in patients with antibody deficiency. To examine the quality of this response in hypogammaglobulinemia we first tested patients adherent MNC for the uptake of labelled antigen. The proportion of virus ingested by monocytes was similar to that we previously found using radiolabelled varicella zoster virus (7) but in the case of poliovirus the addition of antibody did not enhance uptake. This result does not suggest that the T cell responses to poliovirus of antibody deficient patients would be impaired by lack of opsonising antibody.

The frequency of responder T cells we found in our healthy controls and in our varied hypogammaglobulinemia patients was only 1:60,000 or less. This is lower than the 1:10,000 to 1:20,000 frequency we found for latent viruses such as herpes-viruses (5) and is similar to the frequency of tetanus toxoid responsive T cells in children at 12 or more months after their last boost (4). Both the X-linked agammaglobulinemia patients we studied had higher poliovirus RCF's despite the fact that they had not knowingly been exposed to poliovirus since infancy. More of this subgroup of patients will have to be studied to determine whether this is a chance finding or whether it is related to their antibody deficiency. Our results suggest that T cell proliferative responses to enteroviruses are measurable. The state of ECHO virus immunity in antibody deficient patients will be of interest, especially in those who develop chronic encephalitis.

Aknowledgements

We are grateful to Karen Dunn for patient care and contacts, Mark Herberger for invaluable technical assistance and Kerry Morimoto for typing the manuscript. The study was supported by NIH grants HD13733 and RR0069 from the Division of Research Resources.

REFERENCES

1. Abo, W., Chiba, S., Yamanaka, T., Nakao, T., Hara, M., Tagara, I. (1979): Paralytic poliomyelitis in a child with agammaglobulinemia. *Eur. J. Pediatr.* 132:11.
2. Church, J.A., Clay, S. (1979): Agammaglobulinemia and poliomyelitis-like illness. *Ann. Allergy* 42:86.
3. Douglas, S.D., Anolik, R. (1981): Postvaccination paralysis in a 20-month-old child. *Hosp. Pract.* 16:40A, 40F.
4. Hayward, A.R., Glode, M. (1985): Tetanus toxoid responder T cell frequencies following booster immunization in childhood. *Clin. Res.* 33:123A (Abstract).
5. Hayward, A.R., Herberger, M., Groothius, J., Levin, M.R. (1984): Specific immunity after congenital or neonatal infection with cytomegalovirus or herpes simplex virus. *J. Immunol.* 133:2469.
6. Henry, C., Marbrook, J., Vann, D.C., Kodlin, D., Wojsy, C.: Limiting dilution analysis. In: *Selected Methods in Cellular Immunology.* Mischell, B.B., Shiigi, S.M., editors: Freeman Press, San Francisco.
7. Pontesilli, O., Laszlo, M., Levin, M., Hayward, A. (1985): In vitro processing of membrane bound VZV antigens for presentation to T cells. FASEB meeting.
8. Sankano, T., Kittaka, E., Tanaka, Y., Yamaoka, H., Kobayashi, Y., Usui, T. (1980): Vaccine-associated poliomyelitis in an infant with agammaglobulinemia. *Acta Paediatr. Scan.* 69:549.
9. Van Oers, M.H.J., Pinkster, J., Zeijlmaker, W.P. (1978): Quantification of antigen reactive cells among human T lymphocytes. *Eur. J. Immunol.* 8:477.
10. Wright, P.F., Hatch, M.H., Kasselberg, A.G., Lowry, S.P., Waslington, W.B., Karzon, D.T. (1977): Vaccine-associated poliomyelitis in a child with sex-linked agammaglobulinemia. *J. Pediatr.* 91:408.
11. Wyatt, H.V. (1973): Poliomyelitis in Hypogammaglobulinemics. *J. Infect. Dis.* 128:802.
12. Zaia, J.A., Leary, P.L., Levin, M.J. (1978): Specificity of the blastogenic response of human mononuclear cells to herpesvirus antigens. *Infect. Immunol.* 20:646.

Abnormalities of T Cell Subsets and Lymphokines (IL-2 and gamma IFN) in Immunodeficiencies

F. Aiuti, R. Paganelli, B. Ensoli, A. Cabello, M. Cherchi,
S. Venuta, M.R. Capobianchi and F. Dianzani

Department of Clinical Immunology, University of Rome «La Sapienza», Rome, Italy
Department of Biochemical Science, 2nd Faculty of Medicine, University of Naples, Italy
Institute of Virology, University of Rome, «La Sapienza»

INTRODUCTION

Primary and acquired immunodeficiencies have usually been defined by a combination of in vivo and in vitro tests aimed at T and B lymphocyte function measurement, and investigation of phenotypic markers of lymphomonocytes and their subpopulations (11). A good agreement between skin tests to recall antigens and lymphoproliferative in vitro responses has been observed, and stimulation of peripheral blood mononuclear cells (PBMC) with mitogens is commonly used to assess T cell function. Recently the process of T cell activation has been revised after the discovery of soluble mediators (interleukins) capable of regulating the cellular interactions leading to T lymphocyte proliferation. In particular, interleukin-2 (IL-2) can maintain the growth of activated cells and is the antigen non-specific final mediator of replication. It is released by T cells after exposure to antigens or mitogens. The action of IL-2 is exerted on T and NK cells expressing a specific receptor. This receptor is strictly associated to a molecule on the surface of T and NK cells identified by the monoclonal antibody (MoAB) anti-Tac (12). The expression of the putative IL-2 receptor (Tac) as well as the production of IL-2 represent early events in T cell activation leading to proliferative events. Gamma-Interferon (IFN) is also released by T cells, and it appears to have immunoregulatory activity. Its production is enhanced by IL-2 (5).

We measured the presence of IL-2 and gamma IFN by conventional tests after mitogen-induced stimulation, in several patients with immunodeficiencies who show severely defective T lymphocyte function in vivo and in vitro. The study of both IL-2 and gamma-IFN production in these patients is of great importance for potential in vivo applications.

MATERIALS AND METHODS

Selection of Patiens

Patients were diagnosed according to published WHO (11) and CDC-NIH (1) criteria respectively for primary immunodeficiency and lymphoadenopathy syndrome (LAS). Their follow-up observation ranged from 3 months to several years, and repeated immunological estimations of their laboratory parameters were carried out, including skin tests to common recall antigens, serum Ig levels, MoAb phenotyping, mitogen responses. The patients included 20 cases of common variable immunodeficiency (CVI), 3 cases of severe combined immunodeficiency (SCID), 3 with Wiskott-Aldrich (WA) syndrome, 3 with Ataxia-Telangiectasia (A-T), two with hyper IgE syndrome, one with combined immunodeficiency (CID) with hyper-IgM, and 12 patients with LAS, according to CDC-NIH criteria. The patients with hypogammaglobulinemia (including those with A-T) were under continuous treatment with intravenous gammaglobulins. Normal controls were checked by the same methods.

Phenotyping of peripheral blood mononuclear cells (PBMC)

PBMC were isolated by Ficoll-Hypaque sedimentation, washed three times and stained with the following MoAbs: OKT3 (total T cells), OKT4 (helper/inducer), OKT8 (suppressor/cytotoxic) (Ortho, Raritan, NJ, USA).

Tac antigen expression

After 72 hours culture in the presence of phytohemagglutinin (PHA, 1 ug/ml) PBMC were stained with anti-Tac MoAb (a gift of Dr. T. Waldmann) and positive cells identified by indirect immunofluorescence as for other MoAb. Preliminary tests indicated this time of culture as optimal for the highest percentage of cells expressing the Tac antigen.

Cell cultures and IL-2 production

PBMC obtained as indicated were cultured in triplicate wells of microculture plates, with or without the addition of optimal or suboptimal amounts of PHA (1 or 0.5 ug/ml) and recombinant IL-2 (Genentech). Thymidine (3HT, Amersham) (1 uci/well) was added in the final 5 hrs of culture, cells harvested and 3HT uptake assessed by liquid scintillation counting. Results are reported as net cpm (counts/min stimulated - background). Macrocultures of 10^6 PBMC in 1 ml with optimal amount of PHA were also set up in parallel to microcultures. After 24 hrs, the surnatant was removed and stored for IL-2 and IFN determination in separate aliquots at $-70°C$. The IL-2 assay was performed according to published methods (4, 13). Briefly, 4000 murine CTLL cells were grown in the presence of log dilutions of putative IL-2 containing medium in

96-well microtiter plates. Twenty-four hours later, 0.5 uCi of 3HT were added to each well. After 4 hr, the cells were harvested on glass fiber strips and 3HT incorporation measured in a liquid scintillation counter.

The IL-2 concentration in the experimental sample was than calculated by probit analysis using the Jurkat reference standard, and expressed as reference units/ml. The standard error for replicate determination was less than 15%.

Effect of IL-2 on mitogen response

This was assessed by 3HT incorporation by cultured PBMC after 72 hrs with/without purified IL-2 (a gift of Dr. Welte, N.Y.) at 1-10 U/ml, or recombinant IL-2 at the same concentration. The differential cpm count was expressed as percent change from baseline PHA response.

IFN production and titration

Alpha-IFN was induced by incubating PBMC with Newcastle disease virus (NDV), 10 HA/10^6 cells/ml in culture medium (RPMI 1640 with fetal calf serum, FCS) and incubated at 37°C. Supernates were collected after 20 h culture and pH2 treated for 48 h before titration. Gamma-IFN was induced either with staphylococcal enterotoxin B (SEB), 0.2 ug/ml/10 cells, with galactose oxidase (GO), 10 U/ml/10^6 cells for 30 min at 24°C, or with the calcium ionophore A23187 (Calbiochem) at a concentration of 5 uM/10^6 cells, as described (4). Supernatants of both unstimulated (to evaluate spontaneous production) and stimulated PBMC were titrated on human WISH cell cultures in microplates, by Sindbis virus hemagglutinin yield reduction after a single growth cycle. Activity was measured in units/ml against a standard of gamma-IFN as previously described. The antiviral activity found in the sample was identified as alpha- or gamma-IFN according to current criteria (2).

RESULTS

T cell subpopulations

Total T lymphocytes, identified by OKT3 reactivity, were low in patients with SCID, CID with hyper IgM, A-T, WA and hyper IgE syndrome. Variable levels were found in patients with CVI (51-84%) and LAS (46-81%), but all within 2 SD of normal mean. OKT4/T8 ratio was abnormal or reversed in some patients with cellular immunodeficiency but all the subsets were greatly diminished when expressed as absolute figures - since lymphopenia was present in all cases. Low or inverted OKT4/OKT8 ratios were found in 15/20 patients with CVI, although absolute numbers of T4+ cells were normal in some of them. An inverted OKT4/OKT8 ratio with absolute decrease ot T4+ lymphocytes was detected in 9 out of 12 cases of LAS. This finding substantiated the diagnosis in most LAS patients.

Lymphoproliferative responses to PHA

PHA at 1 ug/ml was found to be the optimal stimulus for mitogen-induced lymphoproliferative responses. Normal subjects had an average mean of 39000 ± 16000 cpm (SD). Patients with CVI exhibited a mean response of 28000 ± 21000 cpm, showing a decrease compared to normals. Three cases had 3HT incorporation below 7,000 cpm.

In vitro responses of patients with impaired cell mediated immunity (CMI) were grossly abnormal, with cpm values below 10,000 except 4 patients who showed some degree of lymphoproliferation, within 2 SD of controls' mean. LAS patients were very heterogeneous, showing normal responses in 4 cases (range 18,000-40,000 cpm), low normal (10,000) in 2, and very low in another 2 (4-5,000).

IL-2 Production

PBMC from normal subjects, stimulated with optimal doses of PHA, produced an average of 5.9 ref. U of IL-2/ml (range 0.8-18 ref. U/ml). 16 out of 20 CVI patients had IL-2 production within this normal range, with four cases showing only 0.3-0.4 ref. U/ml in the cell supernatant. The average mean production was 4.7 ± 5.2 ref. U/ml (statistically not significant vs controls).

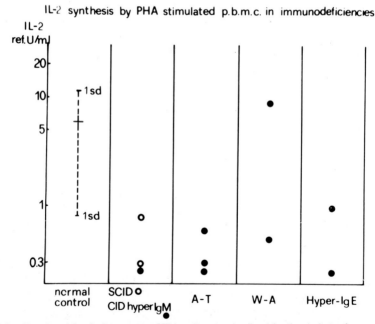

FIG. 1. Results of the IL-2 assay on CTLL cells, standardized for the Jurkat reference, on 24 h PHA-stimulated supernatants from lymphomononuclear cells (pbmc) of normal subjects (n=12) and patients with primary immunodeficiencies. Results are expressed as reference U/ml. For details, see Materials and Methods.

IL-2 production was severely depressed in patients with SCID, CID with hyper IgM, A-T, WA syndrome and hyper IgE syndrome: the levels observed ranged between 1 and less than 0.3 ref. U/ml (detection limit by our assay) (Fig. 1). One patient with WA exhibited normal IL-2 production and his lymphoproliferative response to PHA was also normal, compared to controls.

We measured IL-2 production after PHA induction only in 6 cases of LAS, and found normal levels in all six (mean = 5.9 ± 5.1) with range well within normal limits (0.8-20 ref. U/ml) (Fig. 2).

IL-2 receptor (Tac) expression

Experiments with anti Tac MoAb demonstrated a high percentage of PBMC expressing the IL-2 receptor after 3 days'culture with PHA (mean = 67 ± 11) in normal subjects. Lower percentages were present in CVI cases, tested at least twice on separate occasions: six patients had Tac positive cells values below 2SD of controls. Tac expression was even lower in CMI deficient

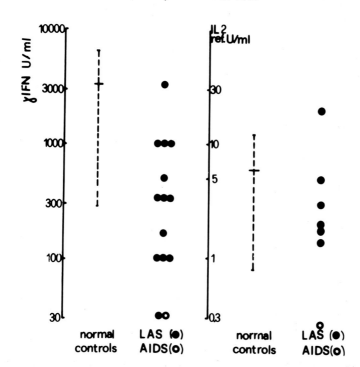

γIFN and IL 2 synthesis by p.b.m.c. after PHA stimulation in patient with LAS

FIG. 2. Results of gamma (γ) IFN and IL-2 production in PHA-stimulated culture supernatans from lymphomononuclear cells (pbmc) of patients with lymphoadenopathy syndrome (LAS=0) and 1 casedof AIDS (0). Normal controls are indicated as mean ±1 S.D. in broken line.

patients: values reported for 12 such cases are all below 2 SD of controls (1 case is just 1% below the limit). Patients with LAS had in all but one case, % Tac values within the normal range.

Gamma IFN and Alpha IFN productions

When stimulated with NDV, all patients showed a normal high production of alpha IFN (i.e. 3000 U/ml). Different inducers for gamma IFN gave different results with respect to absolute values. However, taking into account the relative potency of these inducers (PHA, GO, SEB and Calcium Ionophore A23187) we were able to confirm the lack of major defects of gamma IFN production in most patients with CVI or LAS (Fig. 2, 3). In contrast, patients with severe T cell defects were either grossly defective (3/3 SCID, 3/3 A-T, 1/3 WA, 2/2 hyper IgE) or impaired producers of gamma IFN (in 3 patients). Seven low responders were selected for induction with Calcium Ionophore which was ineffective in all of them, and restoration by addition of exogeneous recombinant IL-2 (10 U/ml) gave no enhancement in 7 out of 7 patients' PBMC tested.

Effect of IL-2 addition

The main effect of IL-2 is to maintain lymphoproliferation, so we tried its addition to PBMC of controls and patients in vitro, and measured its effects on 3HT uptake after 3 days' culture. We divided the case studied into normal PHA responders and defective ones (Fig. 4). Upon addition of 10 U/ml of recombinant or purified IL-2 we measured the percent change in cpm responses and subdivided the defective group into IL-2 responders and non responders (i.e. below or over 100% increase of cpm response). Results are depicted in Fig. 4, showing the range of responses to IL-2 in normals, CVI patients and primary immunodeficiencies of CMI. Most SCID patients had no response to IL-2, as well as 2/3 A-T, 3/3 WA, 2/2 Hyper IgE; responders included primary T cell defects, CID with hyper IgM and occasional other T cell deficiencies.

DISCUSSION

Our studies revealed the presence of defects of mitogen responses due to different defective activation steps in patients with primary deficiencies of cell-mediated immunity. These were largely independent of total number of T lymphocytes and relative percentages of OKT4+ or T8+ subsets, since alterations of these T cell subsets were also present in the majority of patients with CVI or LAS, whose in vitro responses and interleukin 2 synthesis were generally normal.

There is no doubt that patients with SCID and related syndromes have defective T cell activation, besides that the majority of them have some degree of circulating mature T cells. The defect might be explained by the detection of absent or very low production in vitro of IL-2 in SCID and other syndromes with T cell deficiency such as A-T, WA and hyper IgE syndrome.

In patients with SCID the response is not corrected by exogeneous purified or recombinant IL-2 addition, perhaps due to the lack of functionally mature T cells capable of responding to IL-2. This ability is reflected by the restoration of mitogen induced lymphoproliferation after IL2 supplementation, and by the normal expression of IL2 receptors by activated T and NK cells. In fact most patients with defective CMI have a low percentage of cells expressing the IL-2 receptor after mitogen stimulation, identified by the anti-Tac MoAb.

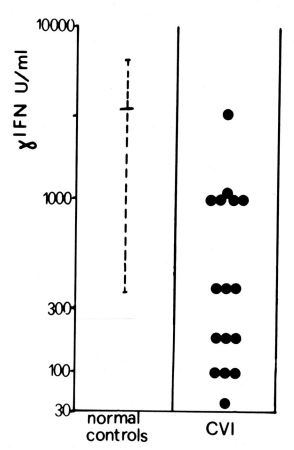

FIG. 3. Results of gamma (γ) IFN synthesis after PHA stimulation in 6 cases of Lymphoadenopathy syndrome (LAS), compared to 12 healthy subjects (broken line indicating mean ± 1 S.D. of the mean).

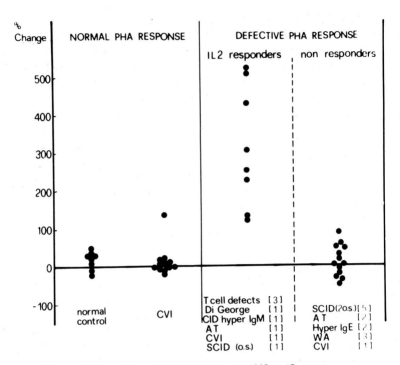

Effect of IL2 addition on PHA response of PBMC in ID patient

FIG. 4. Percent (%) change of the lymphoproliferative response to PHA after addition of 1.10 U/ml of IL-2 in primary immunodeficiency patients (for anonyms refer to Materials and Methods). The subjects were discriminated for the PHA response inferior 1 S.D. of the mean (normal PHA response) or below (defective). IL-2 responders showed an increase over 100% of baseline PHA values. Numbers in parentheses indicate the number of cases for each group. In the SCID group, patients with Ommen Syndrome (O.S.) are also indicated.

However most cases of T cell deficiency responded to PHA when appropriate amounts of exogeneous (recombinant or purified) IL-2 were added (Fig. 4). We subdivided the patients with defective mitogen responses into two groups, IL2 responders and non responders, the latter being the patients with low Tac expression and poor response to IL2.

Kruger et al (6) found a similar pattern of response to purified IL-2 in CVI patients, but our CVI cases seemed to have a less severe defect of mitogen responses and very little restoration with IL-2 could be observed. The findings in SCID and T cell defective patients confirm and expand the results previously reported by us as well as by other investigators (7, 10). Here we add direct evidence of deficient quantitative expression of IL2 receptors on T cells, identified by anti-Tac, and the simultaneous measurement of gamma IFN in addition to IL2 in a large series of patients with primary or acquired ID. So far we know of no other report covering such a large number of cases and embracing so many different primary syndromes.

In cases with A-T low mitogen response, low IL-2 production and defective Tac expression were demonstrated. These cases also had an associated defect of gamma IFN production. Since the addition in vitro of IL-2 was incapable of modifing the immunological aberration, other unknown mechanisms may be postulated. These patients probably represent a subgroup of AT cases with absolute T cell deficiency, although the helper/suppressor balance has been found to be heterogenous in functional studies (3).

We found normal alpha IFN production in all our cases, as previously reported (8). Gamma IFN was reduced in SCID and other T cell deficiencies and this defective production was not due to lack of IL-2 synthesis, since recombinant IL-2 did not correct gamma IFN production in 7 deficient cases. The use of calcium ionophore as IFN inducer, ruled out a defect of calcium influx into the cells after mitogen stimulation. No other membrane defect was in fact found since prior treatment of PBMC with neuraminidase did not restore IFN production. Gamma IFN production by lymphocytes is induced by mitogens through the release of a macrophage mediator after oxidation of molecules on the macrophage membrane. Therefore there is an absolute need for accessory cells in the process of gamma IFN induction which is bypassed only by calcium ionophores acting directly on T cell surfaces and inducing calcium influx into the cells. This event leads to gamma IFN release even in absence of monocytes or macrophages. Therefore our data seem to indicate a defect of transmembrane signalling or a lack of response to calcium influx into T lymphocytes, suggesting either a genetic defect or an aberration at mRNA level/transcription.

No major defects of IFN production were observed in LAS patients, which may differentiate them from AIDS cases who show a severe deficiency of gamma IFN (9) or of IL-2.

More studies on IL-2 responsive T cells in man are therefore clearly required and important in order to propose this immunoregulatory lymphokine in the therapy of selected immunodeficiencies.

The production and response to interleukins, as well as the interactions between these mediators, regulate the expression of immune functions. Therefore their study could be essential for the understanding of illness of the immune system. Our results have indicated that an altered regulation of IL-2 and gamma IFN can be present in primary and acquired immunodeficiencies.

Acknowledgements

This paper has been supported by a grant from Ministero Pubblica Istruzione (40-60%) and Fondazione Cenci-Bolognetti.

REFERENCES

1. Aiuti, F., Allen, J.R., Bijerk, K.J., et al (1984): AIDS in Europe 'status quo' 1983. *Eur. J. Cancer Clin. Oncol.* 20:155-173.

2. Dianzani, F., Monahan, T.M., Schupham, A., Zucca, M. (1979): Enzymatic induction of interferon production by galactose oxidase treatment of human lymphoid cells. *Infect. Immunity* 26:879-882.

3. Fiorilli, M., Businco, L., Pandolfi, F., Paganelli, R., Russo, G., Aiuti, F. (1983): Heterogeneity of immunological abnormalities in ataxia-telangiectasia. *J. Clin. Immunol.* 3:135-139.

4. Gillis, S., Smith, K.A. (1978): T cell growth factor: parameters of production and quantitative microassay for activity. *J. Immunol.*, 120:2027-2032.

5. Kasahara, T., Hooks, J.J., Dougherty, S.F., Oppenheim, J.J. (1983): Interleukin-2 mediated immune interferon (IFN-γ) production by human T cells and T cell subsets. *J. Immunol.* 130:1784-1789.

6. Kruger, et. al. (1984): Interleukin-2 correction of defective in vitro T-cell mitogenesis in patients with common varied immunodeficiency. *J. Clin. Immunol.*, 4:295-303.

7. Lopez-Botet, M., Fontan, G., Rodriguez, M.C., De Landazur, M.D. (1982): Relationship between IL-2 synthesis and the proliferative response to PHA in different primary immunodeficiencies. *J. Immunol.*, 128:679-694.

8. Matricardi, P.M., Capobianchi, M.R., Paganelli, R., et al. (1984): Interferon production in primary immunodeficiencies. *J. Clin. Immunol.*, 4:388-394.

9. Murray, H.W., Rubin, B.Y., Masur, H., Robert, R.B. (1984): Impaired production of lymphokines and immune (gamma) interferon in the acquired immunodeficiency syndrome. *N. Engl. J. Med.* 310:883-889.

10. Paganelli, R., Aiuti, F., Beverley, P.C.L., Levinsky, R.J., (1983): Impaired production of interleukins in patients with cell-mediated immunodeficiency. *Clin. Exp. Immunol.* 51:338-344.

11. Rosen, F.S., Wedgwood, R.J., Aiuti, F., Cooper, M.D., Hitzig, W.J., Matsumoto, S., Good, R.A., Seligmann, M., Hanson, L.A., Soothill, J.F., Waldmann, T.A. (1983): Meeting report: Primary Immunodeficiency Diseases. *Clin. Immunol. Immunopathol.*, 28:450-475.

12. Uchiyama, T., Nelson, D.L., Fleischer, T.A., Waldmann, T.A. (1981): A monoclonal antibody (anti-Tac) reactive with activated and functionally mature human T cells. *J. Immunol.*, 126:1398-1403.

13. Venuta, S., Mertelsmann, R., Welte, K., Feldman, S.P., Wang, C.Y., Moore, M.A.S. (1983): Production and regulation of interleukin-2 in human lymphoblastic leukemias studied with T-cell monoclonal antibodies. *Blood* 61:781-786.

Lymphocyte Abnormalities in Patients with IgG Subclass Deficiency

Isabella Quinti*, Raif S. Geha**, Claudia Papetti*,
Fernando Aiuti*.

*Department of Allergy and Clinical Immunology, University of Rome «La Sapienza», Rome, Italy, and **Division of Allergy, Children's Hospital, Boston, MA, USA

INTRODUCTION

Quantification of the levels of the 3 main serum immunoglobulins, IgG, IgA, IgM, is the most common parameter used in medical practice to assess the immunological competence of an individual.

Serum immunoglobulin levels vary with age and environment, so that appropriate local age-matched normograms should be used in the definition of a pathological concentration. Furthermore, normal immunoglobulin (Ig) levels do not exclude an antibody deficiency and thus, the relative proportions of IgG subclasses and the antibody response to antigenic stimulation should be tested if a humoral iummunodeficiency is suspected.

Selective deficiency of one or more of the IgG subclasses has been rarely reported in the literature in children with recurrent bacterial infections (7, 14, 19, 23), and in patients with well defined immunodeficiencies, such as IgA deficiency (16), Ataxia-teleangectasia (17) and Wiskott-Aldrich syndrome (15). To better clarify the clinical picture and the nature of cellular defects in patients with IgG subclass deficiency, we selected a group of 35 patients (27 children and 8 adults) with: 1) recurrent bacterial infections, 2) no obvious abnormalities in T cell number and function, 3) normal total Ig levels, 4) a deficiency of an Ig subtype: IgG2 and/or IgG3. The clinical characteristics and lymphocyte abnormalities of these patients are reported.

MATERIALS AND METHODS

Patients

27 children (17 males and 10 females) aged 6.2 ± 3.1 years (range 2-14), were diagnosed as selective IgG subclass deficiency: 10 patients had IgG2 deficiency, 10 had IgG3 deficiency and 7 IgG2+IgG3 deficiency.

Serum levels of Ig classes and IgG subclasses

Levels of IgG, IgA, IgM were measured with single radial immunodiffusion method, as previously described (10). Concentrations of IgG subclasses were tested with a modified single radial immunodiffusion assay using polyclonal monkey anti-human IgG subclasses as described (20), or monoclonal antibodies: JL512 (anti-IgG1), GOM-1 (anti-IgG2), ZG4 (anti-IgG3) and RJ4 (anti-IgG4) (9). These monoclonal antibodies were used at concentrations of 6,8,6,6 microliters/ml, respectively, of 0.1M barbitone acetate pH 8.6, buffered 1% agarose with 4% PEG 6000. 3 microliters samples of serum were applied into 2 mm wells and allowed to diffuse at room temperature for 72 hr. The standard used was W.H.O. reference serum 67/97, using the subclass content as defined by Morell and Skvaril (12).

Separation and culture of lymphocytes

Lymphocytes from 17 patients with IgG subclass deficiency and from 10 normal age-matched controls were separated from heparinized venous blood by density sedimentation on Ficoll-Ipaque (4). For the separation of T and B cells, the neuroaminidase-treated sheep erythrocyte rosette formation method was used (3). Equal number of T and B lymphocytes (5×10^5 cells/ml) from patients were cocultured toghether or with counterpart lymphocytes from controls in RPMI 1640 containing 10% FCS, alone or in the presence of PWM (GIBCO, Grand Island, New York, USA, final dilution 1/250) at 37°C for 7 days in a humidified atmosphere of 5% CO_2. The supernatants of single cultures were collected and the IgG subclass content was measured by an enzyme-linked-solid immunoassay (ELISA).

ELISA for IgG subclasses

Polystyrene microtitration plates with 96 flat-bottomed wells (Nunc Lab., Roskilde, Denmark) were coated with 100 µl of a predetermined concentration of each monoclonal antibody to human IgG subclass in carbonate buffer 0.05M, pH 9.6, overnight at room temperature. After 3 washes with PBS-Tween 20 (0.05%) the plates were filled with PBS containing 0.1% gelatin and incubated at 37°C for 1 hr; then, washed again with PBS-Tween. 100 µl of supernatants undiluted, diluted 1/5 and 1/50 were added to wells in duplicate. Each plate included the standard serum 67/97 at 6 different concentrations to establish a calibration curve in every experiment; plates were incubated overnight at 37°C and washed again with PBS-Tween. 100 µl of goat anti-human IgG Alkaline-Phosphatase conjugated (Tago, Burlingame, CA, USA) diluted 1/1000, were added to wells and incubated for 1 hr at 37°C. After 3 washes with PBS-Tween and 1 with 0.1M Tris-HC1 pH 8.6, bound conjugate was revealed by adding 100 µl of paraphenilnitrophosphate (1 mg/ml) in Tris HC1 as substrate. Optical densities were read on microplate reader (Titertek Multiskan, McLean, VA, USA) after 15 and 30 minutes.

RESULTS AND DISCUSSION

We selected a patient population presenting: 1) recurrent bacterial infections, 2) normal Ig levels and no obvious abnormalities in T cell number and function, 3) a deficiency of an IgG subclass: IgG2 and/or IgG3. All patients presented a clinical history of recurrent sinusitis, bronchitis, otitis and approximately 50% of them of pneumonia and bronchopneumonia. The onset of symptoms was within the first 2 years of life in the pediatric group. In some patient we noted an high incidence of allergic manifestations, asthma and rhinitis, confirmed by the positivity of immediate skin test. The association of atopy in immunodeficient patients is well documented in patients with other immunodeficiencies, in particular in patients with IgA deficiency (24), although the pathophysiological mechanisms explaining this association are not completely clarified. Regarding therapy, we treated all our patients with multiple courses of antibiotics and found that this was not sufficient to improve the clinical condition in a group of them. In these patients we then initiated replacement therapy with human gammaglobulins with good results (Tab. 1).

TABLE 1.   *Clinical characteristics of patients with IgG subclass deficiency*

	Deficient subclass					
	IgG2		IgG3		IgG2+IgG3	
	C	A	C	A	C	A
Number of patients	10	—	10	6	7	2
Sex (M:F)	5:5		7:3	2:4	5:2	1:1
Age	4.4 ± 3.6		8 ± 2.5	31 ± 18	7 ± 3.2	35 ± 19
Recurrent infections:						
— otitis and sinusitis	100%		100%	100%	100%	100%
— pneumonia	40%		60%	66%	42%	50%
Atopy:						
— allergic rhinitis	01%		10%	16%	26%	50%
— asthma	40%		40%	33%	57%	10%
Therapy						
— antibiotics	100%		100%	100%	100%	100%
— gamma-globulins	45%		40%	24%	56%	50%

C: children; A: adults.

Immunoglobulin levels were within the normal limits in all our patients with the exception of 5 patients, who presented IgA deficiency. This observation confirms the data of Oxelius on the association between IgA and IgG subclass deficiencies (16).

Quantification of IgG subclasses levels allowed us to make a diagnosis (Tab. 2). While many were low (in comparison to normal values of the corresponding age), none of our patients lacked entirely any of the IgG subclasses, IgG1, IgG2, IgG3. In this study, we have not considered IgG4 subclass, because of the difficulty of defining a clinical status of IgG4 defi-

TABLE 2. *Laboratory evaluation*

	Deficient subclass		
	IgG2	IgG3	IgG2+IgG3
CHILDREN			
IgG1 (mg/dl)	643 ± 317	528 ± 228	512 ± 116
IgG2 (mg/dl)	32 ± 19	134 ± 48	36 ± 21
IgG3 (mg/dl)	50 ± 32	19 ± 13	15 ± 10
IgG4 (mg/dl)	21 ± 18	43 ± 47	72 ± 69
ADULTS			
IgG1 (mg/dl)	—	565 ± 159	600 ± 141
IgG2 (mg/dl)	—	203 ± 64	50 ± 15
IgG3 (mg/dl)	—	21 ± 7	16 ± 11
IgG4 (mg/dl)	—	21 ± 14	27 ± 2

ciency. Many authors reported, in fact, very low or absent IgG4 levels in a high percentage of normal subjects (2).

In order to identify the nature of cellular defect related to the selective IgG subclass deficiency, we studied the in vitro IgG synthesis by lymphocytes from 17 patients and 10 normal controls. We analyzed all supernatants with an ELISA assay, using monoclonal antibodies to human IgG subclasses.

First, we studied a group of 10 normal subjects between the ages of 5 to 40 years to assess their lymphocytes ability to synthesize IgG subclasses during in vitro cultures. The percentages of IgG subclasses in supernatants were similar to those reported in studies from other laboratories (11, 13, 18, 21, 22) using immunofluorescence or immunoassy. B cells from most individuals were found to differentiate into immunoglobulin secreting cells when cocultured with purified autologous T cell preparations, although there was considerable variability observed among individual donors (Tab. 3). This variability causes

TABLE 3. *Immunoglobulin G subclasses synthesis by normal PBL in vitro*

Cellular composition of cultures	Ig determinations in supernatants			
	IgG1	IgG2	IgG3	IgG4
	(mean values in ng/ml and in % of total IgG ± SD)			
UNSTIMULATED				
T + B (ng/ml)	162 ± 155	65 ± 49	8 ± 12	3 ± 5
(%)	40 ± 38	50 ± 38	3 ± 4	0.7 ± 1.1
T + (T + B) (ng/ml)	148 ± 183	130 ± 104	3 ± 7	0.2 ± 0.4
(%)	45 ± 37	53 ± 38	1 ± 2	0.4 ± 0.8
PWM				
T + B (ng/ml)	1195 ± 510	338 ± 340	47 ± 40	32 ± 85
(%)	74 ± 15	22 ± 15	4 ± 3	2.3 ± 4.5
T + (T + B) (ng/ml)	1025 ± 713	209 ± 176	53 ± 33	30 ± 48
(%)	75 ± 18	22 ± 18	4 ± 6	0.8 ± 1.7

the wider S.D. we had compared to that of data reported in literature. One possible explanation is the wide range in ages in the normal donors in our series. In fact, it has been reported that the IgG1/IgG2 ratio decreases during the first years of life (1). Due to this, we performed our experiments of cocultures comparing results obtained with cells from patients with those from an age-matched control. The results we obtained confirmad that PWM, a T-dependent polyclonal B cell activator, induces IgG secretion with a subclass distribution similar to that found in normal sera. Additionally, in unstimulated cultures the proportion of secreted IgG1 and IgG2 is similar (about 50% of IgG1 and 50% of IgG2). IgG3 and IgG4 were secreted only in the presence of mitogen. Only low levels of IgG subclasses were detectable before the 4th day of incubation. The Ig in supernatants indicated actually synthesized new protein because less than 5% of these IgG were present in cultures treated with ciclohexemide.

We then analyzed the cooperation between 1) patient's T and B cells; 2) patient's T cells and normal B cells; 3) normal T cells and patient's B cells, in the synthesis of IgG subclasses in vitro, spontaneously or in a PWM driven system. Results of these experiments were expressed as percentages of values obtained coculturing normal T and B cells. Fig. 1 shows IgG subclasses secreted in supernatants of cultures of cells from a patient with IgG2 defi-

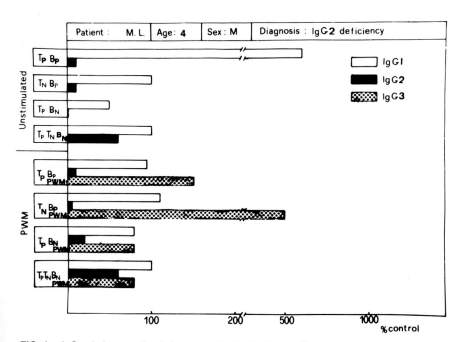

FIG. 1. IgG subclass synthesis in supernatants of cultures of lymphocytes from a patient with IgG2 subclass deficiency (results expressed as percentages of values obtained in culture of normal cells).

ciency. Lack of IgG2 synthesis by the patient B cells in the presence of normal
T cells and PWM reflects an intrinsic defect in IgG2 B cell activation: this
resulted in a selective deficiency of IgG2 synthesis or in a selective secretory
deficit. We have not measured the IgG content of B cell lysates, so we cannot
rule out a defect in IgG subclass secretion. Moreover, the defective synthesis
by the normal B cells in the presence of patient T cells strongly suggests a T
cell immunoregolatory dysfunction, since IgG secretion by B cells is largely T
cell dependent. The failure of the patient T cells to support IgG synthesis by
normal B cells (but their ability to support IgG1 synthesis) could result from
a lack of IgG2 specific helper T cells or alternatively from the presence of an
excess of IgG2 specific suppressor T cells. In order to distinguish between the
two possibilities, T cells from the patient were assayed for their ability to
specifically suppress IgG subclass synthesis when added to normal T and B
cells. T cells from the patient were added to normal T and B cells at a 2:1:1
ratio and the subclass synthesis was compared to that of cultures containing
equal number of irradiated allogeneic T cells, normal T and B cells at a 2:1:1
ratio. In this patient the failure of T cells to support the IgG2 synthesis by
normal B cells was due to lack of specific T helper cells and not to the presence
of an excess of specific suppressor T cells.
In patient with IgG3 deficiency (Fig. 2) we could demonstrate that the failure

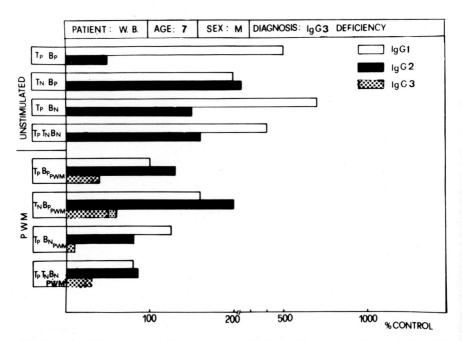

FIG. 2. IgG subclass synthesis in supernatants of cultures of lymphocytes from a patient with
IgG3 subclass deficiency (results expressed as percentages of values obtained in culture of
normal cells).

TABLE 4.   IgG subclass deficiency: analysis of IgG 1-2-3 production in vitro (summary)

In Vivo Defect	No of patients	In vitro defect			
		B cell defect	Excessive suppressor T cell activity and/or failure of T helper cell activity	B and T cell dysfunction	Unclear
IgG2 deficiency	4	IgG2 (2 pts.)	—	IgG2 (1 pt.)	(1 pt.)
IgG3 deficiency	4	—	—	IgG3 (2 pts.)	(2 pts.)
IgG2+IgG3 deficiency	4	IgG2+IgG3 (1 pt.) IgG3 (1 pt.)	—	IgG2+IgG3 (1 pt.) IgG2 (1 pt.)	(1 pt.)
Hypogammaglobul.	5	IgG1+IgG2 (2 pts.)	IgG1+IgG2 (1 pt.) IgG2 (1 pt.)	IgG1+IgG2 (1 pt.) IgG1+IgG2 (1 pt.)	—

of patient T cells to support IgG3 synthesis was mainly due to an excess of IgG3 specific T suppressor cells. The normal synthesis of IgG subclasses by the patient B cells in the presence of normal T cells suggests that the defect is not due to an intrinsic B cell defect.

In almost all our patients we ascertained that the IgG1 response is intact and more often increased in comparison to the synthesis by normal B cells. This could be considered an expression of a compensatory mechanism by the cells of patients with IgG2 or IgG3 deficiency.

Tab. 4 summarizes the results obtained in experiments done with 17 patients. We have demonstrated the presence of a defect intrinsic to the B cells in the majority of our patients. In some cases this defect is associated with an increase of suppressor and/or a decrease in T cell helper function, specific for IgG subclass. In about 25% of patients the in vitro study did not allow us to identify a clear cellular defect.

CONCLUSIONS

In patients with recurrent bacterial infections, with normal serum levels of total IgG and no obvious abnormalities in T cell number and function, IgG subclass deficiency may be the responsible defect. In children, we noted an early onset of symptoms and in some cases a familial incidence of immunodeficiencies. In vitro cell culture studies revealed that the pathophysiological mechanisms underlying the selective IgG subclass deficiency are heterogeneous. In some patients we demonstrated a defect in B cell function required for the IgG subclass synthesis. In others the B cell defect was associated with 1) an increase in T suppressor and/or 2) a decrease in T cell helper function, specific for IgG subclass.

Acknowledgements

Supported by Fondazione "Istituto Pasteur-Fondazione Cenci-Bolognetti and U.S.P.H.S. grants AM31925, AI21163 a grant from the National Foundation, March of Dimes and an Allergic Disease Academic Award (to R.S.G.) K07 AI-0440-02.

REFERENCES

1. Anderson, U., Bird, A.G., Britton and Palacios, R. (1981): Humoral and Cellular Immunity in Human Studies at the Cell Level from Birth to Two Years of Age. *Immunological Rev.* 57:5-33.
2. Aucouturier, P., Danon, F., Daveau, M., Guillou, B., Sabbah, A., Besson, J., and Preud'homme, J.L. (1984): Measurement of serum IgG4 levels by a competitive Immunoenzymatic Assay with monoclonal antibodies. *Journal of Immunological Methods*, 74:151-162.
3. Bentwich, S., Douglas, S.D., Siegal, F.P., Kunkel, H.G., (1973): Human lymphocyte sheep erytrocyte rosette formation: some characteristics of the interaction. *Clin. Immunol Immunopathol.* 1:511-522.
4. Boyum, A., (1968): Isolation of leucocytes from human blood. *Scand. J. Clin. Invest.*, 21 Suppl. 97:9-89.

5. Geha, R.S., Schneberger, E., Merler, E., and Rosen, F.S. (1974): Heterogeneity of "acquired" or common variable agammaglobulinemia. *New Engl. J. Med.* 291:1-6.
6. Haaijman, J.J., Deen, C., Krose, J.M., Zijlstra, J.J., Coolen, J., and Radl, J. (1984): A jungle full of pitfalls. *Immunology today*, 5:3:56-58.
7. Isaacs, D., Webster, D.B. and Valman, H.B. (1984): Immunoglobulin levels and function in pre-school children with recurrent respiratory infections. *Clin. Exp. Immunol.* 58, 335-340.
8. Jefferis, R., Ling, N.R. (1984): More pitfalls in the use of monoclonal antibodies. Immunol. Today, 5,127.
9. Lowe, J., Bird, P., Jefferis, R., and Ling, N.R. (1982): Monoclonal antibodies to human IgG subclasses. *Immunology* 47,329.
10. Mancini, G., Carbonara, O., and Heremans, J. (1965): Immunochemical quantitation of antigen by single radial immunodiffusion. *Immunochemistry* 2:235.
11. Mysumi, M., Kuritani, H., Kubagawa, H., and Cooper, M.D. (1983): IgG subclass expression by human B lymphocytes and plasma cells: B lymphocytes precommited to IgG subclass can be preferentially induced by policlonal mitogens with T cell help. *J. Immunol.* 30,2,671-677.
12. Morell, A., and Skvaril, R. (1971): A modified radioimmunoassay for quantitative determination of IgG subclass in man. *Protides of the Biological Fluids*, 19:533-540.
13. Morell, A., Van Loghem, E., Nef, M., Theilkases, L., and Skvaril, F. (1981): Determinatin of IgG subclasses and Gm Allotypes in culture supernatans of pokeweed mitogen-stimulated human blood lymphocytes. *J. Immunology*, 127,3,1099-1102.
14. Oxelius, V.A. (1974): Chronic infections in a family with hereditary deficiency of IgG$_2$ and IgG$_4$. *Clin. Exp. Immunol.* 17:19-27.
15. Oxelius, V.A. (1979): Quantitative and qualitative investigation of serum IgG subclasses in immunodeficiency disease. *Clin. Exp. Immunol.* 36:112-116.
16. Oxelius, V.A., Laurell, A.B., Lindquist, B., Golebiowska, H., Axelssan, U., Bjorkanden, J., and Larson, L.A. (1981): IgG subclasses in selective IgA deficiency. *New Engl. J. Med.* 304:1476-1477.
17. Oxelius, V.A., Izzet Berkel A., Hanson L.A. (1982): IgG$_2$ deficiency in ataxia-telangectasia. *New Engl. J. Med.*, 306:9,515-517.
18. Partidge, L., Jefferis, R., Hardie, D., Ling, N.R. and Richardson P. (1984): Subclasses of IgG on the surface of human lymphocytes: a study with monoclonal antibodies. *Clin. Exp. Immunol.* 56:167-174.
19. Schur, P., Borel, H., Gelfand, E.W., Alper, C.A., and Rosen, F.S. (1970): Selective gamma-G globulin deficiencies in patients with recurrent pyogenic infection. *New Engl. J. Med.* 283:631-634.
20. Schur, P.H., Rosen, F.S., Norman, M.E. (1979): Immunoglobulin subclasses in normal children. *Pediat. Res.* 13:181-183.
21. Scott, M.G., Nahm, M.H. (1984): Mitogen-induced human IgG subclass ex pression. *J. Immunology.* 135:5:2454-2460.
22. Simmons, J.G., Fuller, C.R., Buchanan, P.D., and Yount, W.J. (1981): Distribution of surface, cytoplasmic and secreted IgG sublass in human lymphoblastoid cell lines and normal peripheral blood lymphocytes. *Scand. J. Immunol.* 14:1-13.
23. Smith, T.H., Morris, E.C., and Bain, R.P. (1984): IgG subclasses in non allergic children with chronic chest symptoms. *J. Pediatrics.* 105:896-900.
24. Southill.

Defective Synthesis of HLA Class I and II Molecules Associated with a Combined Immunodeficiency

C. Griscelli, A. Fischer, B. Lisowska-Grospierre, A. Durandy
C. Bremard, N. Cerf-Bensussan, F. Le Deist, A. Marcadet*
and C. de Preval**

Unité d'Immunologie pédiatrique Inserm U 132, Départment de pédiatrie
Hôpital des Enfants Malades, Paris
*Inserm U 93 Hôpital St. Louis, Paris, France
**Département de microbiologie Université de Geneve, Suisse

It has been established that major histocompatibility complex (MHC) products play a central role in the antigen recognition by T lymphocytes (2, 10). MHC class I molecules are expressed on all cells, MHC class II molecules are expressed on B lymphocytes and monocytes and both are required for cellular interactions leading to antigen-specific activation of all types of immune effect on cells.

An inherited immunodeficiency syndrome associated with a defective expression of HLA class I molecules has been described in 1978 by Touraine et al. (13) and in 1979 by Schuurman et al. (12). We then observed several immunodeficient patients in whom are observed a defective membrane expression of both HLA class I and II molecules on bone marrow derived cells (3, 5). This immunodeficiency appeared unique in its expression since it is characterized by a complete lack of cellular and humoral immune response to foreign antigens. We herein report a study of 15 patients including clinical, immunological, genetic, and biochemical aspects of the disease. The results provide a strong suggestion for the existence of a regulatory gene, located outside the MHC complex region and governing the transcription of HLA class I and II genes, that is abnormal in this autosomal recessive disease.

CASE REPORTS

Fifteen patients were referred to us because of repeated infections and/or protracted diarrhoea and were found to have severe immunodeficiency associated with a defective expression of membrane HLA antigens. All patients

(10 males and 5 females) were of North African origin and belonged to 13 families. The parents were related in 9 of them. Thirteen out of thirty five related siblings died within the first years of life usually with infections and chronic diarrhoea. First clinical manifestation in the fifteen reported patients were noted between the first weeks and the eight month of life. The frequency of the major sings is shown on Table 1. Infections due to various types of

TABLE 1.   *Clinical manifestations in combined immunodeficiency with defective synthesis of MHC products in 15 patients*

Protracted diarrhoea	14	
Lower respiratory tract infections	11	
Upper respiratory tract infections	13	
Severe viral infections	9	
Failure to thrive	12	
Sclerosing cholangitis	2	
Autoimmune hemolytic anemia	1	
Autoimmune neutropenia	1	
Fatal outcome (age of death)	5	(14 to 66 months)
Follow up of alive patients (years)	1 to 13	

microorganisms, including bacterias, fungi, parasites such as cryptosporidia (3 patients) and viruses. Viral infections were especially frequent and severe as shown on Table 2. It is striking to note than none of the 5 patients who

TABLE 2.   *CID with defective HLA molecules synthesis. Viral infections*

Viruses	Patients affected	Clinical manifestations
Polio V.	3	Encephalomyelitis (1) Myelitis (2)
Coxsackie V.	2	Meningoencephalitis (1) Pneumopathy (1)
Adeno V.	2	Meningoencephalitis (2) Pneumopathy (1)
Herpes simplex V.	2	Recurrent skin and mucous lesions
Cytomegalovirus V.	4	Pneumopathy (2) Hepatitis (2)

received BCG did develop a BCG sepsis. Five patients died from chronic, disseminated infections. Nine patients are receiving prophylactic antibiotics, gammaglobulins and for 4 of them, parenteral nutrition. One patient has been successfully transplanted with an HLA matched bone marrow.

RESULTS

Immunological investigations

As depicted on Tables 3 and 4 the main immunological characteristic consisted in a complete defect in cellular and humoral immune responses to

TABLE 3.

	Normal	Diminished	Absent
Total blood lymphocytes (1)	14	1	0
$T_3(+)$ lymphocytes (2)	12	3	0
Mitogen-induced proliferation (3)	14	1	0
Response to allogeneic leukocytes (4)	12		1
Cell mediated lymphocytotoxicity (4)	3	0	1
Antigen-induced proliferation (5)	0	0	15
Delayed type skin reactivity to antigens (6)	0	0	15

(1) Normal > 1500 lymphocytes/mm³, 500 < Dimished < 1500/m³
(2) Normal > 50% T_3 (+) lymphocytes, 10 < Diminished < 50%
(3) Mitogen induced proliferation were studied using PHA, Con A and PWM Normal > 50% of control response, 5 < Diminished, < 50%
(4) Normal > 50% or control response, Absent < 5% of control response
(5) Antigen induced proliferation were studied using candida-, tetanus toxoid, PPD (in BCG vaccinated patients) CMV (in CMV infected patients) antigens. Absent < 5% of control response.
(6) Skin tests were performed with candida-, tetanus toxoid and PPD antigens. Absent: no erythema and no induration after 48 hours.

TABLE 4.

	Normal	Diminished	Absent
SIg(+) lymphocytes (1)	13	2	0
Serum immunoglobulin levels (2)			0
— IgG	11	4	0
— IgA	2	10	3
— IgM	12	3	0
Serum antibody to:			
— Blood group substances (A and/or B)	8	0	0
— Vaccinal antigens	0	0	15
— Infections microorganisms:			
Candida albicans	2	0	8
Enteroviruses (3)	0	1	4
Herpes group virus (3)	4	0	2
Adenovirus (3)	0	0	2

(1) Normal > 5% surface immunoglobulins(+) cells (s Ig) < Dimished < 5%
(2) Normal > age-matched values minus 2S-D. 5% of age-matches values < Diminished < age-matched values minus 2S-D.
(3) See Table II

vaccinal antigens. Cellular immune responses to infections antigens (candida and CMV) were absent as well, whereas an antibody response was observed in a few occasions to blood group substances, candida and herpes virus group antigens (CMV and HSV) but not to enteroviruses and adenovirus.

Serum immunoglobulin levels were variable from patient to patient. An IgA deficiency (complete or partial) appeared to be a rather common feature. T lymphocyte membrane markers tested (T_3, T_4, T_8, T_{11}) were normally expressed. B lymphocytes normally bore surface immunoglobulins (μ, δ, γ, α) and Fc γ receptor. The Tac expression on 3 day-PHA-induced blast cells was found normal (Data not shown). Cell-to-cell interaction for immunoglobulin and antibody production was studied in two different specific in vitro antibody production assays. No or very small numbers of immunoglobulin containing cells were generated in PWM-stimulated cultures. Whereas no IgG antibodies to influenza virus and to mannan of candida albicans were produced, IgM antibodies in the PWM-driven system and in the mannan system were found.

Membrane HLA molecules expression

As shown on Table 5, HLA class II expression on leucocytes was found profoundly defective in all patients whatever the method of detection used. HLA class II antigens were completely lacking on cell surface in 12 patients

TABLE 5.

	Technique used	Absent	Low	Normal
HLA Class I				
Leukocytes	CT	6	7	2
	IF	0	11	2
Platelets	CF	4	1	0
IL2-dependent T blasts	IF	0	0	4
β_2 microglobulins				
Leukocytes	IF	0	11	2
IL2-dependent T blasts	IF	0	0	4
HLA Class II				
Leukocytes	CT	14	1	0
	IF	12	3	0
B Lymphocytes	IF	10	3	0
Monocytes	IF	8	3	0
EBV transformed B cells	IF	2	0	1
PHA-induced blasts	IF	11	0	0
IL2-depedent T blasts	IF	4	0	0

HLA class I and II molecules expression.
HLA class I and/or II were studied by cytotoxicity (CT) and complement fixation (CF) using antisera specific fro polymorphic determinants and by immunofluorescence (IP) using various monoclonal antibodies specific for monomorphic determinants.
(1) Low exxpression of HLA antigens as studied by CT was defined as possible but difficult HLA typing.
Low expression of HLA antigens as defined by IF studies was characterized by the detection of positive cells with a intensity of fluorescence.

as detected by immunofluorescence that appeared more sensitive than C.T. In the last 3 patients, HLA class II expression was found on a small percentage of cells with a faint fluorescence intensity. These data did include HLA-DR, DQ and DP molecules for the 4 patients tested with the relevant monoclonal antibodies (Data not shown). The defective expression of the three types of HLA class II antigens was also observed on purified B lymphocytes, monocytes and activated T lymphocytes. It is striking to note that no HLA class II antigens no cell could be detected on PHA-induced or IL2-dependent-T cells. In 8 patients out of 11, a mild or normal ability to stimulate in MLR was found (Data not shown). HLA class I expression was found reduced or normal but not absent in all patients tested using the IF technique. The HLA class I typing of nine patients could be achieved by the C.T. method. There was a marked reduction of HLA class I expression on platelets in the 5 patients investigated. In contrast to the profound defect of HLA class II expression, HLA class I molecules and β_2 microglobulin were normally found on T blasts. Expression of class I antigens on non hematopoïetic cells was found normal on cultured fibroblasts, keratinocytes and enterocytes as seen on biopsy samples using specific monoclonal antibodies. HLA class II expression on Langerhans cells revealed by anti T_6 monoclonal antibody was found absent on skin biopsies as well as on macrophages located in the lamina propria of the intestinal mucosa. Taking advantage of the possibility to detect the defective membrane HLA class I and II molecules expression by indirect immunofluorescence, the disease has been excluded in three fetuses at rish on blood samples obtained under foetoscopy. This has been confirmed at birth.

HLA class III molecules detection

In all patients serum C_2, C_4 and Bf complement fractions were normally detected (Data not shown).

Effects of interferons on membrane HLA molecules expression

As seen in cytofluorometry studies, the incubation of patients mononuclear cells with α or γ interferon did enhance the membrane expression of HLA class I molecules and β_2 microglobulin resulting in an higher percentage of positive cells detected by immunofluorescence under microscopy. Similar data were observed after in vivo administration of α_2 interferon in one patient (Data not shown). In contrast γ-interferon incubation of PHA-induced blasts, monocytes and B lymphocytes had no effect on the expression of membrane HLA class II molecules as judged by cytofluorometry and microscope immunofluorescence.

HLA class I and II gene products

The biosynthesis of HLA class I and class II molecules was studied on PHA-induced blasts from 8 patients labelled with ^{35}S methionine. The cell lysates were immunoprecipitated using anti class I or II monoclonal antibodies in one (one D) or two dimensional (two D) SDS-PAGE. Heavy chain of class I molecules was found in decreased amounts in contrast with a normal presence of β_2 microglobulin in all patients tested. Immunoprecipitates of HLA class II molecules analysed on one-D (8 patients) or two-D (4 patients) failed to reveal α and β chain of HLA DR molecules using several distinct anti HLA DR mab and mab to non assembled α and β chain polypeptides. In contrast, the Ii variant chain was readily detected. HLA class II mRNA were studied after extraction of RNA from PBM of two patients by analysis on a Northern blot hybridization using specific cDNA probes. In the patients cells no mRNA for HLA-DR α and β chains can be detected whereas the mRNA for the Ii chain was present similarly to control (data not shown) (8).

Genetic studies

Using an HLA class I cDNA probe and an HLA class β DQ cDNA probe, DNA fragments from 4 patients, their parents and siblings were analysed by the Southern blot hybridization technique. Polymorphic restriction fragments found in the parents could be normally found in the patients according to the segregation of paternal and maternal haplotypes (Data not shown) (9). Studies of segregation of HLA genotypes in the 13 families has shown that in two families, two affected children were found to have inherited two distinct HLA haplotypes. More over in 3 other families healthy siblings or father were found to have inherited the same HLA haplotypes.

Bone marrow transplation

Three patients who did have an HLA matched donor as shown by HLA typing (class I antigens) and DNA polymorphism studies received a bone marrow transplantation. They have been prepared by a conditioning regimen consisting of CCN U (300 mg/m^2) procarbazine and cyclophosphamide (200 mg/kg) in 1 patient, of Busulfan (16 mg/kg) and cyclophosphamide (200 mg/kg) in 2 patients. The first patient had a poor engraftment and died from CMV infection. The second patient experienced a full engraftment but died early (D 50) from a disseminated adenovirus infection. In both cases, the causal viruses have been detected in patients prior to transplant. In the third patient who was free from infection at time of transplantation (11 months of age) a mixed chimerism developed for erythrocytes (10% donor cells), monocytes, T and B lymphocytes (around 40% donor cells as shown by HLA class I and II molecules expression). Immunologic functions appeared to be entirely normal both for cell-mediated and humoral immunity 2 and a half years post-transplant. No GVHd occured.

DISCUSSION

We herein report the defective expression of membrane HLA molecules in 15 patients with a combined immunodeficiency. In all patients HLA class II molecules expression was found virtually absent on bone marrow derived cells, B lymphocytes, activated T lymphocytes, monocytes and Langerhans cells. This defects was shown by cytotoxicity, immunofluorescence as well as biosynthetic labelling using various antibodies specific for monomorphic epitopes of HLA DR, DQ and DP molecules and for polymorphic epitopes of HLA DR and DQ. A deficiency in HLA class I expression was found as well, however variable from patient to patient and in a given patient.

In this respect, we observed in one family, a 6 months old patient free of infection in whom neither HLA class II nor HLA class I molecules were expressed on PBM and a 3 year old brother with protracted diarrhoea and preunoritis in whom HLA class II molecules were not detected while HLA class I were nearly normally detected.

These data together with in vitro and in vivo effects of interferon on HLA class I expression suggest that the HLA class I expression defect can be overcome by exogenous factors inactive on HLA class II molecules expression. In contrast, this defective expression of HLA molecules was not found in 45 patients with various types of severe combined immunodeficiencies (Adenosine deaminase deficiency, SCID with B cells, SCID with abnormal T cells).

Other patients with combined immunodeficiency have been so far reported in the literature (3, 5-7, 12-14). In seven of them a similar defect in both HLA class I and II molecules expression was described (3, 5, 6, 7, 14) while in the two patients originally reported by J.L. Touraine et al. (13), a defect in HLA class I expression only has been described as Bare lymphocyte syndrome. Two other subjects in one family have been described by Payne et al. (11) with a selective deficiency in HLA class I molecules expression but with normal immune functions, one of them being affected with an aplastic anemia. It is striking to note that despite profound deficiency in HLA class II expression, patients' PBM were able, in several cases, to stimulate allogeneic PBL. HLA class I like molecules such as T_6 appeared not to be affected. Since HLA class III serum products (C_2, C_4, B) result from both hepatic and bone marrow-derived cells, one cannot exclude a defective production by bone-marrow-derived cells only.

The defective expression of HLA class I and II molecules has been shown to be secondary to a decrease synthesis of these molecules. The magnitude of this defect appears far more pronounced for HLA class II molecules that are not detected than for HLA class I molecules. Furthermore evidence is given that this abnormal biosynthesis of MHC class II products is a consequence of a defective transcription of HLA class II genes since no mRNA for HLA class II products could be detected in patients PHA activated T blasts. Altogether, these data could suggest a primary abnormality located within the MHC gene complex. This hypothesis is unlikely for the following reasons. DNA/DNA hybridisation of class I and class II genes did not reveal any gross abnormality and above all segregation studies in several families have shown the absence of linkage between the disease expresison and the MHC gene complex. Thus, one is left with the possibility of a regulatory defect responsible for an abnormal HLA class II gene transcription. γ interferon could have been a good candidate since this lymphokine has been shown to induce HLA class II molecules expression at the transcriptional level. However, interferon production by patients PBM was found normal (Data not shown), incubation of monocytes, B and activated T lymphocytes with γ interferon did not restore their HLA class II molecules expression and the Ii chain, previously shown to be coregulated with HLA class II α and β chains by γ interferon was normally synthetised in patients PBM. These data strongly argue against interferon-mediated defective HLA class II molecules expression. One showed this postulate the existence of a transactive plenotropic MHC regulatory gene located outside of the MHC complex which is abnormal in this disease. The situation in these patients resembles the HLA DR-negative variants obtained experimentally (1, 4), in which an absence of HLA-DR mRNA with a presence of Ii chain mRNA was described.

The main feature of the combined immune deficiency observed in these patients is characterized by the lack of in vivo and in vitro immune response to exogenous antigens. In contrast, proliferation and cytotoxicity towards allogeneic cells in preserved. Lymphocytes together with monocytes are present in patients blood, expressing normally differentiation membrane molecules such as T_3, T_4, T_8, T_{11}, membrane immunoglobulins, complement receptor type 2, LFA-1 and Fc-receptor. The expression of activation-associated molecules (IL2-receptor, T_{10} and T_9) a part of HLA class II on lectin-stimulated T cells was found normal.

An obvious explanation accounting for this immunodeficiency consists in a defective antigen presentation in the context of poor or no expression of HLA class II molecules. This hypothesis is supported by the normal response towards allogeneic cells which is known to be independent of antigen presentation by autologous antigen presenting cells and by results from Kuis et al. showing that patients monocytes are unable to present ovalbumin or sheep red cells to normal T cells in an in vitro antibody production assay (7, 14). A few positive antibody responses toward fungi or viruses have been observed in some patients. This might be due to the persistent expression of microorganism antigens on cell membranes associated to a few residual HLA class II or class I molecules. However, no firm conclusion about the causal relationship between HLA expression deficiency and the immunodeficiency can be drawn from the above date. Another mechanism unless improbable responsible for the immunodeficiency cannot yet be excluded.

The clinical consequences of this immunodeficiency appear severe since all these patients have repeated infections caused by a variety of pathogenic and opportunistic microorganisms. The noteworthy frequency and severity of viral infections might be partially explained by the inability of patients cells to be an adequate target in cytotoxic T cell activity assays. This suggests that patients cells infected by a virus will not be killed appropriately by effector cells because of the defective HLA molecules expression. It is noticeable that despite the poor expression of HLA molecules, auto-immune manifestations can occur as observed in two patients. The chronic infections observed in this disease are clearly life threatening, justifying attempts at curing the disease by allogeneic bone marrow transplantation. In two of our patients as well as two others such a treatment was not successfull because of the severity of infections prior to transplant and/or inadequate conditioning regimen. In one patient, who was transplanted within the first year of age, a mixed chimerism was achieved leading to normal and stable immune functions. Thus, the C.I.D. with defective HLA molecules expression can be corrected by normal bone marrow stem cells indicating that there is no inhibitory process of HLA molecules expression. The C.I.D. with defective expression of HLA molecules represents a newly recognized example of I.D. in which well defined membrane glycoproteins deficiency could lead to abnormal cell to cell interactions required for immune responses. This type of I.D. as well as the recently described deficiency of adhesive proteins brings new sight into the physiological role of these membrane molecules and in the regulation of their biosynthesis.

REFERENCES

1. Accolla, R.S. (1983): Human B cell variants immunoselected against a single Ia subset have lost expression of several Ia antigens subsets. *J. Exp. Med.* 157:1053.
2. Benacerraff, B. (1981): In: *The Role of the Major Histocompatibility Complex in Immunobiology*. M.E. Dorf, editor. Garland, New York. 255.
3. Durandy, A., Virelizier, J.L., and Griscelli C. (1983): Enhancement by interferon of membrane HLA antigens in patients with combined immunodeficiency with defective HLA expression. *Clin. Exp. Immunol.* 52:173.
4. Gladstone, P., and Plous D. (1978): Stable variants affecting B cell alloantigens in human lymphoid cells. *Nature.* 271:459.
5. Griscelli, C., Durandy, A., Virelizier, J.L., Hors, J., Lepage, V., and Colombani, J. (1980): Impaired cell to cell interactions in partial immunodeficiency with variable expression of HLA antigens. In: *Primary Immunodeficiencies*, M. Seligman and H. Hitzig, editors, Elsevier/North-Holland, Biochemical Press. 499.
6. Hadam, M.R., Dopfer, R., Peter Hans-Hartmut and Niethammer, D. (1984): Congenital agammaglobulinemia associated with lack of expression of HLA-D-region antigens. In: *Progress in Immunodeficiency Research and Therapy I*, C. Griscelli and J. Vossen editors, Elsevier Science Publishers B.V.
7. Kuis, W., Roord, J.J., Vossen, J.M., Ballieux, R.E., Stoop, J.W. (1981): Clinical and immunological studies in a patient with the «Bare lymphocyte» syndrome. In: *Bone Marrow Transplantation in Europe*. J.L. Touraine, E. Gluckman, C. Griscelli, eds., Excerpta Medica/Amsterdam. 201.
8. Lisowska-Grospierre B., Charron, D.J., de Préval, C., Durandy, A., Griscelli, C. and Mach B.: A defect in the regulation of MHC class II gene expression in HLA-DR negative lymphocytes from patients with combined immunodeficiency syndrome. *J. Clin. Inv.* (in press.).
9. Marcadet, A., Cohen, D., Dausset, J., Fischer, A., Durandy, A., Griscelli C.: Genotyping using DNA probes in combined immunodeficiency syndrome with defective expression of HLA. *N. E. J. Med.* (in press.).
10. McDevitt, H.O. (1976): Functional analysis of Ia antigens in relation to genetic control of the immune response. In: *The Role of the Products of the Histocompatibility Gene Comples in Immune Responses*. D.H. Katz, and B. Benaceraff, editors. Academic press, Inc., New York. 257.
11. Payne, R., Brodsky, F.M., Peterlin, B.M. and Young, L.M. (1983): *Human Immunol*, 6:219.
12. Schuurman, R.K.B., Van Rood, J.J., Vossen, J.M., Schellekens, P.A., Felkampvroom, T.M., Doyer, E., Gmelig-Meyling, F., and Visser, H.K.A. (1979): Failure of lymphocytes membrane expression in two siblings with combined immunodeficiency. *Clin. Immunol. Immunopathol.* 14:18.
13. Touraine, J.L., Betuel, H., Suillet, G., and Jeune, M.J. (1978): Combined Immunodeficiency disease associated with absence of cell surface HLA A and B antigens. *J. Pediatr.* 93:47.
14. Zegers, B.J.M., Heynen, C.J., Roord, J.J., Kuis, W., Stoop, J.W., and Ballieux, R.E. (1984): Combined immunodeficiency with defective expression of HLA-antigens: analysis of the nature of defective monocyte-T cell interaction. In: *Progress in Immunodeficiency Research and Therapy I*, C. Griscelli and J. Vossen editors, Elsevier Science Publishers, B.V.

Congenital Agammaglobulinaemia associated with Malabsorption: No Expression of MHC-Class-II-Antigens due to a Regulatory Gene Defect?

D. Niethammer[1], R. Dopfer[1], G. Dammer[2], H. Peter[3],
C. de Preval[4], B. Mach[4], M.R. Hadam[5]

[1]Department of Pediatric Hematology, University of Tübingen, Rümelinstrasse, D-7400 Tübingen, FRG
[2]Rudolf-Virchow-Hospital, Reinickedorfer Strasse, D-1000, Berlin 65 FRG
[3]Department of Clinical Immunology, University of Freiburg, Hogstetter Strasse, D-7800, Freiburg
[4]Department of Microbiology, University of Geneva, Avenue de Champel, CH-1211, Geneva 4, Switzerland
[5]Department of Pediatric Surgery, Medical School, Konstanty-Gutschow-Strasse, D-3000, Hannover 61, FRG

INTRODUCTION

In 1978 a combined immunodeficiency disease characterized by the lack of HLA-ABC-antigens has been described by Touraine et al (20) and termed "Bare-Lymphocyte Syndrome" (BLS). Later, additional cases were found by Schuurman et al (14), Griscelli et al (4) and Kuis et al (8), some of which were also to some extent lacking HLA-D-region products. Two affected siblings without overt immune deficiency were contributed by Payne et al (13). Recently we have reported on four patients having congenital agammaglobulinaemia associated with malabsorption who did not express MHC-class-II-antigens (6, 7). Attempts have been made to cover all these diverging aspects as subtypes of BLS (18). However on grounds to be discussed here we do not favour this interpretation.

CASES AND INVESTIGATIONS

Our four patients have been detailed previously (6, 7). Briefly, all presented with upper respiratory tract and other infections before the age of six months. Agammaglobulinaemia of all isotypes was diagnosed and replacement therapy instituted. Subsequent infectious episodes were primarily of bacterial origin and could be controlled by appropriate treatment. During that time diarrhea became clinically prevalent, was not influenced by any therapeutical measure and remained so up to date resulting in malabsorption and marked failure to thrive. Lymphocytes and lymphoid tissue were consistently found. BCG vaccination performed routinely in two patients (RS, FH) did not cause systemic disease as often seen in severe combined immunodeficiency (SCID); skin testing in patient RS demonstrated positive reactions. Laboratory investigations indicated the presence of both T- and B-lymphocytes, low-normal responses to mitogens in vitro and a proliferative response to alloantigens. In contrast, pokeweed mitogen or Epstein-Barr-virus stimulation never resulted in immunoglobulin production in vitro. However some helper T-cell function was demonstrable in mixing experiments with semiallogeneic B-cell preparations.

The principal abnormalities in our patients are readily apparent from a flow cytometric analysis of peripheral blood mononuclear cells. Figure 1 and 2 display representative FACS dot plots from two affected siblings AH (male) and FH (female). In all our four cases mature T-lymphocytes as measured by Leu4 are found in approximately normal numbers. Unique to this type of immunodeficiency is the continuing presence in the circulation of immature B-cells characterized by the expression of multiple immunoglobulin isotypes and a high density of surface IgM. This phenotype is normally seen in cord blood and never in peripheral blood beyond the age of one year. Pathognomonic for this syndrome is the complete absence of MHC-class-II-antigens of all three subregions i.e. HLA-DR/DQ/DP as shown by the negative result with antibodies TÜ-22 (HLA-DQ), TÜ-35 (HLA-DR) and DA6.231 resp. CR3.43 (HLA-DR/DQ/DP; data not shown). The class-II-antigens are lacking from the surface of both lymphocytes and monocytes. They are also not detected after activation by PHA in vitro though receptors for interleukin-2 are induced to normal levels. The complete absence of class-II-antigens has been consistently reproduced. It extends also to endothelial cells and Langerhans' cells in the skin; only in two of our patients a very small proportion of those cells is found positive (6). Some heterogeneity exists at the level of expression of HLA-ABC-antigens. The two male patients are represented by the distribution shown in Figure 1 whereas the two female patients reproducibly had a pattern exemplified in Figure 2. Though never being negative, cells from AH (Fig. 1) always display considerably lower levels of class-I-antigens compared to his sister (Fig. 2: FH). The sex-linkeage observed may be coincidental but certainly warrants further attention. Two-colour immunofluorescence studies have, in addition demonstrated that levels of class-I-antigens are considerably higher on B- as compared to T-lymphocytes (6) in analogy to what is observed in normal human cord blood. There is only a minor T-cell subset in our female patients which expresses lower than average levels of class-I-antigens, whereas in the two males there is no such clearcut distinction. These results emphasize the importance of quantitative immunofluorescence assays on single cells using a fluorescence activated cell sorter

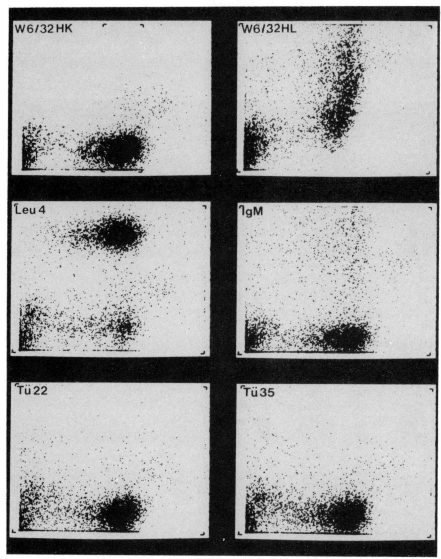

FIG. 1. Flow cytometric analysis of peripheral blood mononuclear cells of patient AH. Displayed are representative dot plots with 4032 events. *Abscissa* is forward light scatter; *ordinate* denotes log fluorescence spanning 2.5 decades. The rectangular marker positions in the dot plot of W6/32 HK indicate the lymphocyte peak. Indirect immunofluorescence labelling and flow cytometry on a FACS IV cell sorter was performed as described (7); numerical evaluation by flow cytometry was done only after gating on forward versus right angle light scatter. Antibodies used are indicated in the upper left corner.

Specificities are: W6/32HK: negative control;
                       W6/32HL: HLA-ABC;
                       Leu4: mature T-lymphocytes (CD3);
                       IgM: surface IgM;
                       Tü-22: HLA-DQ;
                       Tü-35: HLA-DR.

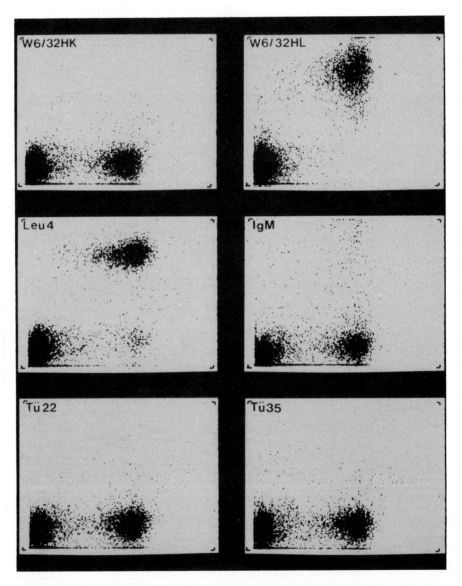

FIG. 2.   FACS analysis of peripheral blood mononuclear cells of patient FH assayed in parallel to patient AH (compare Figure 1). Conditions identical to Figure 1. *Horizontal axis*: forward light scatter; *vertical axis*: log fluorescence, 2.5 decades.

since, from our own experience, microscopic evaluation might have led to a different interpretation.

In order to facilitate in vitro investigations on this immune deficiency disease, lymphoblastoid cell lines (LCL) were sought to be established from peripheral blood by transformation with Epstein-Barr-virus. This task however proved to be unusually difficult since multiple attempts were required for each patient. Moreover cells were growing very slowly initially. After approximately 12 weeks, cultures grew at rates comparable to other LCL. We have now established LCL from all four patients; at present some are in continuous culture for more than 16 months. Initial investigations for immunoglobulin production by these cell lines revealed typical lymphoplasmocytoid blast cells with cytoplasmic immunoglobulins which were unusually restricted in terms of light/heavy chain expression. Most remarkably, as on fresh cells, there was no expression of MHC-class-II-antigens either initially or after prolonged culture of these LCL. Levels of class-I-antigens were variable between different sublines but lower than normal (M.R. Hadam et al., in preparation).

The LCL allowed the unequivocal delineation of the defect involved in the non-expression of MHC-class-II-antigens (C. De Preval, B. Mach et al., in preparation). Thus the genes for class-II-antigens were detected by southern blot analysis in the three patients studied so far (RS, SM, AH). This rules out major structural abnormalities at the DNA level and renders minor ones unlikely, but does not exclude epigenetic mechanisms. The LCL from the same three patients were also tested for the presence of mRNA by northern blot analysis. No mRNA of all three HLA-D-subregions (DR/DQ/DP) was found in patients RS and AH even on overloaded gels; there were traces in patient SM. When LCL were cultured in the presence of recombinant gamma-interferon prior to analysis no additional class-II-specific message was found. However, levels of mRNA for class-I-antigens were increased in response to gamma-interferon indicating that the cells are not unresponsive to interferon. This absence of mRNA focuses our attention to possible defects acting at the transcriptional level.

BARE-LYMPHOCYTE-SYNDROME: A SINGLE ENTITY?

There are three lines of argument which favour a different classification of BLS or HLA-class-I-defects compared to our cases of congenital agammaglobulinaemia with malabsorption of MHC-class-II-defects: (i) the clinical course, (ii) the phenotypic evaluation and (iii) molecular evidences.

First, cases of BLS have been summarized in a registry supported by the WHO (17). The patients described originally for BLS presumably had a more profound alteration of cellular immunity than ours, especially number and functions of T-lymphocytes appear to severly lowered. Moreover lymphoid tissue was scarce and reactions to antigen in vitro or skin reactions were weak if present at all. In contrast, our patients do not exhibit a defect in T-cell maturation as described for BLS (19), at least not at the phenotypic level.

Sizable T-cell function is available in our patients since postpartal BCG vaccination was uneventful and skin reactions were documented. Common to all is the manifestation of persistent diarrhoea and a marked failure to thrive which is also shared with some SCID patients. However on clinical grounds, our patients have always been classified as having congenital, albeit atypical agammaglobulinaemia with complete absence of all isotypes; there were few occasions to consider a combined immune deficiency disease. Similar to Shuurman et al (14) our patients respond favorably to plasma infusions which might substitute yet non-identified factor(s) other than immunoglobulin. Puzzling in the clinical records and hard to classify are the two patients with BLS without immunodeficiency (13). It may indicate, that BLS or class-I-deficiency in its "pure" form, does not necessarily constitute a life-threatening disease.

The current WHO classification (15) lists BLS under the heading of SCID in the group of "predominantly cell-mediated immunity defects". This is conceivable for the cases originally described. However in view of the rather operational WHO grouping, on clinical and functional grounds, our four patients should be considered as "predominantly antibody defects".

Second, on the phenotypic level we have provided evidence for the immaturity of the circulating B-lymphocytes in our patients. So far this unique phenotype characterized by high density surface IgM and the expression of multiple immunoglobulin isotypes has not been observed in other immune deficiencies including BLS. The presence of HLA-class-I-antigens on peripheral blood cells at all times was documented. The use of flow cytometry has allowed their quantitation which is not biased by individual thresholds in the distinction of positive vs. negative cells as is fluorescence microscopy. Hence different class-I-levels could be attributed to T- and B- cells, a finding comparable to normal human cord blood. In conclusion both surface immunoglobulin patterns and class-I-levels demonstrate a maturational arrest at the stage of the normal neonate. Conversely this fact may be viewed as if differentiation during fetal life takes place normally despite the absence of class-II-antigens. Our phenotypic results are not easily compared to those of others. The different methodologies applied for detection cause ambiguities on this issue. In addition the stable patterns of class-I-antigens seen on lymphoid cells of our patients in an apparent sex-linked fashion may provide a clue for a more detailed analysis of this syndrome. We have provided evidence for the complete absence of class-II-antigens of all three subregions on peripheral blood mononuclear cells by means of phenotypic analysis. We could not confirm other observations on variable expression of those determinants (4, 5) nor did we observe phenotypic chimeras even at high numbers of B-cells (10). Moreover, monocytes were always negative in our patients as opposed to others (5). A general defect in lymphocyte activation was excluded by the expression of IL-2-receptors upon stimulation with phytohemagglutinin, despite the continuing lack of class-II-antigens. We have also provided evidence that Langerhans' cells and endothelial cells are negative for class-II-antigens (6). Most importantly all cell lines established from our patients retain this deficiency: upon prolonged culture they continue to lack all class-II-antigens and retain lower levels of class-I-antigens. This constant block of class-II-expression contrasts to the readily observed upregulation of class-I-levels seen in cell lines from patients with BLS. The ease of transformation with Epstein-Barr-Virus in BLS (13, 19) is opposed to our own difficulties mentioned earlier. No published data are available for the class-II-levels on LCL from BLS; however B.M. Peterlin (1984, personal communication) found that with fresh cells and cultured lymphoblasts from their patients (13, 16), levels of class-II-antigens were always normal. Thus on phenotypic grounds BLS may be considered a transient regulatory abnormality in class-I-expression which is normalized in vitro. In contrast, our patients with agammaglobulinaemia and malabsorption consistently fail to express class-II-antigens and so far have not reverted to a positive phenotype. It can be envisaged that combinations of both phenotypic traits occur; however their delineation deserves rigorously controlled phenotypic evaluations on both fresh cells and LCL.

Third, evidence from molecular biology points to a defect at the transcriptional level in our patients, which is stably inherited in more than 200 estimated population doublings in culture. The data are resembling immunoselected B cell variants which have coordinatively lost expression of the whole HLA-D-region (1, 2). Some of these variants were clearly shown to express wild-type levels of class-I-antigens (1). Pivotal for a model of class-II-regulation was the production of somatic cell hybrids reexpressing the missing determinants (3). Moreover non-expression in the variant was due to the absence of mRNA (11, 12). The ensuing model proposed a regulatory gene acting in trans (3, 9). The properties of the LCL established from our patients are compatible with a similar "experiment of nature". This concept is supported by the fact that gamma-interferon and other inducers of class-II-antigens were unable to augment those structures both at the phenotypic and mRNA levels. Likewise the small proportion of Langerhans' cells in the skin found in two patients may be taken as evidence for intact class-II-structural genes. However, reexpression of class-II-antigens in somatic cell hybrids prepared from our patients' LCL is required to formally prove this hypothesis. Molecular data for BLS are sparse (10, 16). The absence of class-II-mRNA in fresh peripheral blood mononuclear cells has been reported (10) as well as small amounts of class-I-mRNA (10, 16). However information from stably transformed lines is lacking. To firmly settle this point it would be of utmost importance to evaluate the LCL from the original patients (19) by the means available today.

CONCLUSIONS

One may derive two separate models for MHC-class-I- and class-II-defects: Class-I-defects (or genuine BLS) are characterized by drastically lowered class-I-levels and normal class-II-levels. The abnormal class-I-expression is subject to regulatory influences and normalized in vitro. Class-II-defects display lowered class-I-levels and a complete lack of class-II-antigens. This stable class-II-phenotype does not revert in vitro and may be due to the lack of a trans-acting regulatory gene. Clinically, original cases of BLS appear to have a more profoundly affected cell mediated immunity in contrast to our predominantly agammaglobulinaemic patients. Thus due to the distinctive pathogenetic mechanisms involved an independent classification of these patients seems warranted.

Acknowledgements

The generous gift of monoclonal antibodies by Dr. A. Ziegler, Tübingen, FRG and Dr. M. Steel, Edinburgh, Great Britain is greatfully aknowledged. Supported by the Deutsche Forschungsgemeinshaft (SFB 120: B3; Pe151/8), the Swiss National Found for Scientific Research and the Robert-Bosch-Foundation.

REFERENCES

1. Acolla, R.S. (1983): Human B cell variants immunoselected against a single Ia antigen subset have lost expression of several Ia antigen subsets. *J. Exp. Med.*, 157:1053-1058.
2. Gladstone, P. and Pious, D. (1978): Stable variants affecting B cell alloantigens in human lymphoid cells. *Nature*, 271:459-461.
3. Gladstone, P. and Pious, D. (1980): Identification of a transacting function regulating HLA-DR expression in a DR-negative B cell variant. *Som. Cell Gen.*, 6:285-298.
4. Griscelli, C., Durandy, A., Virelizier, J.L. (1980): Impaired cell to cell interactions in partial combined immunodeficiency with variable expression of HLA antigens. In: *Primary immunodeficiencies*, edited by M. Seligman and W.H. Hitzig, pp. 499-503. Elsevier, Amsterdam.
5. Griscelli, C., Durandy, A., Virelizier, J.L., Grospierre, B., Dury, C., de Saint-Basile, G., Coullin, P., Niaudet, P., Betuel, H., Hors, J., Lepage, V., and Colombani, J., (1981): Impaired cell to cell interaction in partial combined immunodeficiency with defective synthesis and membrane expression of HLA antigens. In: *Bone marrow transplantation in Europe, Volume II*, edited by J.L. Touraine, E. Gluckman and C. Griscelli, pp. 194-200. Excerpta Medica, Amsterdam.
6. Hadam, M.R., Dopfer, R., Dammer, D., Peter, H.H., Schlesier, M., Müller, C., and Niethammer, D. (1984): Defective Expression of HLA-D-region determinants in children with congenital agammaglobulinemia and malabsorption: a new syndrome. In: *Histocompatibility Testing 1984*, edited by E.D. Albert, M.P. Baur, and W.R. Mayr, pp. 645-650. Springer, Heidelberg.
7. Hadam, M.R., Dopfer, R., Peter, H.H., and Niethammer, D. (1984): Congenital agammaglobulinaemia associated with lack of expression of HLA-D-region antigens. In: *Progress in immunodeficiency research and therapy I*, edited by C. Griscelli and J. Vossen, pp. 43-50. Elsevier, Amsterdam.
8. Kuis, W., Roord, J., Zegers, B.J.M., Schuurman, R.K.B., Heijnen, C.J., Baldwin, W.M., Goulmy, E., Claas, F., van der Griend, R.J., Rijkers, G.T., van Rood, J.J., Vossen, J.M., Ballieux, R.E. and Stoop, J.W. (1981): Clinical and immunologial findings in a patient with the "bare lymphocyte" syndrome. In: *Bone marrow transplantation in Europe, Volume II*, edited by J.L. Touraine, E. Gluckman, and C. Griscelli, pp. 201-208. Excerpta Medica, Amsterdam.
9. Levine, F. and Pious, D. (1984): Revertants from the HLA class II regulatory mutant 6.1.6: implications for the regulation of Ia gene expression. *J. Immunol.*, 132:959-962.
10. Lisowska-Grospierre, B., Charon, D.J., de Preval, C., Durandy, A., Turmel, P., Griscelli, C., and Mach, B. (1984): Defect of expression of MHC genes responsible for an abnormal

HLA class I phenotype and the class II negative phenotype of lymphocytes from patients with combined immunodeficiency. In: *Histocompatibility Testing 1984*, edited by E.D. Albert, M.P. Baur, and W.R. Mayr, pp. 650-655. Springer, Heidelbger.

11. Long, O.E., Mach, B., and Acolla, R.S. (1984): Ia-negative B-cell variants reveal a coordinate regulation in the transcription of the HLA class II gene family. *Immunogenetics*, 19:349-353.

12. Loosmore, S., Gladstone, P., Pious, D., Jerry, L.M., and Tamaoki, T. (1982): Control of HLA-DR antigen gene expression at the pretranslational level: comparison of an HLA-DR-positive B lymphoblastoid cell line and its HLA-DR-negative variant. *Immunogenetics*, 15:139-150.

13. Payne, R., Brodsky, F.M., Peterlin, M.B. and Young, L.M. (1983): Bare lymphocytes without immunodeficiency. *Human Immunol.*, 6:219-227.

14. Schuurman, R.K.B., van Rood, J.J., Vossen, J.M., Schellekens, P.T.A., Feltkamp-Vroom, Th.M., Doyer, E., Gmeylig-Meyling, F., and Visser, H.K.A. (1979): Failure of lymphocyte-membrane HLA-A and -B expression in two siblings with combined immunodeficiency. *Clin. Immunol. Immunopathol.*, 14:418-434.

15. Rosen, F.S., Wedgwood, R.J. (1983): Meeting report. Primary immunodeficiency diseases. *Clin. Immunol. Immunopathol.*, 28:450-475.

16. Sullivan, K.E., Stobo, J.D., and Peterlin, B.M. (1984): Molecular analysis of the bare lymphocyte syndrome. *J. Clin. Immunol.*, in press.

17. Touraine, J.L. (1981): The bare-lymphocyte syndrome: report on the registry. *Lancet*, i:319-321.

18. Touraine, J.L. (1984): Le syndrome des lymphocytes denudes. Deficit immunitaire combiné par absence d'expression des antigenes IILA. *Presse Med.*, 13:671-674.

19. Touraine, J.L., Betuel, H., and Philipe, N. (1980): The bare lymphocyte syndrome. I. Immunological studies before and after bone marrow transplantation. *Blut*, 41:198-202.

20. Touraine, J.L., Betuel, H., Souillet, G., and Jeune, M. (1978): Combined immunodeficiency associated with absence of cell-surface HLA-A and -B antigens. *J. Pediatr.*, 93:47-51.

DNA-Mediated Gene Transfer into Ataxia-Telangiectasia Cells

M. Crescenzi, S. Pulciani*, M. Carbonari, L. Tedesco, G. Russo
C. Gaetano and M. Fiorilli

*Department of Clinical Immunology, University of Rome "La Sapienza", and *Istituto Superiore di Sanità, Rome Italy.*

INTRODUCTION

Ataxia-telangiectasia (AT) is a rare autosomal recessive disorder characterized by cerebellar ataxia, oculocutaneous telangiectasias, variable immunodeficiency, high incidence of cancer, increased chromosomal breakage, and hypersensitivity to DNA damaging agents (1).

The genetic lesion leading to defective DNA repair and to the pleiotropic clinical manifestations of AT is still obscure. Recently, heterogeneity of AT has become apparent on the basis of genetic complementation studies (16, 17) and of clinical data (1, 9, 26). Further heterogeneity within this syndrome is suggested by the identification (11) of a distinct subset of patients characterized by low-level radiosensitivity. These patients are different from those with "classical" AT for the lower frequency of spontaneous or bleomycin-induced chromosomal breakage, for their cells ability to normally inhibit DNA synthesis following ionizing irradiation (19), and for the minimal immunological impairment. The latter point suggests a direct relationship between the DNA-repair defect and the damage to the immune system in this disease. A clue to understanding this relationship is provided by the knowledge of the molecular events which underlie the diversification and maturation of lymphoid cells.

T and B lymphocytes are remarkably similar in the way they generate their antigen receptor structures. In fact, both types of cells use somatic rearrangement and mutation of limited germ-line genetic information encoded by variable (V), diversity (D), joining (J) and constant (C) regions (2, 21, 25). These rearrangements require the cutting and ligation of specific sequences flanking V, D, J and C genes. Clearly, these recombinational events must be regulated by a set of specific enzymes. While a V-J region-specific nuclease activity has been partially characterized (7), virtually nothing is known about the enzymes involved in the rearrangements of other immunoglobulin or T-cell receptor genes. Lymphocytes from AT patients show spontaneous breaks occuring nonrandomly at specific regions, namely 14q32, 14q11-12, 7q35 and 7p14 (1, 15). Interestingly enough, the recent mapping of the T-cell receptor alpha — and gamma — chain genes at 14q11 and 7p15 (5, 18), respectively, confirmed the suggestion (10) that these nonrandom breaks occur at regions encoding for genes which undergo rearrangements in lymphoid cells. It can be reasonably argued that the AT mutation affects a rejoining enzyme (4) involved both in the repair of at least one type of radiogenic damage and in the physiological rearrangements of lymphocyte receptor genes. Defective ligation might, therefore, lead to an increased frequency of faulty rearrangements of T and B cell receptor genes in AT, resulting in immunodeficiency due to the death or dysfunction of the majority of lymphocytes.

The complete description of the genetic lesion(s) undelying the AT mutation might, therefore, highlight not only a DNA-repair pathway, but also an important aspect of the physiology of lymphocytes. This description probably will not be achieved before the AT genes(s) will be molecularly cloned. In the following paper we will, therefore, briefly describe our preliminary efforts aimed at cloning one of these genes.

DNA-mediated gene transfer into eukaryotic cells has proved a powerful tool for the molecular cloning of certain mammalian genes (13, 27, 29). The possibility to clone a given gene using this technology depends, basically, on the availability of a selectable marker associated with the expression of the transfected gene in the recipient cell. Recently, a human DNA repair gene has been cloned in CHO mutant cells by taking advantage of the increased resistance to ultraviolet radiation of the transformants (22, 28).

As a preliminary step toward the molecular cloning of the AT gene(s), we have attempted to confer radioresistance to AT cells by transfection with normal human DNA.

MATERIALS AND METHODS

AT5BIVA cells, a SV40-transformed fibroblast strain derived from an AT patient (kindly provided by S.A. Harcourt, Brighton, U.K.), were used as recipient cells for gene transfer experiments. The human, repair proficient WISH and Hep-2 cells were used as controls.

Cells were cultured in MEM with Eagle's salts supplemented with 10% FCS and antibiotics. To determine survival following exposure to DNA damaging agents, cells were plated at 3-5.000/60 mm Petri dish; after 24 hours cells were either irradiated with X-rays, at a dose rate of 4 rad/sec, or exposed to bleomycin. For pulse-treatment with bleomycin, cells were washed and resuspended in drug-containing medium for 60 minutes, then washed twice in phosphate buffered saline and resuspended in fresh medium. For double-pulse experiments, the above procedure was repeated after 24 hours. Chronic exposure to bleomycin was started 24 hours after cell plating, and drug-containing medium was replaced every 3-4 days. Surviving colonies were scored 10 days following the beginning of selection using a dissection microscope. For DNA-mediated gene transfer, cells where plated at $10^5/100$ mm Petri dish, in Dulbecco's modified MEM containing 10% FCS. On the following day, DNA transfection was performed by the calcium-phosphate precipitation technique (13). Each plate was transfected with 2 μg of pSV2neo DNA and 80 μg of high molecular weight (HMW) DNA extracted from WISH cells. After 24 hours cells were washed twice and given fresh medium. Two days later selection with geneticin (Grand Island Biological Co.), at 750 μg/ml, was started. X-radiation selection was applied three weeks after transfection.

RESULTS AND DISCUSSION

Survival curves of AT5BIVA, WISH and Hep-2 following exposure to Rx or bleomycin are reported in Fig. 1. Treatment protocols included single or double pulses with different doses of Rx or bleomycin, or chronic exposure to bleomycin. Overall, no significant differences in the selection efficiency (i.e. ratio between the surviving fraction of AT5BIVA and of repair proficient cells) were found between single or double pulses with either Rx or bleomycin. There were no surviving AT5BIVA colonies after chronic exposure to as low as 0.3 μg/ml of bleomycin, while approximately 60% of Hep-2 survived at the same concentration. Nevertheless, surviving Hep-2 colonies showed a completely altered morphology and extremely slow growth rate. We concluded that the best protocol for selecting radioresistant transformants in transfection experiments was the exposure to a single initial dose of 400 rad of X-radiation. This selection procedure kills more than 99.9% of AT5BIVA cells, and approximately 50% of repair proficient cells.

The competence of AT5BIVA cells to incorporate foreign DNA into their genome as shown by the observation of geneticin-resistant colonies following transfection with pSV2neo DNA. Transfection of 2 μg of pSV2neo DNA into 10^5 AT5BIVA cells gave a frequency of geneticin-resistant transformants of approsimately 2×10^{-3} (data not shown). This indicates that AT5BIVA cells are highly competent for incorporating exogenous DNA. Debenham et al. reported recently (6) the transfection of a plasmid containing the Eco-gpt gene into untrasformed AT fibroblasts, with a transfer as high as 10^{-4}. Their choice for untrasformed cells was dictated by the consideration that these cells are generally preferred for investigating cell functions, such as DNA repair, which can be modified by viral transformation (12, 23). However, the limited life span and the long generation time of untransformed fibroblasts preclude their use for the molecular cloning of repair genes by DNA transfection. For this reason we decided to use SV40-transformed cells for our experiments.

The final step of our study was an attempt to obtain radioresistant transformants by co-transfection of AT5BIVA cells with pSV2neo and HMW genomic DNA from repair proficient human cells (WISH). A total of 4×10^6 cells were transfected. After geneticin selection, each Petri dish, containing approxi-

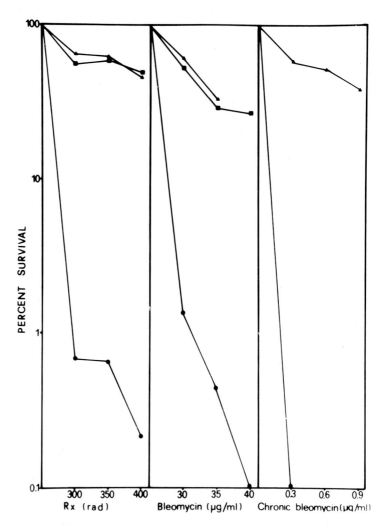

FIG. 1.   Survival of AT5BIVA (●), WISH (▲) and Hep-2 (■) cells exposed to different doses of Rx (single pulse) or of bleomycin (single pulse or chronic exposure).

mately 200 colonies, was trypsinized, cells were replated at $3\times10^3/60$ mm Petri dish, and exposed to 400 rad of X-radiation. After ten days, surviving colonies were reirradiated, without further subplating, with 300 rad. Following the second irradiation, three out of 40 dishes contained significantly ($p < 0.01$, Chi-square test) higher numbers of surviving colonies. Cells from these three dishes were tested for radiosensitivity in comparison to untreated or preirradiated (400+300 rad) AT5BIVA cells (Fig. 2.) No preirradiated AT5BIVA cells survived after exposure to as low as 100 rad, while transfected cells had a survival curve similar to that of non-preirradiated AT5BIVA cells.

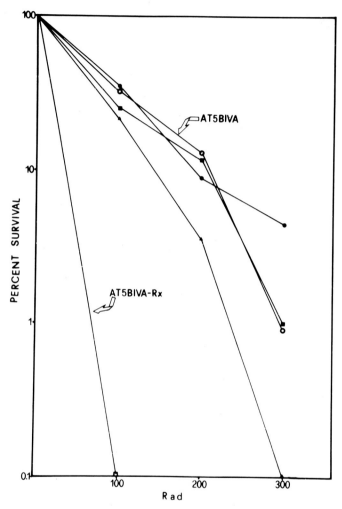

FIG. 2. Survival of untreated AT5BIVA cells (AT5BIVA), of untrasfected AT5BIVA cells which had been pre-irradiated with 400+300 rad (AT5BIVA-Rx), and of three derivatives of transfected AT5BIVA cells. The latter cells, obtained after transfection with human DNA from repair-proficient cells, were those (out of 40 transfection plates) surviving to selection with Rx (400+300 rad).

A major problem in identifying radioresistant transformants following gene transfer was the relatively little difference in radiosensitivity of SV40-transformed AT fibroblasts in comparison to normal cells (12). A large part of our present work was, therefore, devoted to assess the optimal selection conditions. We choose to select transformants by exposing cells to a single dose of 400 rad x-rays, followed by reirradiation with 300 rad after ten days. The results of one transfection experiment, in which AT5BIVA cells were given pSV2neo DNA plus HMW DNA from normal human cells, and selected as described above, were puzzling. When cells from dishes containing significantly higher numbers of surviving colonies were tested for radiosensitivity, they appeared significantly more resistant than control AT5BIVA cells previously exposed to the same irradiation procedure (i.e. 400+300 rad), but similar to unirradiated AT5BIVA cells. These results suggest that the cumulative damage induced by the selection procedure itself might decrease the radioresistance of otherwhise fully corrected transformants, or that the incorporation of a repair gene into these cells did not result in full reversion to wildtype resistance. The latter event has been observed for a UV repair gene (28). These two hypotheses are, clearly, not mutually exclusive. A third possibility is that we did not select true transformants, but less radiosensitive revertants of AT5BIVA cells. The chance that the rare spontaneous revertants incorporated foreing DNA (pSV2neo) is, however, exceedingly low.

Acknowledgements

This work was supported by a grant from the Italian Ministry of Education (Fondi 60%).

REFERENCES

1. Bridges, B.A., Harnden, D.G. (eds.) (1982): Ataxia-telangiectasia: a cellular and molecular link between cancer, neuropathology and immunodeficiency. J. Wiley and Sons, Chichester.
2. Chien, Y., Becker, D.M., Lindsten, T., Okamura, M., Cohen, D.I., Davis, M.M. (1984): A third type of murine T-cell receptor gene. *Nature* 312:31-35.
3. Colbere-Garapin F., Horodniceanu, F., Kourilsky, P., Garapin, A.C. (1981): A new dominant hybrid selective marker for higher eukaryotic cells. *J. Mol. Biol.* 150:1-14.
4. Cornforth, M.N., Bedford, J.S. (1985): On the nature of a defect in cells from individuals with ataxia-telangiectasia. *Science*, 227:1589-1591.
5. Croce, C.M., Isobe, M., Palumbo, A. Puck, J., Ming, J., Tweardy, D., Erikson, J., Davis, M.M., Rovera, G. (1985): Gene for alpha-chain of human T-cell receptor: location on chromosome 14 region involved in T-cell neoplasms. *Science*, 227:1044-1047.
6. Debenham, P.G., Webb, M.B.T., Masson, W.K., Cox, R. (1984): DNA-mediated gene transfer into human diploid fibroblasts derived from normal and ataxia-telangiectasia donors: parameters for DNA transfer and properties of transformants. *Int. J. Rad. Biol.* 5:525-536.
7. Desiderio, S., Baltimore, D. (1984): Double-stranted cleavage by cell extracts near recombinational signal sequences of immunoglobulin genes. *Nature* 308:860-862.
8. Edwards, M.J., Taylor, A.M.R. (1980): Unusual levels of (ADP-ribose) and DNA synthesis in ataxia-telangiectasia cells following gamma irradiation. *Nature*, 287:745-747.
9. Fiorilli, M., Businco, L., Pandolfi, F., Paganelli, R., Russo, G., Aiuti, F. (1983): Heterogeneity of immunological abnormalities in ataxia-telangiectasia. *J. Clin. Immunol.* 3:135-141.
10. Fiorilli, M., Carbonari, M., Crescenzi, M., Russo, G., Aiuti, F. (1985): T-cell receptor genes and ataxia-telangiectasia. *Nature*, 313:186.
11. Fiorilli, M., Antonelli, A., Russo, G., Carbonari, M., Crescenzi, M., Petrinelli, P. (1985): Variant of ataxia-telangiectasia with low-level radiosensitivity. *Human. Genet.* 70:274-277.
12. Gatti, R.A. (1984): Ataxia-telangiectasia: immune dysfunction is one of many defects. *Immunol. Today*, 45:121-123.
13. Graham, F.L., van der Eb, A.J. (1973): A new technique for the assay of infectivity of human adenovirus 5 DNA. *Virology* 52:456-467.
14. Hayday, A.C., Saito, H., Gillies, S.D.,. Kranz, D.M., Tanigawa, G., Eisen, H.N., Tonegawa, S. (1985): *Cell*, 40:259-269.

15. Hecht, F., Morgan, R., Hecht, R.K.M., Smith, S.D. (1984): Common region on chromosome 14 in T-cell leukemia and lymphoma. *Science* 226:1445-1447.
16. Jaspers, N.G.J., Bootsma, D. (1982): Genetic heterogeneity in ataxia-telangiectasia studied by cell fusion. *Proc. Natl. Acad. Sci. USA*, 79:2641-2644.
17. Murnane, J.P., Painter, R.B., (1982): Complementation of the defects in DNA synthesis in irradiated and unirradiated ataxia-telangiectasia cells. *Proc. Natl. Acad. Sci. USA*, 79:1960-1963.
18. Murre, C., Waldmann, R.A., Morton, C.C., Bongiovanni, K.F., Waldmann, T.A., Shows, T.R., Seidman, J.G. (1985): Human gamma-chain genes are rearranged in leukaemic T cells and map to the short arm of chromosome 7. *Nature*, 316:549-552.
19. Painter, R.B., Young, B.R. (1980): Radiosensitivity in ataxia-telangiectasia: a new explanation. *Proc. Natl. Acad. Sci. USA*, 77:7315-7317.
20. Paterson, M.C., Smith, B.P., Lohman, P.H.M., Anderson, A.K., Fishman, L. (1976): Defective excision repair of gamma-ray damaged DNA in human (ataxia-telangiectasia) fibroblasts. *Nature*, 260:444-447.
21. Patten, P. Yokota, T., Rothbard, J., Chien, Y., Arai, K., Davis, M.M. (1984): Structure, divergence and expression of T-cell receptor beta-chain variable regions. *Nature*, 312:40-46.
22. Rubin, J.S., Joyner, A.L., Bernstein, A., Whitmore, G.F. (1983): Molecular identification of a human DNA repair gene following DNA-mediated gene transfer. *Nature*, 306:206-208.
23. Shiloh, Y., Tabor, E., Becker, Y. (1983): Similar repair of 06-methylguanine in normal and ataxia-telangiectasia fibroblast strains: deficient repair capacity of lymphoblastoid cell lines does not reflect a genetic polymorphism. *Mutat. Res.*, 112:47-58.
24. Spector, B.D., Filipovich, A.H., Perry, G.S., Kersey, J.H. (1982): Epidemiology of cancer in ataxia-telangiectasia. In: Bridges, B.A., Harnden, G.D., eds. *Ataxia-telangiectasia. A cellular and molecular link between cancer, neuropathology and immune deficiency.* Chichester and New York: John Wiley and Sons, 103-138.
25. Tonegawa, S. (1983): Somatic generation of antibody diversity. *Nature*, 302:575-581.
26. Waldmann, T.A., Broder, S., Glodman, C.K., Frost, K., Korsmeyer, S.J., Medici, M.A. (1983): Disorders of B cells and helper T cells in the pathogenesis of the immunoglobulin deficiency of patients with ataxia-telangiectasia. *J. Clin. Invest.* 71:282-295.
27. Weinberg, R.A. (1981): Use of transfection to analyze genetic information and malignant transformation. *Biochim. Biophys. Acta*, 651:25-35.
28. Westerveld, A., Hoeijmakers, J.H.J., van Duin, M., de Wit, J., Odijk, H., Pastink, A., Wood, R.D., Bootsma, J., (1984): Molecular cloning of human DNA repair gene. 310:425-429.
29. Wigler, M., Sweet, R., Sim, G.K., Wold, B., Pellicer, A., Lacy, E., Maniatis, T., Silverstein, S., Axel, R. (1979): Transformation of mammalian cells with genes from procaryotes and eucaryotes. *Cell* 16:777-785.

Instability of the Immunoglobulin Coding Region in a Patient with Ataxia-Telangiectasia, T-cell Leukemia and Chromosome 14 Translocation

J.P. Johnson, R.L. White and R.A. Gatti

Department of Pediatrics, University of Utah Medical Center, 50 N. Medical Drive, Salt Lake City, UT 84132
Departments of Human Genetics and of Cellular, Viral and Molecular Biology; and Howard Hughes Medical Institute, University of Utah, 50N. Medical Drive, Salt Lake City, UT 84132.
Department of Pathology, UCLA School of Medicine, Center for the Health Sciences, Los Angeles, CA 90024, USA.

INTRODUCTION

Ataxia-telangiectasia (AT) is a rare (1/40,000), autosomal recessive condition which produces multisystem aberrations. Because of this pleiotropy, the disorder has been diversely classified as a neurocutaneous syndrome or phakomatosis, as an endocrinopathy, as a neurodegenerative disease, and as a primary immunodeficiency. The syndrome also includes premature aging, defective DNA repair or processing, cancer predisposition, and chromosomal instability (5).

About 10-20% of AT patients develop a T-cell translocation involving the band 14q32 where immunoglobulin genes are located (16, 17, 21, 28, 32). Such translocations involve both #14 homologues with a break on one at 14q11 or 12 and on the other at 14q32. The exchange is presumably reciprocal resulting in formation of one #14 with tandem partial duplication and the other with interstitial deletion. The formal designation is trcp (14;14) q12q32 although the exact position of the proximal breakpoint is not yet clearly defined (3). (See Figure 1). In serial karyotypes of a few patients the percentage of T-cells with the translocation increased from 5-10 to 80-100% (1, 17, 28, 32), and concurrently the deleted (14q-) chromosome was often lost (1). Some individuals with these rearrangements have subsequently developed T-cell leukemia (27, 28, 36).

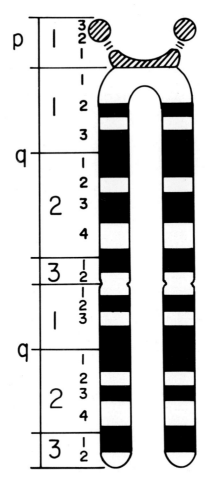

FIG. 1.   The chromosome 14 tandem translocation typical of AT, with breakpoints at 14q11 and 14q32.

A similar translocation of the c-myc oncogene from 8q24 to 14q32 occurs in Burkitt lymphoma (8, 9, 39) and is presumably causally related to malignant transformation of B cells with the rearrangement. Although the mechanism is still not entirely clear, juxtaposition of c-myc with the immunoglobulin heavy chain gene locus alters c-myc expression (13). By analogy, a similar activation process may be involved in the 14q11 (2) - 14q32 T-cell translocation in AT (25, 28). Perhaps a gene in 14q11 (2) is affected by translocation to the 14q32 region (18, 37). The converse is also possible (7).

In the T-cells of an AT patient with a 14-14 translocation we address the question of whether this rearrangement involves the same immunoglobulin region and switch sequences implicated in many of the B-cell (Burkitt) lymphoma rearrangements.

METHODS AND MATERIALS

DNA Samples

The patient was a 48-year-old woman with AT (MP) who developed the characteristic chromosome 14 translocation about 10 years before dying of leukemia (15). When initially evaluated, 100% of her T-cells had 45 chromosomes with the tandemly duplicated #14 chromosome present and the deleted #14 chromosome absent (15, 28). By the time T-cell leukemia developed, the leukemic cells had acquired a number of additional rearrangements: 44 XX, –14, t(14;14), –12, 6q, 12p–, 20p+, iso 8q (37). The peripheral leukocyte population consisted of 70-90% T-cells (by sheep red-cell rosetting) and these were initially shown to exhibit both helper (Tμ) and suppressor (Tγ) cell surface markers (10). Recent retesting of the T-cells reveals that they are a uniform population of helper cells (Leu 4+, Leu 3+, Leu 8–) (14). The DNA used in this study was isolated from frozen lymphocytes collected during the leukemic phase and is therefore predominantly (90+%) of T-cell origin (37). Likewise, the majority of the frozen lymphocytes contained only the rearranged #14 chromosome.

DNA was also isolated from a second AT patient having the chromosome 14 translocation, absence of the deleted chromosome, but no T-cell leukemia. (This patient's affected sister died of T-cell leukemia) (27). The DNA was derived from T-cells (by rosetting) and from polymorphonuclear leukocytes (by Ficoll separation).

Control samples included peripheral leukocyte DNA collected from random unrelated normal subjects, lymphocyte DNA from 11 AT families in which none of the affected AT patients was known to have a chromosome 14 translocation, and leukocyte DNA from a patient with suppressor phenotype acute T-cell leukemia (not karyotyped) (22).

High molecular weight nuclear DNA was isolated using standard lysis procedures (26). The DNA was purified by cesium gradient ultracentrifugation, phenol/chloroform extraction, and ethanol precipitation. It was then resuspended in Tris 10mM pH8 and 1mM EDTA and stored at 4°C.

Probes

CH 4-38, a 12 kilobase (kb) genomic fragment including part of the J region (J$_H$), the IgM switch (Sμ) and the IgM coding region (Cμ), was the major clone used in this study (24). (See Figures 4-6 for all probes). A 5' 3.3kb EcoR1 to Hind III fragment was subcloned into pBR 322 (p3.3) and a 3' 1.4kb EcoR1 to EcoR1 fragment was subcloned into pBR 325 (pl. 4). CH 28-6, an overlapping phage clone including the full J$_H$ region and some 5' flanking sequence, was also used (24). From this, a 5' 3.4kb Bam HI-Bam HI fragment was subcloned into pBR 322 (p3.4). Another pBR 322 subclone of a 5.7kb Bam HI-Hind III fragment including the entire J$_H$ region (HuJ$_H$) was used mainly for mapping (24).

Restriction Enzyme Digests, Electrophoresis, and Southern Blotting

Digestion of DNA was carried out in a 5-10 fold excess of the enzyme in buffers recommended by the manufacturer. The restriction enzymes included Sst I, Bam HI, Hind III, EcoR1, Bgl II, Pst I, and Rsa I. The extent of digestion was assayed by adding prokaryotic DNA to an aliquot of the digest mixture and visualizing ethidium bromide stained prokaryotic restriction fragments under ultraviolet light after agarose gel electrophoresis. Five to six micrograms of digested human DNA were then precipitated or evaporated to an appropriate volume and subjected to agarose gel electrophoresis in Tris acetate buffer. The agarose percentage of the gel, the voltage and current utilized, an the length of time of electrophoresis were varied to optimize restriction fragment separation in the molecular weight range desired for DNA digested with each particular enzyme. After electrophoresis, the gels were denatured in .2N NaOH, .6M NaCl and neutralized with .5M Tris pH 7.5, 1.5M NaCl before blotting in 20xSSC (3M NaCl, .3M sodium citrate), onto Zetapore (AMF) filtration membranes. After overnight blotting, the membranes were washed with 2xSSC, baked in a vacuum oven at 80°C for 1-3 hours, and then washed with .1xSSC and .5% SDS (lauryl sulfate) at 65°C. The membranes were packaged in plastic bags with 5 ml/100 cm^2 of 5xSSC, 10x Denhardt's (.2% polyvinyl prolidone, .2% Ficoll 400, .2% bovine serum albumin), .05 M NaPO$_4$, 500 micrograms/ml sonicated, boiled salmon sperm DNA, 2.5% dextran sulfate, and 50% formamide, and placed at 42°C overnight. They were stored at 4°C.

Probe Labelling, Hybridization, and Autoradiography

The probes were nicked for 15 minutes at 15 °C with DNAase I (Sigma, 20pg) in a buffer containing 1 M Tris pH 7.5, .1M MgCl, 1% gelatin, and .4M beta-mercaptoethanol. For the translation reaction, deoxynucleoside triphosphates in a final concentration of 30 µM (dATP, dTTP, dGTP) and 1.6 µM 32-P-dCTP (3000 Ci/mmol, New England Nuclear), 10 units of DNA polymerase (New England Biolabs), and .25 µg of nicked DNA were incubated for 1/2 hour at 37°C. After this, a 20 fold excess of Tris 10 mM, EDTA 1 mM and 40 µg of salmon sperm DNA were added to the mixture. The DNA was precipitated by adding spermine to a concentration of 500 µM, ultracentrifuged, and the pellet was washed with 1 mM spermine. The labelled DNA was resuspended in Tris 10 mM, 1 mM EDTA, .5 M NaCl, denatured in a 1/2 hour incubation with .4 N NaOH at 37°C, and neutralized with 1/3 volume 2 M Tris pH. 7.6. After assaying for efficiency (usually 10^7 - 10^8 cpm/µg DNA), 4×10^6 cpm/100 cm^2 were added to the membranes in a solution of 50% formamide, 5xSSC, .02M NaPO$_4$ pH 6.7, 100 µg/ml sonicated, boiled salmon sperm DNA, and 10% dextran sulfate. Incubations varied from 12 to 42 hours at 42° to 49°C. The membranes were washed successively in 2xSSC/.1% SDS and .1xSSC/.1% SDS, and the latter wash repeated at 65°C. The membranes were then packaged into a casette with Kodak XAR-5 film and a Dupont Lightning Plus Cronex intensifying screen and stored at –80°C for 24-240 hours. The films were developed in a Kodad RP X-OMAT processor.

Restriction Mapping

The molecular weights of hybridizing restriction fragments detected by autoradiography were calculated by comparison to the electrophoretic migration of standards of known molecular weight after plotting the migration distance of the standards on semi-log paper. These estimates were compared with those published for this region (4, 8, 12, 13, 31, 33-35, 38). The map was constructed by hybridizing to doubly digested DNA (Bam HI/Hind III, Bam HI/EcoR1, Xba 1/Hind III, Sst I/Bam HI, Sst I/Hind III) and by estimating the molecular weight of ethidium stained restriction fragments visualized with ultraviolet light after digesting the probes with single and multiple enzymes.

Densitometry

The density of visualized hybridizing fragments (bands) on autoradiograms was estimated by scanning the films with a Beckman DU-8 spectrophotometer and calculating integrated areas under absorbance curves generated by a plotter attached to the spectrophotometer. Affected and control lanes were selected for comparable background and quality, and the equivalence of DNA content was estimated by internally comparing band intensity for different probes including a control probe derived from chromosome 4 (19).

RESULTS

Hybridization and Restriction Mapping

Digested DNA from MP was initially hybridized to CH 4-38. For 3 enzymes, Sst 1, EcoR1, and Xba 1, no abnormal bands were detected in the leukemic AT T-cell DNA (data not shown). However, abnormal bands were detected with 2 other enzymes — Bam HI and Hind III. No living relative or other tissue (eg, fibroblasts) was available to evaluate whether the abnormal reflect restriction site (fragment length) polymorphism or whether the DNA is rearranged. To evaluate the question of polymorphism, leukocyte DNA from 40 controls was digested with both enzymes, blotted, and hybridized to CH 4-38. Although the probe detects more than one band (due to the switch sequences present 5' to the other immunoglobulin genes and perhaps elsewhere in the genome) (20), and some polymorphism is observed (31), the 26.6kb Bam HI band and the 5.7kb Hind III band in the AT patient (MP, Figure 2) were not observed in the control population. Normal 16.15kb Bam HI and 9.2 and 10.6 kb Hind III bands were also present in the AT patient. (The 10.6kb Hind III band is not shown in Figure 2). Given that there are two copies of the 14q32 region in normal individuals and in the AT patient (one in the region of

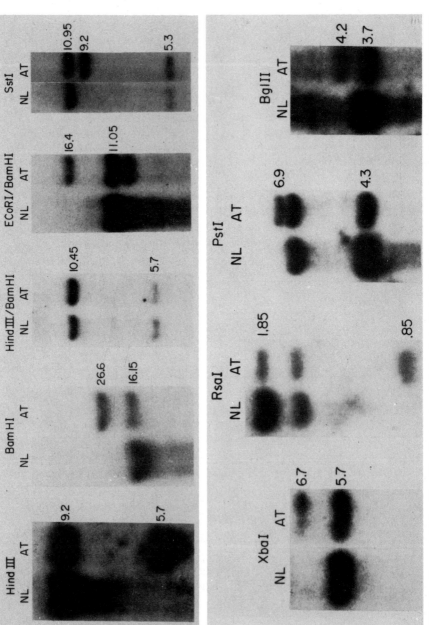

FIG. 2-3.   Genomic blots of the AT patient and control digested with the indicated enzymes and probed with p3.3. Molecular weight estimates were derived as described in the methods section. (Bam HI/Hind III blot probed with CH 4-38).

translocation and one in the telomeric area), it seemed possible that one of these regions was rearranged and one was maintained in control configuration. The T-cell leukemia DNA (digested with Hind III and Bam HI) and that from the other AT patients with the translocation (digested with Hind III and Bam HI) and without the #14 translocation (digested with EcoR1) exhibited normal hybridization patterns.

To map the apparently abnormal restriction sites in the AT patient, a blot of Hind III/Bam HI double-digested DNA was hybridized to CH 4-38. Curiously, as in the case of some of the single enzyme digests, the AT and normal DNA revealed the same hybridization pattern — the expected bands of 5.7 and 10.45kb. (See Figure 2 and Figure 6). Given that an abnormal 5.7kb fragment is observed in a Hind III digest, the simplest explanation of the normal finding in the double digest is that the normal Bam HI-Hind III 5.7kb fragment comigrates with a Hind III-Hind III fragment in the AT patient. (The palindromic recognition sequences for these two enzymes are sufficiently different that base pair mutations cannot account for this change. However, the resolution of molecular weights in this size range is such that a novel Hind III site could be 100 base pairs away from the absent Bam HI site). To further test this hypothesis, the 5' and 3' plasmid subclone probes p3.3 and p1.4 were hybridized to the Bam HI and Hind III digested DNA. Potential positions of novel Hind III sites to account for an abnormal 5.7kb fragment hybridizing to CH 4-38 are illustrated in Figure 4. The top line is the normal IgM restriction map followed by the probe CH 4-38 and the subclones. Of the three possible rearrangements, the second (B) is unlikely given that none of the probes (CH 4-38, p3.3, or p1.4) have homology with the abnormal 5.7kb fragment. In the third possibility (C) two fragments of size 4.9 and 5.7kb would be produced

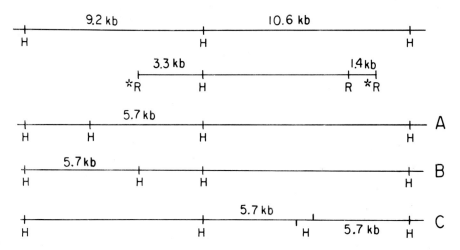

FIG. 4. Hind III (H) restriction maps for the normal IgM and region (line 1), the probes p3.3 and p1.4 (line 2), and three potential rearrangements in the AT patient (A, B, and C, see text).

which might separate or might comigrate and appear as one hybridizing band. However, only the 3' subclone p1.4 would have homology to a 5.7kb band in this situation. In (A), only the 5' subclone p3.3 would have homology to a 5.7kb band. The results of the hybridization supported interpretation (A), as the 5.7kb band was only revealed with p3.3. (This Hind III results is shown in Figure 2). This map interpretation is compatible with the Bam HI-Hind III double-digest result as well.

Both subclones hybridized to the abnormal 26.6kb Bam HI band and thus no information was gained in this experiment. As was mentioned previously, hybridization of CH 4-38 to EcoR1 digested DNA revealed only a normal 16.4kb fragment suggesting that both EcoR1 sites in both 14q32 regions are in normal positions in the AT patient. Figure 5 illustrates potential positions

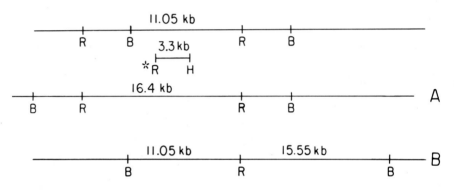

FIG. 5. EcoR1 (R)/Bam HI (B) restriction maps for the normal IgM region (line 1), the probe (line 2), and 2 potential rearrangements in the AT patient (A and B, see text).

of novel Bam Hi sites in the AT patient relative to EcoR1 sites in the normal positions. Again, the normal configuration is depicted first and the probe used in this experiment, p3.3, is shown below. An 11.05kb fragment is expected with hybridization of p3.3 to EcoR1-Bam HI doubly digested DNA. The AT patient should exhibit this fragment which derives from the normal, unrearranged 14q32 region. For the second of the possible rearrangements (B), only an 11.05 kb band would be expected as the change of the 3' Bam HI site to a position further 3' generating a larger 26.6kb fragment is outside the region of homology for this probe. Conversely in (A), if the 5' Bam HI site is replaced by a site further 5' to generate the larger fragment, the hybridization in the AT patient should reveal 2 fragments - an 11.05kb Bam HI - EcoR1 fragment from the unrearranged 14q32 region and the «normal» 16.4kb EcoR1 band in the rearranged region due to loss of the 5' Bam HI restriction site. The two fragments visualized in Figure 2 support interpretation (A).

Changes in restriction fragment lenghts not apparently attributable to restriction site polymorphism suggest the possibility of a DNA rearrangement. However, with three enzymes no such changes were apparent. To resolve this discrepancy, the blots showing no abnormalities were rehybridized with p3.3 to simplify the resulting hybridization pattern. For Sst 1, hybridization with CH 4-38 reveals 13-14 restriction fragments (27). With p3.3, (Figure 2) only a 10.95kb fragment from the J_H region and a 5.3 kb fragment from an unknown location were visualized. (p3.3 apparently also hybridizes to another region of the genome as bands not expected from the map of the immunoglobulin region were detected consistently with several enzymes. The band below the 11.05kb Bam Hi-EcoR1 band in Figure 2 is an example). In the AT patient (MP), an addition 9.2kb hybridizing fragment was present and was not seen in any of the controls. This fragment was also present in the CH 4-38 hybridization but was obscured by the presence of 9kb fragments detected with this probe. This abnormal 9.2kb AT band was not detected with p1.4, again suggesting a 5' alteration of restriction sites.

The same approach was utilized for the Xba 1 blot which had revealed only expected 5.7 and 6.9kb fragments in the AT patient with use of CH 4-38. Hybridization with p3.3 detected the 5.7kb band but also revealed 6.7kb band not seen in controls. Again this band had been obscured in the CH 4-38 hybridization by the presence of a normal band of similar molecular weight -6.9kb. The abnormal band was not detected with p1.4 suggesting a 5' rearrangement of Xba 1 sites (see Figure 3).

A series of double digests and hybridizations with CH 4-38 were then completed to confirm the assignment of novel 5' Hind III, Sst 1, and Xba 1 sites in one 14q32 region in MP. The results (not shown) were consistent with the relative order of these sites suggested by the fragment lenghts detected in the p3.3 hybridizations. Adding these sites to the Bam HI site already mapped, the order of novel sites 5' → 3' is Bam HI - Sst 1 - Xba 1 - Hind III, and the 5' → 3' order of subsequent normal sites is Hind III - Xba - Sst 1 - Bam HI. In fact, these sites appear in mirror image order and the distances between them (carefully calculated from the blots and from the size of restriction fragments produced by digest of the probe clones) are likewise symmetric. (See Figure 6). The midpoints of each fragment coincide and this is shown by an arrow in the AT 14q32 sequence (bottom line). The marked variation of 5' restriction sites from those in the normal 14q32 region is apparent.

Data from several subsequent experiments supported the interpretation of a mirror image duplication suggested by the preliminary restriction map. Digestion of the DNA with three more enzymes - Bg1 II, Pst 1, and Rsa 1, followed by hybridization with p3.3 again produced abnormal hybridizing fragments in the AT patient. The size of these fragments was predicted by the distance of the nearest 3' restriction site to the point of inversion, with the length of the abnormal fragments equal to twice this distance (See Figure 3. The size of the Rsa 1 fragment is equal to the distance between the 3' site and the midpoint, suggesting that a novel Rsa 1 site is present at this point). To further confirm this aberration of DNA 5' to the putative point of inversion, a probe 5' to this region, p3.4, was hybridized to MP DNA digested with all the enzymes previously tested. Only the normal bands expected from the

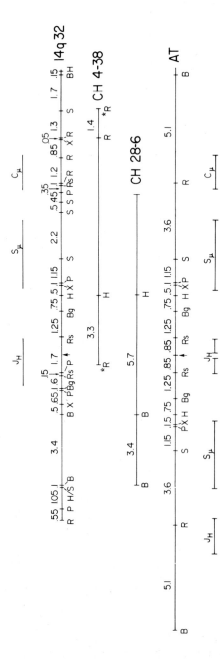

FIG. 6. Derived restriction map of the normal 14q32 region including J$_H$, S$_\mu$, and C$_\mu$ (line 1), the phage clones used in the study (lines 2&3), and the restriction map of the rearranged 14q32 region in the AT patient. Orientation is 5' (telomere) to the left. Only selected sites about the point of inversion are indicated to demonstrate the length of the aberrant fragments and the symmetry of the rearrangement. B=Bam HI, Bg=Bg1 II, H=Hind III, P=Pst 1, R=EcoR1, Rs=Rsa I, S=Sst I, X=Xba I, *R =artificial EcoR1 cloning site.

normal 14q32 region were seen suggesting that this probe has no homology to the abnormal fragments. (Data not shown).

Densitometry

The restriction map (Figure 6) of the AT 14q32 rearrangement predicts that sequences within the Sμ and Cμ coding regions are duplicated, and a third copy is present in the unrearranged, normal 14q32 region. Hybridizing bands 3' to the point of inverted duplication, such as the 10.6kb Hind III fragment spanning Sμ and Cμ, should therefore be 1 1/2 times as intense as the same bands in normal individuals, given that the amount of DNA in each lane of a blot is comparable. Conversely, the 9.2kb fragment spanning the J_H region and the point of inversion sould be only 1/2 as intense, as only one copy of this abnormal sequence is present in tha AT patient. These predictions are based on the assumption that 100% of cells from which DNA was isolated have one normal and one rearranged region. Only 10% of the cells did not contain the translocation, so that for every 100 cells, 90 have only one copy of the normal region and 10 have two, or 110 copies compared to a control of 200 copies (55%). Likewise for the region of triplication the value is 290/200, or 145%. For these predictions we also assume that the percentage of cells with the translocation is equivalent to the percentage with the mirror image duplication. In fact, the data fit these predictions quite well. (Not shown). In Figure 2 and 3, normal bands spanning the point of inversion, such as the 9.2kb Hind III, 16.15kb Bam HI, 11.05kb Bam HI/Eco R1, 10.95kb Sst 1, 5.7kb Xba 1, 3.7kb Bgl II, 4.3kb Pst 1, and 1.85kb Rsa 1 bands are all less intense than normal, whereas the 10.45kb Hind III/Bam HI band is more intense. Of interest is the fact that band densities from fragments hybridizing to p3.4 are about 50% of normal suggesting that the inverted duplication has resulted in deletion of at least some normal DNA in the 5' flanking region. (Densitometry data are available upon request).

An unexplained finding was the absence of rearranged EcoR1 fragments in the AT patients. The restriction map predicts that the normal fragment is 16.15kb and that the fragment from the rearranged region is 16.4kb, as the 3' EcoR1 site is 8.2kb from the point of inverted duplication. These predicted size differences would not be discernable in this high molecular weight region of the gels. However, the presence of two different bands is supported by the densitometry data, as the 16kb unrearranged band hybridizing to p3.4 is only half as intese as the band hybridizing to p3.3. This is because p3.3 hybridizes to both the normal and the rearranged fragments and as they are of very similar size, the combined band intensity is expected to be double that for p3.4.

DISCUSSION

The results of the Southern blot hybridizations and densitometry of hybrizing fragments on autoradiograms indicate that an inverted duplication of H_H

and Cμ coding DNA has occurred within one of the two 14q32 regions in the 14q+ translocated chromosome of a patient with AT and T-cell leukemia. The point of inversion is within the J_H region near J3 and J4 (24), and the length of the mirror-image duplication is at least 26.6kb, the size of the abnormal Bam HI fragment from this region. The mirror image symmetry of restriction sites within this rearranged region argues strongly that the duplicated DNA is inverted. This structural change generates copies of the heavy chain enhancer (29, 30, 34) flanking each side of an inverted region of J_H genes, but functional consequences of this rearrangement would not be expected. However, the deletion of normal 5' DNA as well as the insertion of inverted, duplicated DNA into this region could be functionally significant. The rearrangement appears to involve only one 14q32 region, as hybridizing fragments expected for "germ line" DNA were always visualized on autoradiograms. In addition, the densitometry data (to be published elsewhere) support an equal copy number for rearranged and normal J_H regions in the T-cells. This implies that the AT patient is "heterozygous" for normal and rearranged 14q32 DNA present on the one translocated #14 chromosome. This is analogous to the expectation of one cytogenetically normal 14q32 region from the "donor" #14 involved in the translocation and one rearranged 14q32 - 14q12 region representing the joint-point of the translocation. It is therefore possible to infer that the inverted duplication is associated structurally with the translocation, but this conclusion cannot presently be made as there is no evidence of 14q12 DNA associated with the identified rearrangement. One can conclude, unlike the case in many Burkitt lymphomas (8, 9, 39), that this translocation does not insert into the IgM switch or heavy chain J coding regions. The translocation breakpoint in this AT patient is probably distal to J_H and Cμ, as three copies of this region are present in the AT patient DNA. The presumed deletion of one copy of DNA distal to the point of inversion suggests that the duplicated region rejoins the normal 14q32 region with loss of DNA. Amplification of the restriction map and density data may answer the questions of association of the duplicated region with the translocation and of the extent of duplication and deletion.

Chromosome 14 inversions (14q12-q32) occur in normal T-cells (2), in T-cell leukemias and lymphomas (41-43), and in T-cells of patients with AT (2, 25). One structural rearrangement which could produce an inverted duplication within the J_H region involves a preexisting inversion of one chromosome #14 homologue, with breaks within J_H and 14q12, inverting J_H into the 14q12 region of this chromosome. If the 14q12 point again breaks and the inverted long arm translocates to the other #14 homologue itself broken at 14q32 within the J_H region, a translocated chromosome with J_H inversion at the joint point would be generated. (t (14; inv 14)14p13 → 14q32:q32 → q12:q32 → ter). However, as breaks in J_H occur on both 14 homologues, no normal 14q32 region is retained. There is no deletion in this process, but the 14q12:q32 junction occurs within the same point of the J_H region and would produce novel bands revealed by J_H probes. As MP has one normal 14q32 region, has a deletion, and has no rearrangement corresponding to a $14q12:J_H$ junction, this structural possibility is excluded. A recent revaluation of the patient's karyotype supports this conclusion (37).

If the $S\mu$ and $C\mu$ regions are triplicated, and there is no "donor" chromo-some to account for this (the "lost", deleted 14q- chromosome presumably consists of 14p, 14q to q12, and distal, telomeric 14q32 DNA), the triplication must have arisen during cell division. A meiotic event in a parent of the AT patient giving rise to a constitutional karyotype with the #14 translocation and inverted duplication can be excluded by the fact that a fibroblast karyotype of this patient was normal (37). Therefore, a mitotic event in a T-cell giving rise to a clone with the inverted duplication is the most likely explanation (40). Perhaps during chromosome replication, either both parent strands, or one parent and a daughter strand, or both daughter strands experienced breaks and the rejoining process generated an inverted duplication. Of the many enzymes involved in the process of DNA replication, dysfunction of unwinding enzymes, of DNA binding proteins, or of the ligase necessary to join fragments of the lagging strand seems most likely to contribute to instability resulting in rearrangement. Because the abnormal event occurred in J_H, perhaps the repeated sequences used as recombination signals for V_H - J_H joining in B cells (35) or the enzyme (recombinase) (10) mediating this process were in-volved. Further analysis of breakpoints in AT chromosomes may answer these questions.

Finally, it is interesting that AT rearrangements frequently involve chromosomal regions coding for genes expected to undergo rearrangements, such as the $T\alpha$ receptor gene in 14q12, the $T\beta$ receptor gene in 7q35, the $T\gamma$ receptor gene in 7p14, and the immunoglobulin genes in 14q32 (11). This suggests that normal processes involving gene rearrangement in a local *cis* fashion are exaggerated resulting in abnormal *trans* rearrangements with presumably similar sequences on other chromosomes or in distal *cis* changes such as inversions. Some of this instability, such as the J_H inverted duplication reported here, may not result in fuctional changes for the cells experiencing such a rearrangement. However, as in the case of c-myc amplification as-sociated with the 8:14 reciprocal translocation in B cell lymphomas, exagger-ation of DNA rearrangement processes might occasionally result in juxtapos-ition of a quiescent oncogene with active regions, resulting in a potential for cell transformation (23). In T-cells, a tandem #14 translocation appears to be the primordial event, and perhaps the multiple secondary chromosomal rear-rangements observed in this case and in other AT patients in whom T-cell leukemia subsequently develops are the "second hits" (24) which finally in-itiate the transformation process.

Acknowledgements

The authors thank Philip Leder for supplying clones used in this study, Seth Pincus for cell separations, Blair Bybee for patient samples, Tena Sears for technical assistance, and Stacy Berg for manuscript preparation. This work was supported by N.I.H.-B.R.S.G. Grant RR 05428, A.C.S. Grant IN-154, N.E.H. Grant 2-13650, USPHS Grant CA 35966, and the Ataxia-Telangiectasia Medical Research Foundation. JPJ dedicates this work to the loving memory of Cleo A. Johnson.

REFERENCES

1. Al Saadi, A., Palutke, M., and Komar, G.K. (1980): Evolution of chromosomal abnormalities in sequential cytogenetic studies of ataxia-telangiectasia. *Hum. Genet.*, 55:23-29.
2. Aurias, A., Dutrillaux, B., Buriot, D., and Lejeune, J. (1980): High frequencies of inversions and translocations of chromosome 7 and 14 in ataxia-telangiectasia. *Mutat. Res.*, 69:369-374.
3. Aurias, A., Dutrillaux, V., and Griscelli, C. (1983): Tandem translocation t(14;14) in isolated and clonal cells in ataxia-telangiectasia are different. *Hum. Genet.*, 63:320-322.
4. Battey, J., Moulding, C., Taub, R., Murphy, W., Stewart, T., Potter, H., Lenoir, G., Leder, P. (1983): The human c-myc oncogene: structural consequences of translocation into the IgH locus in Burkitt lymphoma. *Cell*, 34:779-787.
5. Bridges, B.A. and Harnden, D.G., editors (1982): *Ataxia-Telangiectasia. A Cellular and Molecular Link Between Cancer, Neuropathology, and Immune Deficiency*, John Wiley & Sons, New York.
6. Croce, C.M. (1985): Chromosomal translocation, oncogenes, and B-cell tumors. *Hosp. Pract.*, 20:41-48.
7. Croce, C.M., Isobe, M., Palumbo, A., Puck, J., Ming, J., Tweardy, D., Erikson, J., Davis, M., and Rovera, G. (1985): Gene for α-chain of human T-cell receptor: location on chromosome 14 region involved in T-cell neoplasms. *Science*, 227:1044-1047.
8. Dalla-Favera, R., Bregni, M., Erikson, J., Patterson, D., Gallo, R.C. and Croce, C.M. (1982): Human c-myc onc gene is located on the region of chromosome 8 that is translocated in Burkitt lymphoma cells. *Proc. Natl. Acad. Sci. USA*, 79:7824-7827.
9. Dalla-Favera, R., Martinotti, S., Gallo, R.C., Erikson, J., Croce, C.M. (1983): Translocation and rearrangements of the c-myc oncogene locus in human undifferentiated B-cell lymphomas. *Science*, 219:963-967.
10. Desiderio, S. and Baltimore, D. (1984): Double-stranded cleavage by cell extracts near recombinational signal sequences of immuglobulin genes. *Nature*, 308:860-862.
11. Gatti, R.A., Aurias, A., Griscelli, C., and Sparkes, R.S. (1985): Defective DNA rearrangement in ataxia-telangiectasia: an experiment of nature. Submitted for publication.
12. Gelmann, E.P., Psallidopoulos, M.C., Papas, t.S., and Favera, R.D. (1983): Identification of reciprocal trnaslocation sites within the c-myc oncogene and immunoglobulin μ locus in a Burkitt lymphoma. *Nature*, 306:799-803.
13. Giallongo, A., Appella, E., Ricciardi, R., Rovera, G., Croce, C.M. (1983): Identification of the c-myc oncogene product in normal and malignant B cells. *Science*, 222:430-432.
14. Giorgi, J. (1985): Personal communication.
15. Goodman, W.N., Cooper, W.C., Kessler, G.B., Rishcer, M.D. and Gardner, M.B. (1969): Ataxia-telangiectasia. A report of two cases in siblings presenting a picture of progressive spinal muscular atrophy. *Bull. L. A. Neurol. Soc.*, 34:1-22.
16. Harneden, D.G. (1974): Ataxia-telangiectasia syndrome: cytogenetic and cancer aspects. In: *Chromosomes and Cancer*, edited by J. German, pp. 619-636, Wiley, New York.
17. Hecht, F., McCaw, B.K., and Koler, R.D. (1973): Ataxia-telangiectasia-clonal growth of translocation lymphocytes. *N. Engl. J. Med.*, 289:286-291.
18. Hecht, F., Morgan, R., Hecht, R.K.M., and Smith, S.D. (1984): Common region on chromosome 14 in T-cell leukemia and lymphoma. *Science*, 226:1445-1447.
19. Humphries, S.E., Imam, A.M.A., Robbins, T.P., Cook, M., Carrit, B., Ingles, C., and Williamson, R. (1985): The identification of DNA polymorphism of the fibrinogen gene, and the regional assignment of the human fibrinogen genes to 4q26-qter. (in press).
20. Kirsch, I.R., Ravetch, J.V., Kwan, S.P., Max, E.E., Ney, R.L., and Leder, P. (1981): Multiple immunoglobulin switch region homologies outside the heavy chain constant region locus. *Nature*, 293:585-587.
21. Kirsch, I.R., Morton, C.C., Nakahara, K., and Leder, P. (1982): Human immunoglobulin heavy chain genes map to a region of translocations in malignant B lymphocytes. *Science*, 216:301-303.

22. Kjeldsberg, C.R., Head, D.R., Kadin, M., Pick, T., and Bybee, B. (1985): Childhood pleomorphic T-cell malignancy resembling ATLL. (in press).
23. Klein, G. (1981): The role of gene dosage and genetic transpositions in carcinogenesis. *Nature*, 294:313-318.
24. Knudson, A.G., Jr. (1977): Genetics and Etiology of Human Cancer. In: *Advances in Human Genetics*, edited by H. Harris and K. Hirschhorm, pp. 1-66. Plenum Press, New York.
25. Kohn, P.H., Whang-Peng, J., and Levis, W.R. (1982): Chromosomal instability in ataxia-telangiectasia. *Can. Genet. Cytogenet.*, 6:289-302.
26. Kunkel, L.M., Smith, K.D., Boyer, S.H., Borgaoknar, D.S., Wachtel, S.S., Miller, O.J., Breg, W.R., Jones, J.W., Jr., and Rary, J.M. (1977): Analysis of human Y-chromosome-specific reiterated DNA in chromosome variants. *Proc. Natl. Acad. Sci. USA* 74(3):1245-1249.
27. Levitt, R., Pierre, R.V., White, W.L., and Siekert, R.G. (1978): Atypical lymphoid leukemia in ataxia-telangiectasia. *Blood*, 52:1003-1011.
28. McCaw, B.K., Hecht, F., Harnden, D.G., and Teplitz, R.L. (1975): Somatic rearrangement of chromosome 14 in human lymphocytes. *Proc. Natl. Acad. Sci. USA*, 72:2071-2075.
29. Mercola, M., Wang, X., Olsen, J., and Calame, K. (1983): Transcriptional enhancer elements in the mouse immunoglobulin heavy chain locus. *Science*, 221:663-665.
30. Mercola, M., Goverman, J., Mirell, C., and Calame, K. (1985): Immunoglobulin heavy-chain enhancer requires one or more tissue-specific factors. *Science*, 227:266-270.
31. Migone, N., Feder, J., Cann, H., West, B., Hwang, J., Takahashi, N., Honjo, T., Piazza, A., and Sforza, C.L.L. (1983): Multiple DNA fragment polymorphisms associated with immunoglobulin μ chain switch-like regions in man *Proc. Natl. Acad. Sci. USA*, 80:467-471.
32. Oxford, J.M., Harnden, D.G., Parrington, J.M., and Delhanty, J.D.A. (1975): Specific chromosome aberrations in ataxia-telangiectasia. *J. Med. Genet.*, 12:251-262.
33. Rabbitts, T.H., Forster, A., and Milstein, C.P. (1981): Human immunoglobulin heavy chain genes: evolutionary comparisons of Cμ, Cδ and Cγ genes associated switch sequences. *Nucleic Acids Res.* 9(19):4509-4524.
34. Rabbitts, T.H., Forster, A., Baer, R., and Hamlyn, P.J. (1983): Transcription enhancer identified near the human Cμ immunoglobulin heavy chain gene is unavailable to the trans-located c-myc gene in a Burkitt lymphoma. *Nature*, 306:806.
35. Ravetch, J.V., Siebenlist, U., Korsmeyer, S., et al. (1981): Structure of human immunoglobulin μ locus: characterization of embryonic and rearranged J and D genes. *Cell*, 27:583-591.
36. Saxon, A., Stevens, R.H., and Golde, D.W. (1979): Helper and suppressor T-lymphocyte leukaemia in ataxia-telangiectasia. *New Engl. J. Med.*, 300:700-704.
37. Sparkes, R.S., Como, R., and Golde, D.W. (1980): Cytogenetic abnormalities in ataxia-telangiectasia with T-cell chronic lymphocytic leukemia. *Can. Genet. Cytogenet.*, 1:329-336.
38. Takahashi, N., Nakai, S., and Honjo, T. (1980): Cloning of human immunoglobulin μ gene and comparison with mouse μ gene. *Nucleic Acids Res.*, 8(24):5983-5991.
39. Taub, R., Kirsch, I., Morton, C., Lenoir, G., Swan, D., Tronick, S., Aaronson, S., and Leder, P. (1982): Translocation of the c-myc gene into the immunoglobulin heavy chain locus in human Burkitt lymphoma and murine plasmacytoma cells. *Proc. Natl. Acad. Sci. USA*, 79:7837-7841.
40. Taylor, K.M., Francke, U., Brown, M.G., George, D.L., and Kaufhold, M. (1977): Inverted tandem ("mirror") duplications in human chromosomes: inv dup 8p, 4q, 22q. *Amer. J. Med. Genet.*, 1:3-19.
41. Ueshima, Y., Rowley, J.D., Variakojus, D., Winter, J., and Gordon, L. (1984): Cytogenetic studies on patients with chronic T-cell leukemia/lymphoma, *Blood*, 63(5):1028-1038.
42. Zech, L., Gahrton, G., Hammarstrom, L., Juliusoon, G., Mellstedt, H., Robert, K.H., and Smith, C.I.E. (1984): Inversion of chromosome 14 marks human T-cell chronic lymphocytic leukaemia. *Nature*, 308:858-860.
43. Zech, L., Hammarstrom, L., and Smith, C.I.E. (1983): Chromosomal aberrations in a case of T-cell CLL with concomitant IgA myeloma. *Cancer*, 32:431-435.

The Molecular Basis of Ig Deficiencies

O. Carbonara, N. Migone, S. Oliviero and M. De Marchi

Istituto di Genetica Medica, Università di Torino, e CNR Centro Immunogenetica ed Istocompatibilità, Via Santena, 19, 10126 Torino, Italy

INTRODUCTION

Organization of the immunoglobulin heavy chain (IgCH) genes as a cluster of repeated multiple sequences was first suggested by studies with immunogenetic markers (14, 20) and has recently been confirmed at the DNA level (4, 5, 25). Recurrence of unequal crossing-over events has led to both amplification through gene duplication and contraction through gene deletion (7).

This fluctuation in gene number is also present in the lambda light chain gene cluster on chromosome 22 (26). In the IgCH region, it is rendered more evident by the occasional observations of subjects with lack (or duplication) of some Ig isotypes (10, 14, 15, 20), or with hybrid Ig molecules in their serum (8). In the most common types of immunodeficiency, however, both the genetic and the immunological evidence suggests that other mechanisms not controlled by the IgCH region are involved (15, 24, 27). Apart from Bruton type agammaglobulinemia. with its clear X-linked inheritance, therefore, the familial picture in even the more common selective IgA deficiencies points to segregation independent of Gm allotypes (14, 15). Moreover, investigation of lymphocyte subpopulations after in vitro induction has shown expression of IgA in keeping with an immunoregulatory defect rather than structural gene abnormalities (7, 27). Our molecular investigations of Ig deficiencies in healthy and diseased subjects and their families are here reviewed.

MATERIALS AND METHODS

Subjects

1) Healthy blood donors (n=13770) and selected groups of patients (Celiac Disease (CD) n=140, Insulin Dependent Diabetes Mellitus (IDDM) n=80, various dermatological disorders n= 5625) were screened for IgA1 and/or IgA2 deficiency by an immunoenzymatic assay adjusted to reveal levels of

either IgA subclass higher than 1 μg/ml. Whenever possible, the first-degree relatives of the immunodeficient patients (index cases) were also investigated.

2) A few families were referred independently on the basis of multiple cases of IgA deficiency, associated in one with SLE and in another with pyoderma gangrenosum (3).

3) Randomly selected two — and three — generation families were analyzed during a genetic study of the new restriction fragment length polymorphisms (RFLPs) associated with the switch sequences of the IgCH region defined by one of us (17).

Direct gene analysis of the IgCH region was performed by means of Southern blotting, using genomic probes for the α, γ, and ε structural genes and for the switch sequences, as previously reported (17, 18).

RESULTS

The examples of IgA deficiency found in each group, must be analyzed separately for correct estimation of the respective frequencies.

In group 1, the deficiency of both isotypes in blood donors had a frequency of 0.17%, comparable with that of the literature (24), and a higher frequency (5.3%) in CD and (5.0%) in IDDM. As will be reported in detail elsewhere (3), the main features of this group were: i) presence of low levels of IgA by sensitive RIA test in 50%; ii) anti-α isotype and allotype antibodies in some of those with the lowest IgA levels; iii) no gross abnormality in the IgCH region detected at the DNA levels; iv) association with HLA B14 and B8 (relative risk 5.6 and 2.8 respectively) in blood donors; this was difficult to demonstrate in CD and IDDM, because of the HLA association of these diseases per se; in both cases, however, the IgA deficient patients belonged to the DR3 positive group, suggesting a common susceptibility role of DR3 for both autoimmunity and IgA deficiency.

Multiple case families with deficiency of both IgA subclasses appeared to have a relatively lower frequency and/or to be associated with clinical symptoms, since they were only represented in group 2, and not in any of the first degree relatives of group 1 probands. In two families such deficiency segregated independently from Gm allotypes; studies at the DNA level merely confirmed this, by showing segregation of IgCH RFLPs in agreement with the Gm haplotypes, and the presence of regular bands for both the structrural genes and the switch regions.

Thanks to the use of anti-subclass antisera, rarer individuals with IgA1 deficiency and normal IgA2 levels were occasionally found. Two of them (SAF and FRO, Ref. 18) also showed the absence of IgG2 and IgG4, and one (SAF) of IgE as well. Direct gene analysis of their family members with different DNA probes does not reveal extensive deletions in the IgCH region: proband SAF was homozygous for a deletion encompassing Cα1, ψγ, Cγ2, Cγ4 and Cε (Type I deletion, Fig. 1); proband FRO carried two different deletions: in one chromosome the same type as above, and in the other chromosome a deletion of ψε, Cα1, ψγ, Cγ2 and Cγ4 (Type II deletion, Fig. 1). As expected,

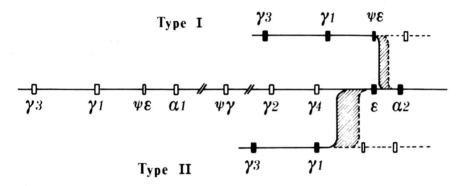

FIG. 1. Schematic representation of unequal homologous cross-over that could account for the deletions of C region genes observed in SAF (Type I) and FRO (Types I and II) families.

all their children were heterozygous for the deletion, as revealed by half intensity signals of the relevant bands (18), but phenotypically showed normal levels of IgA1, IgG2, IgG4 and IgE.

In the third family selective IgA2 deficiency was present in a mother and one of three children (1, 16). The combined serological Gm markers and RFLPs findings did not completely rule out linkage with the IgCH region, but made it very unlikely. Since the blotting patterns did not reveal any abnormality, either point mutations in coding or non-coding sequences of the α-2 gene, or, more likely, a genetic control outside the IgCH region may be assumed.

Group 3 was investigated by means of a μ-switch probe, to analyze the segregation of allelic fragments of at least four IgCH-linked polymorphic loci, three of which map near or within the μ-, α1-, and α2- switch sequences respectively (17, 19). All these switch regions share a high sequence homology based on the content of highly repeated pentanucleotides (2, 21-23). In stringent hybridization conditions, the μ-switch probe cross-hybridizes with the homonymous γ- and ε- regions. The presence of both deleted and duplicated switch- containing fragments was occasionally suggested by the abnormal intensity of a few allelic fragments (Fig. 2).

Within switch α2, whose instability has been shown to be the actual mechanism for the generation of duplication/deletion of "allelic" fragments, a "null" variant lacking almost all α2- switch sequences has been described (17). Analysis of this large family showed five heterozygotes for such deleted haplotypes (Fig. 2).

Nine unrelated subjects showed an unbalanced intensity signal between allelic switch α1- containing segments. DNA analysis of two of them with six addition restriction enzymes strongly suggested that one of their chromosomes

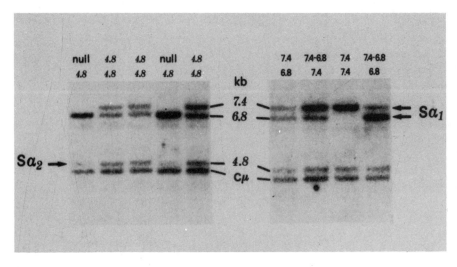

FIG. 2. Southern hybridization of the switch μ probe and Cμ gene to Sst I digested DNA, samples, from families carrying deletions (left panel) or duplications (right panel) of the S-α2 and S-α1 containing fragments respectively. The genotypes at the S-α2 and Sα1 polymorphic "loci" derived by family analysis are indicated at the top of the panels, with the length of the respective fragments in Kb. (The Cμ containing, not discussed here, migrates at 4.4. Kb). The half-intensity signal at the 4.8 Kb position is present in two sisters (lane 1 and 4, left panel) and suggest a "null" S-α2 "allele". Lane 2, 3, and 5 are normal relatives. In the right panel (lane 2 and 4 one parent and her son) a duplicated S-α1 containing haplotype is shown by the unbalanced intensity between allelic fragments compared to a normal heterozygote (lane 1, one parent) or a homozygote (lane 3, a daughter). Segregation analysis on three generations confirmed the genotype reported at top of the figure.

might be carrying a very large DNA duplication spanning several thousands kilobases (kb) (including at least the ψε and α1 genes). Seven out of nine of these duplicated chromosomes carried a different combination of allotypic and/or DNA polymorphic markers, indicating that they were originated by independent events.

DISCUSSION

As in many other fields of human pathology, the introduction of molecular investigations has thrown new light on the study of immunodeficiencies. Thus, a distinct though rare condition due to deletion of Ig structural genes has thus been characterized within the heterogeneous group of immunoglobulin deficiencies. The few reported cases, despite their diversity, are all marked by involvement of several Ig isotypes without overt clinical symptoms. Two Tunisian Berber families reported by Lefranc et al. (11, 12, deletions type *j* and *s* in Fig. 3) and our two Italian families (type I = *p*, type II = *o*) carry on both IgCH haplotypes extensive deletions exist, though they are undetectable by immulogical screening. Their direct identification at the DNA level would

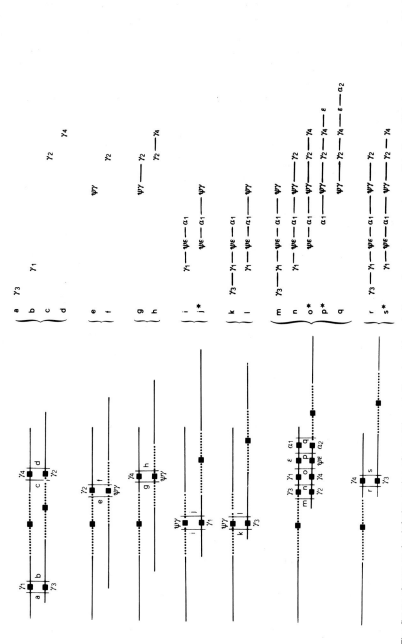

FIG. 3. The figure shows to the left the series of possible meiotic mispairings between homologous regions within the IgCH cluster, together with the schematical location of unequal recombinations, relatively to the IgCH gene map: ahead and behind each mispaired gene. For simplicity intragenic unequal recombination have been omitted, though these events may be expected with a similar frequency to those listed. The genes expected to be deleted or duplicated following each crossover are reported to the right: the asterisks indicate deleted haplotypes whose existence has recently been confirmed by DNA analysis. Deletions j and s ref. 11, 12; deletions p and o ref. 18.

hardly be conceivable in random subjects, due to the unreliable comparison of band intensity between unrelated individuals. An indirect estimate, based on the frequency of the homozygous genotype, and on the assumption of Hardy-Weinberg equilibrium, gives a figure of 1-3% heterozygous carriers of IgCH deletions, including the α1 gene. In the group of random families (group 3), cases with mendelian segregation of unbalanced band intensity ratios, suggesting duplication or deletion of different IgCH segments, were indeed detected; it is interesting to note that their frequency fulfills the requirements of a genetic polymorphism as usually defined (7).

On theoretical grounds, a large number of different, unequal crossing-over types, leading to duplication/deletion of a varying number of genes, can be predicted on the assumption of mispairing between the most homologous regions (Fig. 3, *a* to *s*). This could be verified by immological screening for deficiencies of the Ig isotypes in homozygotes or compound heterozygotes. Moreover, other types of deletions may derive from the instability of the S-sequences (2, 21-23). In our experience, a single instance of deletion of the S-α2 was found, in the heterozygous state, in a healthy random family; for this reason, we could not determine whether, in the homozygous state, this would result in lack of α2 gene expression. Since all the reported homozygotes with Ig deficiencies have deletions of the structural genes, this mechanism would be exceptional, though not impossible.

Acknowledgements

We are indebted to Dr. T. Honjo for the gift of the γ, α2 and Switch-μ probes; to Dr. T. Rabbitts for the ε probe; to Prof. J. P. Vaerman and Dr. D. Delacroix for the anti-IgA1 and -IgA2 reagents; to Dr. Erna van Loghem and Gerda deLange for Gm and A2m typing; to Dr. E.J.E.G. Bast for the samples of IgA2 deficiency; to Mrs. Cleide Boccazzi for excellent technical assistance.

Work supported in part by CNR Progetto Finalizzato «Ingegneria genetica e Basi molecolari delle malattie ereditarie» and MPI 40% and 60%.

REFERENCES

1. Carbonara, A.O., Oliviero, S., Bast, E.J.E.G., Loghem, E. van, De Marchi, M. (1985): Direct gene analysis in a familial case of IgA2 deficiency. *in preparation*.
2. Davis, M.M., Kim, S.K., and Hood, L.E. (1980): DNA sequences mediating class switching in α-immunoglobulins. *Science*, 209:1360-1365.
3. De Marchi, M., Contu, L., Boccazzi, C., Migone, N., Oliviero, S., Delacroix, D., Carbonara, A.O. Immunogenetic and molecular analysis of IgA deficiency. (submitted).
4. Ellison, J., and Hood, L. (1982): Linkage and sequence homology of two human immunoglobulin γ heavy chain constant region genes. Proc. Natl. Sci. USA, 79:1984-1988.
5. Flanagan, J.G., and Rabbitts, T.H. (1982): Arrangement of human immunoglobulin heavy chain constant region genes implies evolutionary duplication of a segment containing γ, ε and α genes. *Nature*, 300:709-713.
6. Ford, E.B. (1965): *Genetic polyporphism*. Faber and Faber, London.
7. Hood, L., Campbell, J.H., and Elgin, S.C.R. (1975): The organization, expression, and evolution of antibody genes and other multigene families. *Ann. Rev. Genet.* 14:305-353.

8. Kunkel, H.G., Natvig, J.B. and Joslin, F.G. (1969): A "Lepore" type of hybrid γ-globulin. *Proc. Natl. Acad. Sci. USA* 62:144-149.
9. Lawton, A.R., Royal, S.A., Self, S. and Cooper, M.D. (1972): IgA determinant on B-lymphocytes in patients with deficiency of circulating IgA. *J. Lab. Clin. Med.* 80:26-33.
10. Lefranc, G., Dumitresco, M., Salier, J.P., Rivat, L., De Lange, G., Loghem, Erna va., and Loiselet, J. (1979): Familial lack of the IgG3 subclass. Gene elimination or turning off expression and neutral evolution in the immune system. *J. Immunogenet.*, 6:215-221.
11. Lefranc, M.P., Lefranc, G., and Rabbitts, T.H. (1982): Inherited deletion of immunoglobulin heavy chain costant region genes in normal human individuals. *Nature*, 300:760-762.
12. Lefranc, G., Chaabani, H., Loghem, Erna van, Lefranc, M.P., De Lange, G. and Helal, A.N. (1983): Simultaneous absence of the human IgG1, IgG2, IgG4 and IgA1 subclasses: immunological and immunogenetical consideration. *Eur. J. Immunol.*, 13:240-244.
13. Lefranc, M.P., Lefranc, G., De Lange, G., Out, T.A., den Broek, P.J. van, Nieuwkoop, J. van, Radl, J., Helal, A.N., Chaabani, H., Loghem, E. van, Rabbitts, T.H. (1983): Instability of the human immunoglobulin heavy chain constant region locus indicated by different inherited chromosomal deletions. *Mol. Biol. Med.*, 1:207-217.
14. Loghem, E. van (1974): La genetique des immunoglobulines A. *Ann. Immunol. (Inst. Pasteur)*, 125 C, 57-62.
15. Loghem, E. van (1974): Familial occurrence of isolated IgA deficiency associated with antibodies to IgA. Evidence against structural gene defect. *Eur. J. Immunol.*, 4:57-60.
16. Loghem, E. van, Zegers, J.M., Bast, E.J.E.G. and Kater, L. (1984): Selective deficiency of Immunoglobulin A2. *J. Clin. Invest.*, 72:1918-1923.
17. Migone, N., Feder, J., Cann, H., West, B. van, Hwang, J., Takahashi, N., Honjo, T., and Piazza, A. (1983): Multiple DNA fragment polymorphisms associated with immunoglobulin μ chain switch-like regions in man. *Proc. Natl. Acad. Sci. USA.* 80:467-471.
18. Migone, N., Oliviero, S., De Lange, G., Delacroix, D.L., Boschis, D., Altruda, F., Silengo, L., De Marchi, M. and Carbonara, A.O. (1984): Multiple gene deletions within the human immunoglobulin heavy-chain cluster. *Proc. Natl. Acad. Sci. USA,* 81:5811-5815.
19. Migone, N., De Lange, G., Piazza, A. and Cavalli Sforza, L.L. (1985): Genetic analysis of eight linked polymorphisms within human IgH region. *submitted.*
20. Natvig, J.B. and Kunkel, H.G. (1973): Human immunoglobulins: classes, subclasses, genetic variants and idiotypes. *Adv. Immunol.*, 16:1-59.
21. Nikaido, T., Nakai, S. and Honjo, T. (1981): Switch region of immunoglobulin Cμ gene is composed of simple tandem repetitive sequences. *Nature*, 292:845-848.
22. Rabbitts, T.H., Forster, A. and Milstein, C.P. (1981): Human immunoglobulin heavy chain genes: evolutionary comparisons of C, C and C genes and associated switch sequences. *Nucleic Acids Res.*, 9:4509-4524.
23. Ravetch, J.V., Kirsch, I.R., Leder, P. (1980): Evolutionary approach to the question of immunoglobulin heavy chain switching: Evidence from cloned human and mouse genes. *Proc. Natl. Acad. Sci. USA*, 77:6734-6738.
24. Rosen, S.R., Cooper, M.D. and Wedgwood, R.J.P. (1984): The primary immunodeficiencies. *New Engl. J. Med.*, 311:235-242; 300-310.
25. Takahashi, N., Ueda, S., Obata, M., Nikaido, T., Nakai, S. and Honjo, T. (1982): Structure of human immunoglobulin gamma genes: implications for evolution of a gene family. *Cell*, 29:671-679.
26. Taub, R.A., Hollis, G.F., Hieter, P.A., Korsmeyer, S., Waldmann, T.A. and Leder, P. (1983): Variable amplification of immunoglobulin light-chain genes in human populations. *Nature*, 304:172-174.
27. Waldmann, T.A. and Broder, S. (1977): Suppressor cells in the regulation of immune response. In: *Progress in Clinical Immunology*, edited by R. Schwartz. Grune Stratton, Inc. New York. 3:155-199.

Assessment of the Humoral Immune Response in Immunodeficiencies

Ralph J. Wedgwood, M.D.* and Hans D. Ochs, M.D.*

*Department of Pediatrics RD-20, School of Medicine,
University of Washington,
Seattle, WA 98195, USA

In the final analysis, the assessment of the humoral immune response requires examination of antibody formation: the entire process that is initiated by the presentation of antigen through the establishment of immunologic memory and the fully mature expression of antibody production with isotype switch. While measurements of immunoglobulin concentrations, even with the inclusion of immunoglobulin subclasses and age specific standards may be informative, they are not in themselves sufficient. Normal immunoglobulins do not exclude defective antibody formation. The same caution must be extended to the enumeration of B lymphocyte by any of various markers. While the absence of B lymphocytes is informative, their presence does not exclude a functional impairment. The most recent report for the WHO (12) recommended the assessment of antibody formation by three general types of tests: (a) the measurement of "natural" antibodies such as A and B isohemagglutinins, heteroagglutinins or heterolysins (for example, those against sheep or rabbit erythrocytes), antistreptolysins, or bactericidal antibodies against Escherichia coli; (b) the antibody responses to usual immunization, such as the response to diphtheria/tetanus toxoid or killed poliomyelitis vaccine; (c) or active immunization against unusual antigens, such as bacteriophage ØX 174, polyribose phosphate Hemophilus influenza polysaccharide (except in infants under the age of one year), monomeric flagellin, pneumococcal polysaccharide, Vi antigen and Keyhole Limpet Hemocyanin (KLH). Of these only two (bacteriophage ØX 174 and KLH) are sufficiently rare as to provide a secure assessment of the primary as well as the secondary response. Since abnormality may be more clearly demonstrable in the primary than the secondary response, the distinction may well be important. Furthermore, with the more common antigens, the variance of prior exposure or dosage may mask abnormality; persons with multiple prior exposure or larger amounts of antigen are far more likely to produce antibody, including IgG antibody. Insensitive assays may suggest normality in persons where more sensitive assessment can demonstrate clearly that there is in fact an immune defect.

For the past twenty years our laboratory has been involved with the assessment of the humoral immune response in man by use of bacteriophage ∅X 174 as the antigen. We have over these years quantitated the responses of hundreds of persons. The experience has demonstrated that it is a safe, potent and useful antigen; and that the assay provides a uniquely sensitive assessment of the humoral immune response.

The 'phage is a single stranded DNA virus; a dodecahedron of about 250 A diameter; its molecular weight around 3×10^6 (14). The protein coat appears to be made up of 180 identical sub-units, a symmetry that may account for its unusual antigenicity, its specificity and the precision found in assay for antibody (9). The specific host strain of bacteria is E. coli C.

For use as an antigen the 'phage is grown and purified by the method of Uhr (15). It is sterilized by filtration through a millipore filter and tested for sterility, pyrogenicity, and antigenicity in accord with FDA regulations. We use a final concentration of 10^{11} pfu/ml: the final protein concentration is about 0.050 mgm/ml. 'Phage is assayed by a standard plaque forming technique. Antibody is determined by a neutralization assay, and is expressed by the rate of 'phage inactivation: the assumption of first order kinetics has been shown to hold if less than 90% of the 'phage is inactivated (9). To assess the relative contribution of IgM and IgG antibody we use 2-mercaptoethanol (5) which we have found to agree reasonably with gel filtration (10). 2-ME sensitive antibody is considered to be IgM, 2-ME resistant antibody to be IgG. While in absolute terms differences in affinity between the two classes of antibody could affect the relative proportions, for purposes of comparison between patients the distinction is sufficient.

The antigen in virtually all normal humans appears to be a true "neoantigen". Pre-existing antibody — that is, antibody before immunization — is rarely found (<3%). In patients with disease we have recently found two exceptions to this general rule: a significant number of persons with active EBV infection (8) and children with juvenile rheumatoid arthritis (6) have low levels of neutralizing antibody prior to immunization. This appear most probably to be due to polyclonal activation. It is perhaps of interest that from the ontogenetic viewpoint bacteriophage ∅X 174 is one of the earliest antigens to which the sheep fetus can respond (13). If the same position holds for man, then in the process of polyclonal activation this antibody might be one of the first expressed.

The antigen is given intravenously at a dose of 2×10^9 pfu/kg. Both the dose and the route are critical for the evaluation of the response (11). Alternate routes or larger doses may obscure distinctions between normal and abnormal responses. The initial volume of distribution is the vascular space. After about 24 hours, rapid clearance of the antigen begins and is generally complete by four days. The clearance appears to be entirely immune clearance; in patients with X-linked agammaglobulinemia who make no antibody, the antigen persist disappearing at the same rate as the biological decay of the 'phage at 37°C (3). When clearance is complete antibody can demonstrated, reaching a peak at about two weeks. This primary response, which reflects a thousand-fold increase in antibody activity over the initial level after clearance, is generally entirely IgM. This serum antibody then gradually decreases slightly over the next four weeks and during this time in some persons small amounts of IgG antibody activity can be found. A secondary immunization, at the same dose and route, is given at six weeks. A rapid response, essentially immediate, is found which peaks at 1 week, with levels usually 2- to 3-fold higher than the peak primary response. The antibody activity at the peak of the secondary response is on average more than 50% IgG. Thus memory, amplification and isotype switch are demonstrable.

The full response is T cell dependent. For man this can be nicely demonstrable in patients with the Third/Fourth Arch, Rudimentary Thymus Syndromes. The response is not entirely ablated, but the primary response is markedly (10- to 100-fold) reduced. The secondary response is likewise diminished and the isotype switch is absent, or incomplete. Thus the T cell dependence is reflected in both the primary and the secondary response.

The full expression of the response appears also possibly to be a sensitive indicator for allogeneic restriction of the interacting cells — as discussed later, presumably macrophage-T cell identity. Patients receiving syngeneic bone marrow transplants demonstrate earlier and more complete immunologic reconstitution when tested with this antigen than patients receiving allogeneic grafts (4): patients with haplo-identical grafts who have minimal GVHD have earlier and more complete recovery of response than patients with more severe GVHD (16). The primary and the secondary response, particularly the isotype switch, is affected.

One can also demonstrate the modulation of the response by the complement (C3b) and the C3 receptor. This was first brought to our attention by studies on a boy with C4 deficiency (7). Subsequent studies in other patients have shown a similar abnormality in patients with deficiency of the second and third, but not subsequent components of the classic pathway. In guinea pigs we have shown that the abnormal humoral immune response can be corrected by restoration of the missing complement component at the time of induction of the primary response. Complement does not appear to be required at the time of the secondary once the primary has been effectively established (11). We have found a similar abnormality of the response to bacteriophage ØX 174 in patients with a glycoprotein membrane defect of their white cells (2) which involves the receptor for C3bi.

Thus the use of this antigen has permitted us to show that in man, as in experimental animals, the initiation of the primary response is critical to the subsequent expression of the secondary response. And that the effective induction of the primary response involves the interaction of complement and (presumably) histocompatible macrophages as well as T and B lymphocytes.

This accords with generally accepted views for the initiation of the humoral immune response based on animal studies, and indicates that this antigen can be used to identify the full range of interacting components in the response. It thus has utility beyond its use in defects involving B lymphocytes alone and permits evaluation of the many factors that regulate the amplitude and the expression of humoral immunity, and some of the factors that enter into the establishment of the isotype switch in this response.

It would be predicted under these circumstances that the response to the antigen would be sensitive to modulation by factors other than those usually associated with humoral immunity. One such is sex. In females the primary response and to a lesser degree the secondary response are greater than that for males. Similarly, we have been able to quantitate a transient diminution of immune function during infectious mononucleosis (8).

Thus the use of bacteriophage ØX 174 antigen has proven in our hands to be an extraordinarily useful tool for the in vivo examination of the humoral immune response in normal and immunodeficient persons, as well as animals. Perhaps fortuitously, the route, dose and timing of the immunizations, as well as the nature of the antigen and the sensitivity of the assay permit demonstration of not only B cell function but also of the regulatory factors which modulate that function.

Because of these findings we have more recently turned our attention to the use of the antigen to examine in vitro antibody sinthesis. For these studies (1) we took peripheral blood lymphocytes from normal human volunteers at intervals after primary and secondary immunization with the bacteriophage and assessed in vitro antibody formation, both in the absence and in the presence of antigen. Shortly following immunization cells appeared in the peripheral blood which spontaneously, in the absence of added antigen, synthesized antibody in culture. The class of antibody was identical to that found in the serum. The amounts of antibody synthesized were small, but significant. The spontaneously formed antibody in vitro peaked at about the same time as that in vivo. The function was inhibited by puromycin and irradiation, and thus presumably represented de novo synthesis. Spontaneous antibody production was independent of T cells and occured within the first 36-72 hours of culture. Cells spontaneously synthesizing antibody in vitro were only found in recently immunized subjects. Spontaneous in vitro antibody synthesis was not found, for example, 90 days or more after immunization.

Peripheral blood mononuclear cells synthesized significantly more antibody after immunization if antigen was added to the culture. The amounts were at least 10-fold higher than the spontaneous antibody formation. Again, the peak of in vitro antigen induced antibody formation matched that found in vivo. But antigen induced in vitro antibody formation persisted for months, and even years after immunization. Initially, both after the primary and secondary immunization, the antibody induced in vitro by antigen was IgM. Indeed, IgM antibody appeared in the antigen induced system in vitro at times when the in vivo antibody was primarily IgG. Presumably the B cells that have undergone isotype switch home first in the lymphoid organs, and only later appear in the circulation. It took 3 months or more for in vitro, antigen induced antibody of peripheral blood mononuclear cells to undergo isotype switch to IgG even though in vivo the switch had occurred many weeks before. Once the switch had occurred, antigen induced in vitro antibody formation remained IgG apparently indefinitely. One subject has been followed now for 16 years, and his peripheral blood mononuclear cell still produce IgG antibody in vitro on antigen stimulation. Late after immunization the number of reactive units in the peripheral blood are very few less than 1:10,000. The antigen induced in vitro antibody formation represents de novo synthesis; it is blocked by puromycin and irradiation. It is T cell dependent, and seems to require the presence of macrophages.

To look further into the nature of the in vitro response we have examined in vitro antibody production in identical twins. This minimizes the problems of allogeneic response and non-specific or polyclonal activation. The work is preliminary (Lindgren, Ochs and Wedgwood, work in progress). However, some informative results are appearing. With identical twins we can make mixes of instructed (post-immunization) and uninstructed cells (pre-immunization). We cal also use cells before and after isotype switch. These studies to date suggest that macrophages are required for the in vitro process. Responses using syngeneic T cells and macrophages produce more antibody than allogeneic mixes. However, no match seems to be needed between B cells and T cells, or B cells and macrophages. Instructed T cells, with matched macrophages and antigen can induce instructed B cells to make antibody in large amounts. If the B cells come from subjects prior to isotype switch, the antibody is IgM. If the B cells are derived from subjects after isotype switch, the antibody is IgG. Thus the class of antibody is B cell determined. It may be T cell determined also. There is suggestive, but not conclusive evidence in some experiments that instructed T cells, presented with antigen by macrophages, may induce IgM antibody formation in naive (uninstructed) B cells. We have not, however, been able to induce a full in vitro primary response, using entirely naive cells throughout.

We have now begun to examine our patient population using in vitro antibody formation to assess B cell function and regulation. The technique is far more sensitive than polyclonal activation with pokeweed mitogen, and we believe will be a most useful adjunct to the in vivo assessment of the response to bacteriophage ØX 174.

Acknowledgements

This work was supported by grants from the National Institutes of Health (AI-07073), and from the March of Dimes Birth Defects Foundation (6-273). A portion of this work was conducted through the Clinical Research Center facility at the University of Washington supported by NIH Grant RR-37.

REFERENCES

1. Bohnsack, J., Ochs, H.D., Wedgwood, R.J., Heller, S.R. (1985): Antibody synthesis to bacteriophage ØX 174 by cultured human peripheral blood lymphocytes. *Clin. Exp. Immunol.*, 59:673-678.
2. Bowen, T.J., Wedgwood, R.J., Ochs, H.D., Henle, W. (1983): Transient immunodeficiency during asymptomatic Epstein-Barr virus infection. *Pediatrics,* 71:964-967.
3. Ching, Y.C., Davis, S.D., Wedgwood, R.J. (1971): Immunologic responses to bacteriophage ØX 174 in immunodeficiency diseases. *J. Clin. Invest.* 45:1593-1600.
4. Fass, L., Ochs, H.D., Thomas, E.D., Mickelson, E., Storb, R., Fefer, A. (1973): Studies of immunologic reactivity following syngeneic or allogeneic marrow grafts in man. *Transplantation* 16:630-640.
5. Grubb, R., Swahn, B. (1958): Destruction of some agglutinins but not of others by two sulfhydryl compounds. *Acta. Pathol. Microbiol. Scand.* 43:305-309.
6. Ilowite, N.T., Wedgwood, R.J., Rose, L.M., Clark, E.A., Lindgren, C.G., Ochs, H.D. (1985): Impaired in vivo and in vitro antibody response to bacteriophage ØX 174 in juvenile rheumatoid arthritis (in preparation).
7. Jackson, C.G., Ochs, H.D., Wedgwood, R.J. (1979): The immune response of a patient with deficiency of the fourth component of complement and systemic lupus erythematosus. *N. Engl. J. Med.* 300:1124-1129.
8. Junker, A.K., Clark, E.A., Ochs, H.D., Puterman, M.L., Wedgwood, R.J. (1985): Transient immune deficiency in patients with acute Epstein-Barr virus infection (in preparation).
9. Krummel, W.M., Uhr, J.H.W. (1969): A mathematical and experimental study of the kinetics of the neutralization of bacteriophage ØX 174 by antibodies. *J. Immunol.*, 102:772-785.
10. Ochs, H.D., Davis, S.D., Wedgwood, R.J. (1971): Immunologic responses to bacteriophage ØX 174 in immunodeficiency diseases. *J. Clin. Invest.* 50:2559-2568.
11. Ochs, H.D., Wedgwood, R.J., Frank, M.M., Heller, S.R., Hosea, S.W. (1983): The role of complement in the induction of antibody responses. *Clin. Exp. Immunol.* 53:208-216.
12. Rosen, F.S., Wedgwood, R.J., Aiuti, F., Cooper, M.D., Good, R.A., Hanson, L.A., Hitzig, W.H., Matsumoto, S., Seligmann, M., Soothill, J.F. & Waldmann, T.A. (1983): Meeting Report. Primary Immunodeficiency Diseases. Report prepared for the WHO by a scientific group on immunodeficiency. *Clin. Immunol. Immunopathol.*, 28:450-75.
13. Silverstein, A.M., Parshal, C.J., Uhr, J.W. (1966): Immunologic maturation in utero: kinetics of the primary response in the fetal lamb. *Science* 154:1675-1676.
14. Sinsheimer, R.L. (1939): Purification and properties of bacteriophage ØX 174. *J. Mol. Biol.*:37-42.
15. Uhr, J.W., Finkelstein, M.S., Baumann, J.B. (1962): Antibody formation III. The primary and secondary response to bacteriophage ØX 174 in guinea pigs. *J. Exp. Med.* 115:655-670.
16. Witherspoon, R.P., Storb, R., Ochs, H.D., Flournoy, N. Kopecky, K.J., Sullivan, K.M., Deeg, H.J., Sosa, R., Noel, D.R., Atkinson, K., Thomas, E.D. (1981): Recovery of antibody production in human allogeneic marrow graft recipients: influence of time post-transplantation, the presence or absence of chronic graft-versus-host disease, and antithymocyte globulin treatment. *Blood*, 58:360-368.

Abnormalities of Humoral Immunity Resulting from Immunoregulatory T-cell Dysfunction

Erwind W. Gelfand and Hans-Michael Dosch

Division of Immunology/Rheumatology, Research Institute,
The Hospital for Sick Children, 555 University Avenue, Toronto, Ontario M5G 1X8

The earliest progenitors of immunoglobulin/antibody-secreting cells are identified within the fetal liver and later in ontogeny, amongst the bone marrow cells. Precursor cells give rise to a rapidly dividing population of pre-B cells that produce μ heavy chains detected in the cytoplasm, but not on the cell surface. The next stage of differentiation is comprised of B-cells expressing surface immunoglobulin of the IgM class. Through the process of heavy chain switching, each B-cell becomes committed to production of one of the five main immunoglobulin isotypes (3). Based on the analysis of leukemic cells of B-lineage and cell lines, a developmental hierarchy of immunoglobulin gene rearrangements has been proposed whereby μ heavy chain rearrangement precedes light (ϰ) chain rearrangement and λ light chain rearrangements follows if both ϰ alleles have been deleted. In this model, the sequential rearrangement of genes for Cμ, Cδ, Cγ, Cα and Cε precedes the expression of the respective immunoglobulin class and subclass.

Once B-cells express surface immunoglobulin, they become antigen-responsive. The development of a full complement of antigen-reactive B-cells appears to arise as a result of genetic events and without a major influence, if any, of cells of T-lineage. The response to specific antigen and the synthesis of specific antibody involves cell division and terminal plasma cell differentiation. The generation of specific immune responses involves a complex cascade of restricted interactions between antigen-presenting cells and antigen-specific and non-specific T-cell subpopulations which play a major role in the regulation of the humoral immune response. Helper and suppressor T-cells recognize antigenic determinants directly or presented in the context of class II determinants on antigen presenting cells. They are stimulated to proliferate and differentiate into effector cells, as well as to secrete soluble mediators which, through interaction with other T-cells, B-cells and other cell types, influence antibody responses.

In view of the complex processes, signals and enzymes involved in B-cell differentiation and immunoglobulin synthesis, it is not surprising that abnormalities of normal antibody production occurr. Many of the disorders described are genetic in origin and specific to B-cell maturation; many do not involve obvious abnormalities of cells of T-lineage. It is similarly not surprising that given the delicate balance between effector/helper and regulatory/suppressor cells in the regulation of antibody production, certain antibody deficiency states would result from abnormalities of T-cell immunoregulatory subsets. The study of immunoglobulin production in diseases with T-cell immunoregulatory defects has been important in our understanding of the biology of human T-cell function in normal and antibody deficiency states.

Over the last decade, a number of laboratories have described a variety of humoral immunodeficient states associated with a functional defect of immunoregulatory T-cell subsets, using *in vitro* assays. In the majority, peripheral blood lymphocytes are stimulated to produce immunoglobulin in culture. Immunoglobulin is detected as IgM anti-sheep red blood cell antibody, in a reverse hemolytic plaque assay for all immunoglobulin classes or may be quantitated by radioimmunoassay or ELISA. Such *in vitro* studies have shown that B-cells differentiate into immunoglobulin-secreting cells *in vitro* and that the synthesis of IgG, IgM and IgA is regulated by T lymphocytes. A second system, used extensively in our own laboratory, has been the *in vitro* generation of antigen-specific plaque-forming cells (PFC) and the demonstration of circulating T-cells in patients, which can suppress the PFC (6). Such circulating suppressor T-cells are reminiscent of the findings in bursectomized chickens where transplantable suppressor T-cells, when injected into normal chickens, render them agammaglobulinemic (1).

In this review, examples of human diseases characterized by abnormal immunoglobulin production and which appear to involve excessive or deficient T-helper and T-suppressor cell activities are discussed (Table 1). The list is not complete and particular attention is paid to only a very few. Nevertheless, they provide a framwork for understanding immunoregulatory abnormalities in man and serve as a stimulus for devising new strategies for therapy.

A. PRIMARY DISORDERS

Failure of T-cell help

Abnormalities of Blocks of T-cell Differentiation. The best example of a disease in this category is severe combined immunodeficiency disease (SCID). The demonstration of circulating B-cells in normal or elevated number in many of these patients argues against the concept of a primary stem cell defect (16). In the presence of functional T-cells, SCID B-cells can generate

TABLE 1. *Abnormalities of Humoral Immunity Secondary to T-cell Immunoregulatory Dysfunction*

A. Primary Disorders
  1. Failure of T-Cell Help
    a) Abnormalities of T-cell differentiation, e.g., SCID
    b) Transient hypogammaglobulinemia of infancy
    c) Congenital agammaglobulinemia
    d) Common variable immunodeficiency
  2. Excess T-Cell Help
  3. Absence of T-Suppressor Cell Activity
    a) Nucleoside phosphorylase deficiency
    b) Atopic dermatitis
  4. Excess T-Suppressor Cell Activity
    a) Cord blood
    b) Common variable immunodeficiency
    c) Congenital agammaglobulinemia
    d) IgA deficiency

B. Secondary Disorders
  1. Failure of T-Cell Help
    a) AIDS
    b) Post bone marrow transplant
    c) Drugs
  2. Excess T-Cell Help
    a) Mucocutaneous lymph node syndrome
  3. Absence of T-Suppressor Cell Activity
    a) Autoimmune disorders
    b) Myasthenia gravis
  4. Excess T-Suppressor Cell Activity
    a) Graft-versus-host disease
    b) Infectious mononucleosis
    c) Drugs

normal Ig responses as specific antibodies *in vitro* (5). The failure of B-cell function in these patients appears to be secondary to a lack of T-cell help which in some of these patients is due to abnormal thymus epithelial cell function. *In vitro* and *in vivo*, restoration of T-cell help and immunoglobulin and antibody production followed provision of normal thymus epithelial cells (5, 14, 15, 20).

Transient Hypogammaglobulinemia of Infancy. Siegel et al. have demonstrated normal B-cell numbers and B-cell function in these patients, whereas their T-cells are deficient in the ability to generate help for immunoglobulin synthesis (33). The deficiency in T-helper activity is associated with a reduced number of circulating T4 cells. With resolution of their disease, the abnormalities disappear.

Congenital or Common Variable Immunodeficiency. Failure of T-cell help has been suggested in a few patients.

Excess T-cell help

To our knowledge, there have been no known primary disorders described in man.

Absence or failure of T-suppressor activity

Nucleoside Phosphorylase Deficiency. Deficiency or purine nucleoside phosphorylase (PNP) was first described in 1975 in a child presenting with an isolated deficiency of T-cell immunity (18). Since them, more than 12 patients have been described with this deficiency. The pattern of T-cell deficiency is rather selective, with what appears to be a deficiency of T-suppressor cell activity (Table 2) manifesting with heightened antibody responses, monoc lonal immunoglobulins and autoimmunity.

TABLE 2.   *T-Cell-Dependent Functions in PNP Deficiency*

Present	Absent or decreased
Pre-thymic and post-thymic T-precursor cells	Lymphocyte count
	Proliferative responses
T-helper cell function	Delayed hypersensitivity
Normal (increased) antibody responsiveness	T-suppressor cell function

The pathogenesis of the disease appears related to the accumulation of deoxyguanosine which is phosphorylated to deoxyGTP (reviewed in 17, 26). Studies in T-lymphoma mutants and T-leukemic cells imply that deoxyguanosine toxicity is the result of the accumulation fo deoxyGTP which leads to the inhibition of ribonucleotide reductase, depletion of deoxyGTP pools and inhibition of DNA synthesis.

The generation of an antigen-specific PFC response is sensitive to the balance between T-helper and T-suppressor cell signals; at supraoptimal antigen concentrations, the PFC response is inhibited as a result of the generation and expansion (proliferation) of the suppressor cell pool size (6). In contrast to the antigen-induced activation of T-helper cells, the differentiation of B-cells to an antibody-secreting stage and the activation of antigen-specific T-suppressor cells requires cell proliferation. We have examined the effects of deoxyguanosine on the cellular components of the PFC response (12). As shown in Table 3, control cells generated a typical bell-shaped antigen dose-dependent PFC response. Suppression of the PFC response is observed at the higher antigen concentrations. In the presence of 2.5 - 250 µM deoxyguanosine, there was no inhibition of the PFC response at high antigen concentrations. These data indicate that in the presence of deoxyguanosine, suppressor cell activity is abrogated, whereas B-cell and the non-proliferating dependent T-helper cell effects proceed normally.

Similar studies have been carried out in mice (7). Following immunization with supra-optimal antigen concentrations, the splenic PFC response, measured 5 days later, was markedly reduced. Animals which received daily intraperitoneal injections of deoxyguanosine (but not guanosine or saline)

TABLE 3. *Effect of Deoxyguanosine on the PFC Response*

µg Ovalbumin/Culture	PFC/Culture (x10^{-2}) Concentration of Deoxyguanosine (µM)				
	0	1	2.5	25	250
0.1	360	375	375	450	570
0.3	880	980	1000	1100	800
1.0	1300	1300	1800	1820	1100
10	680	720	1820	1830	1070
100	250	260	1800	1850	1100

Cultures containg 2x 10^6 B lymphocytes and 1 x 10^6 T lymphocytes, obtained from tonsil, were incubated for 5 days in the presence of different concentrations of the drug and increasing concentrations of ovalbumin. Results are expressed as the mean PFC/culture carried out in triplicate.

demonstrated a normal PFC response, indicating the *in vivo* anti-suppressor cell activity of deoxyguanosine.

Subsequently, a number of laboratories have confirmed these findings in several different systems. Deoxyguanosine has been shown to inhibit cord blood suppressor-cell activity on pokeweed mitogen-induced immunoglobulin synthesis (19). In a murine cytolytic T-cell system, deoxyguanosine reversed the inhibition exhibited by suppressor T-cells in mice infected with malarial parasites (23). Benner et al. have also shown that deoxyguanosine inhibits the generation of murine suppressor T-cell activity, but not delayed type hypersensitivity reactions (2). As discussed elsewhere (17, 26), the differential sensitivity of lymphocyte subsets may reflect the differential expression of purine enzymes during lymphocyte ontogeny.

Atopic Dermatitis. Work by Leung et al. suggests that there is a reduction in numbers of circulating suppressor T-cells and a deficiency of IgE-specific suppressor T-cells (24).

Excess of T-suppressor cell activity

Cord Blood. Heightened activity of a possibly unique suppressor T-cell in human cord blood has been well desribed (11, 19, 28). Various functions of adult T and B cells are inhibited by cord blood lymphocytes, particularly the production of immunoglobulin.

Common Variable and Congenital Hypo- or Agammaglobulinemia. Studies from a large number of laboratories have demonstrated suppression of immunoglobulin synthesis following the addition of T-cells in either the pokeweed mitogen or PFC assay. In our studies, this suppressor cell was identified in the theophylline-sensitive, Fc-γ^+ T-cell subset (4, 6). Enhancement of suppressor cell activity was observed in the presence of drugs which increase intracellular levels of cyclic AMP. Of interest was the ability of lithium to reverse, *in vitro*, the suppressive effect of patient T-cells (13). In one patient treated with lithium, this suppressor-cell activity disappeared and sIg-positive cells appeared in the circulation. Following immunization, specific antibody to bacteriophage ØX 174 was detected, but the antibody persisted as an IgM response without conversion to IgG (8). Recently, H_2-receptor antagonists have been reported to decrease excessive suppressor-cell activity and allow endogenous immunoglobulin production in some patients with common variable hypogammaglobulinemia (36).

Selective Deficiency of IgA. Subclass specific suppressor cells directed against IgA-secreting cells have been identified in some of these patients (31).

B. SECONDARY DISORDERS

Failure of T-cell help

Acquired Immunodeficiency Syndrome. Patients with AIDS have a complicated and variable immunodeficiency. Despite the presence of hypergammaglobulinemia and large numbers of spontaneous immunoglobulin-producing cells, they have poor antibody responses to many specific antigens. This may in part be due to the particular selectivity of HTLV III for the T4 subset (21).

Post Bone Marrow Transplant. Following bone marrow transplantation, there is often a marked delay in functional reconstitution of T-cell immunity, despite the presence of phenotypically normal circulating T-cells. The failure to respond to specific antigens *in vivo* and *in vitro* may include an impairment of T-cell help (9).

Drugs. A number of drugs have complicated effects on immunoregulatory T-cell subsets. Some, such as corticosteroids and cyclosporine may have direct effects on helper T-cells.

Excess T-cell help

Mucocutaneous Lymph Node Syndrome. In patients with Kawasaki's disease, there appears to be an increased number of activated T4 cells in the circulation. Circulating T8 cells are reduced and this is accompanied by a high rate of spontaneous immunoglobulin synthesis and hypergammaglobulinemia (25).

Absence of T-suppressor cell activity

Autoimmune Disorders. In a number of "autoimmune disorders", ranging from multiple sclerosis to the collagen-vascular diseases such as lupus erythematosus, reduced numbers of function of circulating suppressor cells have been identified in some patients. This may be accompanied by a deficiency in the regulation of *in vitro* immunoglobulin production.

Myasthenia Gravis. Myasthenia gravis is a specific autoimmune disorder with altered suppressor cell function. In our studies of patients with this disease (32), a circulating IgG antibody, inhibitable by d-tubocurarine, and therefore presumably binding to the acetylcholine receptor (AchR), has a significant effect on a subset of T cells which mediates suppressor-cell activity in the PFC assay. This antibody interferes with the binding of sheep red blood cells to E-receptors unless the affinity of E-receptor binding is enhanced through the use of E_{AET} (Table 4). The reduction in E-rosette formation

TABLE 4.   *T-Cell Subsets and Effect of Myasthenic Serum*

	% E-rosettes		
	E_{AET}	E	E + Th
Patient 1	68	32	28
2	62	24	23
3	75	21	19
4	60	28	25
Control	76	56	28
Control plus Serum from			
Patient 1	74	39	33
2	72	34	29
3	75	36	27
4	76	32	26

E-rosette formation was enumerated in the presence (E + Th) or absence (E) of theophylline (Th, 3mM) and untreated sheep erythrocytes or with treated erythrocytes (E_{AET}). In studies with patient serum, normal cells were incubated with 30% patient serum for 2 hrs. at 4°C or 37°C, and washed three times prior to assay.

involves a block of the theophylline-sensitive cells only. A similar abnormality can be induced on normal T-cells following incubation with patient serum (Table 4). In the PFC assay, the patients' cells, or normal cells following incubation with patient serum, fail to inhibit the PFC response at supra-optimal antigen concentrations (Table 5). Following plasmapheresis these effects of patient serum were no longer detectable (27).

TABLE 5.   *PFC Response in Patients and Effect of Myasthenic Serum*

	PFC/Culture ($\times 10^{-2}$) µg Ovalbumin/Culture	
	3	100
Patient 1	2100	2000
2	1900	1920
3	1650	1700
Control	2400	400
Control + Patient Serum	1900	1850

PFC response as in legend to Table 3 except that 3×10^6 peripheral blood mononuclear cells/culture were used. All cultures were in 10% normal human serum, except for "control + patient serum" where normal cells were cultured in 10% patient serum.

These data suggested that the IgG antibody has anti-AchR activity and conversely that "theophylline-sensitive" suppressor T-cells have an AchR linked in some way to the expression of E-rosette formation and T-suppressor cell activity. The secretion of anti-AchR antibody would further impair T-suppressor cell activity, perhaps resulting in the production of more antibody (Figure 1).

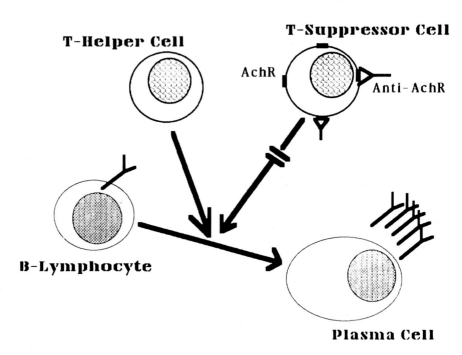

FIG. 1.   Immunomodulatory effects of anti-acetylcholine receptor (AchR) antibody.

Excess T-suppressor cell activity

Graft-versus-Host Disease. Chronic GvHD is associated with an excess of suppressor T-cells. An increased number of activated T8 cells can be detected in the circulation and there is suppression of pokeweed mitogen-dependent immunoglobulin synthesis (30).

Infectious Mononucleosis. In this condition, there is generally a self-limited proliferation of suppressor T cells able to inhibit *in vitro* immunoglobulin synthesis (35). In some families, infectious mononucleosis is followed by hypogammaglobulinemia (29).

Drugs. Drugs can have a number of effects on the immune system. One particular group of drugs, the phenytoins, have been associated with abnormalities of the immune system in up to 70% of patients. The most frequent

TABLE 6. *Evaluation of Humoral Immunity*

	Admission	5 Wks.	10 Wks.
Serum Igs			
IgG (mg/dl)	220	35	500
IgM (mg/dl)	<10	30	70
IgA (mg/dl)	<10	20	40
IgE (mg/dl)	<10	N.D.	165
Schick Test	+	N.D.	−
Isohemmaglutinins	1:2 - 1:4	1:8	1:32
B Lymphocytes			
(% sIg)	0.1	0.4	2.5

TABLE 7. *Evaluation of the* in vitro *PFC Response*

	Admission	PFC/Culture 5 Wk.	10 Wks.
Ovalbumin			
Patient	510 ± 40	880 ± 110	1730 ± 120
Controls	1950 ± 140	1790 ± 120	1860 ± 90
Controls + Phenytoin	1630 ± 100	1810 ± 90	1480 ± 130
Ovalbumin + Pokeweed			
Patient	<200	320 ± 60	2200 ± 40
Controls	2360 ± 110	2510 ± 190	2490 ± 170
Controls + Phenytoin	2100 ± 180	2660 ± 170	2030 ± 220

Numbers indicate ovalbumin-specific PFC generated per culture of 3×10^6 peripheral blood mononuclear cells in the presence of $0.3\mu g$ ovalbumin. Controls given phenytoin had normal serum immunoglobulin levels.

abnormality is the development of IgA deficiency (34). We have observed a patient who, following a dilantin-induced hypersensitivity reaction, developed hypogammaglobulinemia (10) (Table 6). Circulating B-cells were depleted in number and antibody responses were diminished. When studied in the PFC assay, he had low numbers of PFC (Table 7). When his cells were cultured with antigen plus pokeweed mitogen, a response was no longer observed (normal donors generated higher numbers of PFC), similar to patients with congenital or common variable immunodeficiency (4). Following withdrawal of the drug, there was a progressive increase in circulating immunoglobulins and a disappearance of the abnormal suppressor-cell activity.

These findings of drug-dependent antibody deficiency and concomitant expression of abnormal suppressor T-cell activity strengthen the argument for the role of suppressor T cells in the pathogenesis of some disorders of B-cell immunity.

Acknowledgements

This work was supported by the Medical Research Council of Canada, the Muscular Dystrophy Foundation and the National Cancer Institute.

REFERENCES

1. Blaese, R.M., Weiden, P.L., Koski, J., and Dooley, N. (1974): Infectious agammag-lobulinemia: Transmission of immunodeficiency, with grafts of agammaglobulinemic cells. *J. Exp. Med.* 140:1097-1101.
2. Bril, H., van den Akker, T.W., Molendijk-lok, B.D., Bian-Chi, A.T. and Benner, R. (1984): Influence of 2' - deoxyguanosine upon the development of DTH effector T cells and suppressor T cells in vivo. *J. Immunol.* 132:599-604.
3. Cooper, M.D. (1981): Pre B cells; Normal and abnormal development. *J. Clin. Immunol.* 1:81-9.
4. Dosch, H.M., Percy, M.E. and Gelfand, E.W. (1977): Functional differentiation of B-lym-phocytes in congenital agammaglobulinemia. I. Generation of hemolytic plaque-forming cells. *J. Immunol.* 119:1959-64.
5. Dosch, H.M., Lee, J.W.W, Falk, J.A. and Gelfand, E.W. (1978): Severe combined im-munodeficiency disease: A model of T-cell dysfunction. *Clin. Exp. Immunol.* 34:260-7.
6. Dosch, H.M. and Gelfand, E.W. (1979): Specific in vitro IgM responses of human B-cells: A complex regulatory network modulated by antigen. *Immunol. Rev.* 45:243-74.
7. Dosch, H.M., Mansour, A., Cohen, A., Shore, A. and Gelfand, E.W. (1980): Inhibition of suppressor T-cell development following deoxyguanosine administration. *Native*, 285:494-496.
8. Dosch, H.M., Matheson, D., Schuurman, R.K.B. and Gelfand, E.W. (1980): Anti-suppres-sor cell effect of lithium in vitro and in vivo. In: *Effects of Lithium on Granulopoiesis and Immune Function.* Eds. A.H. Rossol and W.H. Robinson. Plenum Press, New York, N.Y., pp. 447-462.
9. Dosch, H.M. and Gelfand, E.W. (1981): Failure of T-B-cell cooperation during graft vs host disease. *Transplantation*, 31:48-50.
10. Dosch, H.M., Jason, J. and Gelfand, E.W. (1982): Transient antibody deficiency and abnormal T-suppressor cells induced by phenytoin. *New Eng. J. Med.*, 306:406-9.
11. Durandy, A., Fischer, A. and Griscelli, C. (1979): Active suppression of B lymphocyte maturation by two different newborn T lymphocyte subsets. *J. Immunol.* 123:2644-9.
12. Gelfand, E.W., Lee, J.J. and Dosch, H.M. (1979): Selective toxicity of purine deoxynuc-leosides for human lymphocyte growth and function. *Proc. Nat. Acad. Sci.* 76:1998-2002.
13. Gelfand, E.W., Dosch, H.M., Hastings, D. and Shore, A. (1979): Lithium: A modulator of cyclic AMP-dependent events in lymphocytes. *Science* 203:365-7.
14. Gelfand, E.W., Dosch, H.M., Shore, A., Limatibul, S. and Lee, J.W.W. (1980): The role of the thymus in human T-cell differentiation. In: *The Biological Basis for Immunodeficiency Disease.* Eds. E.W. Gelfand and H.M. Dosch. Raven Press, New York, N.Y., pp. 39-56.
15. Gelfand, E.W. and Dosch, H.M. (1982): Differentiation of precursor T lymphocytes in man and delineation of the selective abnormalities in severe combined immune deficiency disease. *Clin. Immunol. Immunopath.* 25:303-15.
16. Gelfand, E.W. and Dosch, H.M. (1983): Diagnosis and classification of severe combined immunodeficiency disease. *Birth Defects Original Article Series*, 19:65-72.
17. Gelfand, E.W. and Cohen, A. (1983): Disorders of purine metabolism and immunodefi-ciency. In: *Advances in Host Defense Mechanisms.* Eds. J.I. Gallin and A.S. Fauci. Raven Press, New York, N.Y., pp. 43-68.
18. Giblett, E.R., Anderson, J.E., Cohen, F., Pollara, B. and Meuwissen, H.J. (1972): Adenosine-deaminase deficiency in two patients with severely impaired cellular immunity. *Lancet*, 2:1067-69.
19. Hayward, A.R. (1981): Development of lymphocyte responses and interactions in the human fetus and newborn. *Immunolog. Rev.* 57:39-60.
20. Hong, R., Schulte-Wisserman, H., Horowitz, S., Borzy, M. and Finlay, J. (1978): Cultured thymic epithelium in severe combined immunodeficiency. *Transpl. Proc.* 10:201-4.
21. Klatzmann, D., Champagne, E., Chamaret, S., Gruest, J., Guetard, D., Hercend, T., Gluckman, J.C. and Montagnier, L. (1984): T-lymphocyte T4 molecule behaves as the receptor for human retrovirus LAV. *Nature*, 312:767-8.
22. Korsmeyer, S.J., Heiter, P.A., Ravetch, J.V., Poplack, D.G., Waldmann, T.A. and Leder, P. (1981): Developmental hierarchy of immunoglobulin gene rearrangements in human, leukemic pre-B-cells. *Proc. Nat. Acad. Sci.* 78:7096-100.
23. Lelchuk, R., Sprott, V.M.A. and Playfair, J.H.L. (1981): Differential involvement of non-specific suppressor T cells in two lethal murine malaria infections. *Clin. Exp. Immunol.* 45:433-8.

24. Leung, D.Y.M., Rhodes, A.R. and Geha, R.S. (1981): Enumeration of T-cell subsets in atopic dermatitis using monoclonal antibodies. *J. Allergy Clin. Immunol.* 67:450-5.
25. Leung, D.Y.M., Chu, E.T., Wood, N., Grady, S., Meade, R. and Geha, R.S. (1983): Immunoregulatory T cell abnormalities in muco-cutaneous lymph node syndrome. *J. Immunol.* 130:2002-4.
26. Martin, D.W. Jr. and Gelfand, E.W. (1981): Immunodevelopment Disease. *Ann. Rev. Biochem.* 50:845-77.
27. Mizuno, Y., Humphrey, J., Dosch, H.M. and Gelfand, E.W. (1982): Carbamylcholine modulation of E-rosette formation. Effect of plasmaphoresis in myastenia gravis. *Clin. Exp. Immunol.* 49:209-16.
28. Morito, T., Bankhurst, A.D. and Williams, R.C. (1979): Studies of human cord blood and adult lymphocyte interactions with in vitro immunoglobulin production. *J. Clin. Invest.* 64:990-5.
29. Provisor, A.J., Iacuone, J.J., Chilcote, R.R. and Baehner, R. (1975): Acquired agammaglobulinemia after a life-threatening illness with clinical and laboratory features of infectious mononucleosis in three related male children. *N. Eng. J. Med.* 293:62-5.
30. Reinherz, E.L., Parkman, R., Rappaport, J., Rosen, F.S. and Schlossman, S.F. (1979): Aberrations of suppressor T cells in human graft-versus-host disease. *N. Eng. J. Med.* 300:1061-8.
31. Scwartz, S.A. (1980): Heavy chain-specific suppression of immunoglobulin synthesis and secretion by lymphocytes from patients with selective IgA deficiency. *J. Immunol.* 124:2034-41.
32. Shore, A., Limatibul, S., Dosch, H.M. and Gelfand, E.W. (1979): Identification of two serum components regulating the expression of T-lymphocyte function in childhood myasthenia gravis. *N. Eng. J. Med.*, 301:605-29.
33. Siegel, R.L., Issekutz, T., Schwaber, J., Rosen, F.S. and Geha, R.S. (1981): Deficiency of T helper cells in transient hypogammaglobulinemia of infancy. *N. Eng. J. Med.* 305:1307-13.
34. Sorrell, T.C., Forbes, I.J., Burness, F.R. and Rischbieth, R.H.C. (1971): Depression of immunological function in patients treated with phenytoin sodium (sodium diphenylhydantoin). *Lancet*, 2:1233-5.
35. Tosato, G., MacGrath, I., Koski, I., Dooley, N. and Blaese, M. (1979): Activation of suppressor T cells during Epstein-Barr-virus-induced infectious mononucleosis. *N. Eng. J. Med.* 301:1133-7.
36. White, W.B. and Ballow, M. (1985): Modulation of suppressor-cell activity by cimetidine in patients with common variable hypogammaglobulinemia. 312:198-202.

Ontogeny of T Cell Subsets in the Neonatal Period

A.G. Ugazio*, R. Maccario** and G.R. Burgio**

*Department of Pediatrics, University of Brescia, Italy
**Department of Pediatrics, University of Pavia, Italy

The high susceptibility of the neonate to bacterial, viral and fungal infections is mainly related to incomplete maturation of the immune system at birth.

Immaturity of neonatal lymphocyte functions and active suppressive mechanisms are probably important factors involved in preventing rejection of the fetus and a graft versus host (GvH) reaction generated by transplacental passage of immunocompetent maternal cells.

Though proliferation in response to PHA is present in fetal thymus from the 10th-12th week of gestation and responsiveness to allogeneic stimuli is present in the 11-15th week fetus, neonatal peripheral blood includes a high percentage of immature T cell subsets and some cell-mediated functions are not as efficient as in adult subjects (3, 14, 26).

Neonatal T cell subsets

Evaluation of T cell subsets in neonatal and adult blood has demonstrated some differences between the two groups (Fig. 1).

The main differences characterizing cord blood lymphocytes (CBL) are as follows:

a) low percentage of T lymphocytes forming E rosettes due to the presence of T cell subsets with low avidity for sheep erythrocytes (22);

b) low percentage of OKT3$^+$ cells (9, 19);

c) high percentage of OKT8$^+$ cells (19). However some groups have reported a low number of OKT8$^+$ cells (11, 29). This is probably related to the use of T cell-enriched CBL. In fact, as discussed later, many OKT8$^+$ CBL are found in the T cell-depleted fraction;

d) high percentage of cells bearing the receptor for peanut agglutinin (PNA) (18), which reacts with immature cells such as thymocytes (17, 24)?

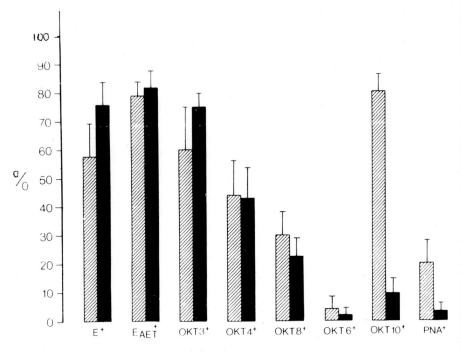

FIG. 1. Lymphocyte subpopulations in adult peripheral blood (■) and in cord blood (□).

e) very high percentage of cells reacting with the OKT10 monoclonal antibody (MoAb), usually reacting with thymocytes, activated T and B cells and some NK cells (5, 13, 23, 25).

Moreover in the neonate the sum of the percentages of lymphocytes reacting with OKT8 and OKT4 MoAb is always greater than the percentage of OKT3[+] cells. Fractionation experiments leading to E-rosette-enriched and E-rosette-depleted populations have shown the presence of an E[-], OKT3[-], OKT8[+] subset in cord blood not detectable in adult blood (tab. 1) (19, 28).

TABLE 1. *Percentage of OKT[+] cells among T cell-enriched and T cell-depleted fractions of cord blood lymphocytes and adult peripheral blood[*]*

	E-RFC		OKT3		OKT4		OKT8	
	CBL	APBL	CBL	APBL	CBL	APBL	CBL	APBL
Unseparated	58	76	59	77	45	42	35	20
E-RFC-Enriched	ND*	ND*	88	93	54	51	23	22
E-RFC-Depleted	2	1	4	5	2	1	29	1

[*] Each value is the mean of six separate experiments. **ND: not done. (J. Immunol. 130: 1129-1131, 1983) (19).

Recently, a high percentage of neonatal cells has been reported to react with the OKT6 MoAb (9), which is known to react with thymocytes; however this phenomenon was not statistically significant in our hands (19).

It has also been reported that OKT4$^+$ cord blood lymphocytes do not express the DR antigen after stimulation with pokeweed mitogen (PWM), while more than 50% of OKT4$^+$ adult cells become DR$^+$ under the same culture conditions (15, 20). This phenomenon could play a crucial role in T cell regulation of the neonatal immune response.

Neonatal T cell function

T cell proliferation. CBL are known to display a high degree of "spontaneous" proliferation *in vitro*, i.e. in the absence of mitogenic stimuli (fig. 2a, b). The mechanism underlying this phenomenon is still obscure: it may be related to "pre-activation" *in vivo* by feto-maternal interaction or to the presence of immature spontaneously-replicating cells among CBL. At birth T cell proliferation in response to PHA and Con A shows remarkable individual variability (fig. 2a, b); some neonates display a normal response and others show a low proliferation (279.

Moreover, it has been shown that in premature infants, with a birth weight < 1250 g, PHA- and ConA-responsiveness is lower than in infants weighing > 2500 g (16). This phenomenon is difficult to relate to the early apparence of PHA- and ConA-responsive cells during fetal life and is probably caused by suppessive factors.

There is disagreement in the literature about the capacity of neonatal lymphocytes to proliferate *in vitro* in response to allogeneic HLA-unrelated cells; some authors describe a low response (7) and others a normal response (8). Using limiting dilution cultures, Hayward et al. have demonstrated that the frequency of T lymphocytes (both OKT4$^+$ and OKT8$^+$) proliferating in response to allogeneic cells is about the same in newborn and adult peripheral blood (12).

T cell cytotoxicity. Experiments on the efficiency of T-cells with specific cytotoxic activity have generated variable results. Many studies have shown that neonatal cells have a limited capacity for specific killing of hapten-modified self, semiallogeneic and allogeneic target cells. Neither PHA nor interleukin-2 (IL-2) added to the cultures increased specific cell-mediated lympholysis (CML) (14, 26). However, other reports have demonstrated a high degree of individual variability with some neonates showing an "adult pattern" of response and others low CML activity (26). These contrasting results may suggest that the stage of maturation of CML function is variable at birth and perhaps related to the high individual variability of the susceptibility of the neonate to viral infections.

Regulatory T cell function. Helper activity, measured as the efficiency to induce *in vitro* immunoglobulin production, is profoundly limited in the neon-

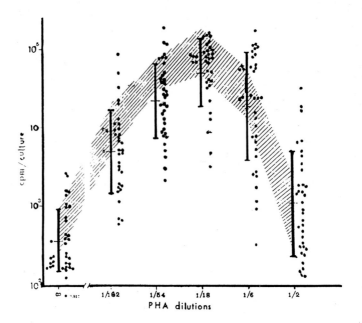

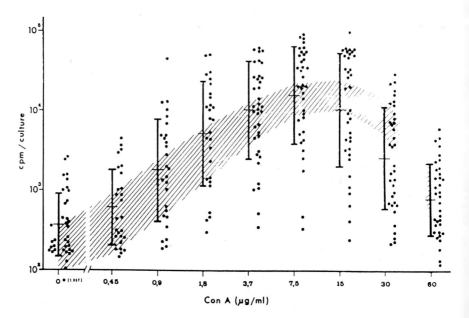

FIG. 2. Dose-response curves of lymphocytes from each of the newborns under study (●) to increasing concentrations of PHA (2a) and ConA (2b). Vertical bars: 1SD of the neonatal mean; shaded area: 1SD of the adult mean (Ugazio et al., *Boll. Ist. Siroter. Milanese,* 1976, 55:455-456) (27).

ate (3, 14, 26). Although irradiated OKT4$^+$ lymphocytes induce significant IgG synthesis (14), helper activity is not detectable under other experimental conditions, probably because it is obscured by OKT4$^+$ radiosensitive suppressor cells. In fact OKT4$^+$ CBL include two subpopulations, a radiosensitive suppressor subset which is very active, and a radioresistent helper subset which is less efficient than in adults (14).

In contrast with helper activity, suppressor function is very active in the neonate, probably in order to inhibit maternal cell proliferation *in vivo* and rejection of the fetus. Neonatal suppressor lymphocytes are radosensitive and, at variance with adult suppressor cells, have been reported to partain exclusively to the OKT4$^+$, OKT8$^-$ subset (14). However, some authors have reported that OKT8$^+$ cells are responsible for the high suppressor activity of neonatal lymphocytes (11).

Neonatal Lymphokine Production

Production of some lymphokines, such as LIF, is detectable in normal amounts at birth (10). Brysol et al. (6) have shown that cord blood leukocytes produce alfa-interferon (α-IFN) but not gamma-interferon (γ-IFN). Nevertheless, Anderson et al. recently reported γ-IFN production by CBL (4). These contrasting results probably derive from the different sensitivities of the techniques used to detect and measure γ-IFN.

IL-2 production in response to the polyclonal activators, PHA and ConA, is comparable in neonatal and adult peripheral blood (tab. 2). As previously

TABLE 2. *PHA and ConA-induced IL-2 production in CBL and A-PBL**

	Medium	PHA	ConA
CBL	<0.15	47.2	8.5
A-PBL	<0.15	52.2	11.4

* Each value is the mean of eleven separate experiments.

mentioned, CBL diplay a high rate of "spontaneous" proliferation and therefore might well be expected to show a high rate of "spontaneous" IL-2 and IL-1 production. There is recent evidence that neonatal leukocytes cultured *in vitro* produce spontaneously detectable amounts of IL-1 (Notarangelo, unpublished results). However, IL-2 activity has never been detected in supernatants from unstimulated cultures. These results do not rule out the possibility that spontaneous proliferation is due to small amounts of IL-2 produced spontaneously in unstimulated neonatal lymphocyte cultures and quickly consumed by lymphocytes expressing the IL-2 receptor.

T and NK Lymphocyte Ontogeny: two interacting Pathways?

As mentioned previosly, neonatal lymphocytes include a sizeable subset of OKT8$^+$, OKT3$^-$ cells, virtually absent among adult lymphocytes (19, 28);

these cells are also E⁻, OKT4⁻, HNK-1⁻, OKM1⁻. Functional studies have shown that these cells diplay NK activity, although lacking the HNK-1 antigen (28). Subsequently we have demonstrated that more than 50% of these cells react with the B73.1 MoAb which recognizes the IgG-Fc receptor present on NK cells; moreover most of them bear the DR antigen and the receptor for PNA and react with the OKT10 MoAb (fig. 3). E⁻, OKT3⁻, OKT8⁺ CBL

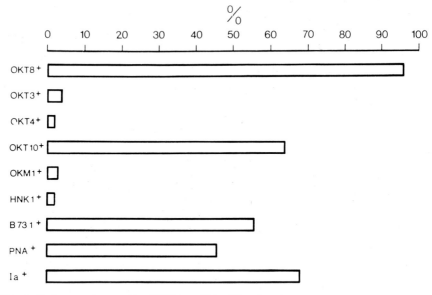

FIG. 3. Surface markers on E⁻, OKT8⁺ cord blood lymphocytes.

do not adhere to nylon wool and represent about 5% of CBL (28). This neonatal subset diplays a higher NK activity than unseparated CBL, which diplay very little NK activity (28). Furthermore, prelminary results show that it is sensitive to boosting effect of β-IFN preincubation (tab. 3). When stimulated with PHA and ConA, E⁻, OKT3⁻, OKT8⁺ CBL both produce IL-2 (fig. 4) and proliferate (fig. 5). Moreover this neonatal subset produces IL-1 both spontaneously and in response to lipopolysaccharide (LPS) (tab. 4).

TABLE 3. *Boosting of NK activity by IFNβ in CBL, A-PBL and E⁻, OKT8⁺, CBL**

	NK activity (LU$_{30}$/10⁶ cells)	
	Medium (2HR)	IFNβ (10³ U/ML) (2HR)
CBL Unseparated	1.3	14.2
E⁻, OKT8⁺	9.5	39
A-PBL	8.3	41.5

* Each value is the mean of seven separate experiments.

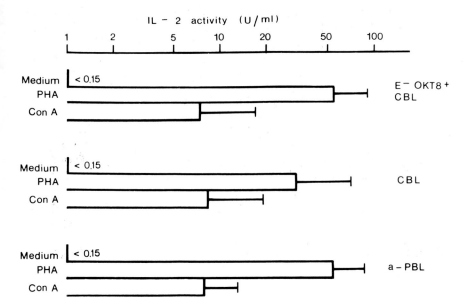

FIG. 4. PHA- and ConA-induced IL-2 production by adult peripheral lymphocytes (a-PBL), cord blood lymphocytes (CBL) and E⁻, OKT8⁺ CBL.

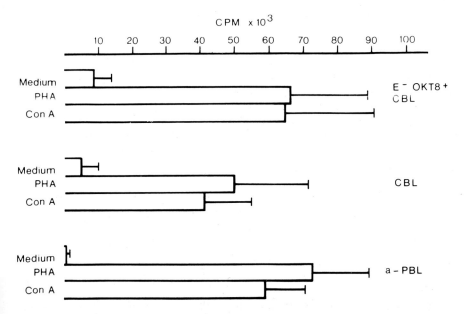

FIG. 5. PHA- and ConA-induced proliferation rates by adult peripheral lymphocytes (a-PBL), cord blood lymphocytes (CBL) and E⁻, OKT8⁺ CBL.

TABLE 4.   *LPS-induced IL-1 and IL-2 production in E⁻, OKT8⁺ CBL**

	IL-1 (U/ML)	IL-2 (U/ML)
Medium	3 ± 3.5	<0.15
LPS	11 ± 5	<0.15

*Each value is the mean of eight separate experiments

Many hypotheses have been formulated as to the pathway of differentiation of NK cells; they may belong to a T-cell or myelomonocyte lineage, or to a separate pathway of differentiation. An alternative possibility is that some NK cells have a common precursor with T lymphocytes, while other NK subsets derive from a myelomonocytic lineage (21).

A relationship between T and NK lymphocytes is suggested by the isolation of various NK clones expressing a T-cell-associated phenotype (E-rosette-receptor, OKT3, OKT8, OKT4, OKT10 antigens) (2) and by the capacity of NK cells to both produce IL-2 and proliferate in response to this lymphokine but not in response to PHA or ConA (21).

Many features of the NK subset identified in neonatal blood further suggest a close interaction between T-cell and NK cell ontogeny. In fact this subset or stage of maturation shares some characteristics with thymocytes, such as OKT8 positivity and OKT3 negativity, presence of a receptor for PNA as well

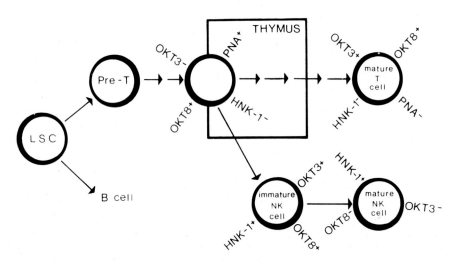

FIG. 6. Hypothetical scheme of the interactions between T cell and NK cell ontogeny. According to the hypothesis, the neonatal subset of OKT3⁻, OKT8⁺ lymphocytes represents an intermediate stage of differentiation between the pre-T lymphocytes and thymocytes. These cells are able either to differentiate in the thymus along the T cell axis or to leave the thymus and, reaching secondary lymphoid compartments as OKT3⁺, OKT8⁺, HNK-1⁺ cells (1), differentiate into "mature" NK cells. The presence of an high percentage of OKT3⁻, OKT8⁺ cells in neonatal peripheral blood could be related to the high rate of recirculating immature cells in the neonatal period.

as capacity to proliferate in response to PHA and ConA and displays the main features of NK cells, such as NK activity, sensitivity to IFN, and capacity to produce IL-1 and IL-2.

As shown in fig. 6 our current speculation is that the neonatal subset of NK cells includes a common precursor of NK cells and T lymphocytes.

REFERENCES

1. Abo, T., Miller, C.A., Gartland, L., and Balch, C.M. (1983): Differentiation stages of human natural killer cells in lymphoid tissue from fetal to adult life. *J. Exp. Med.*, 157:273-284.
2. Alavena, P., and Ortaldo, J.R. (1984): Characteristics of human NK clones: target specificity and phenotype. *J. Immunol.*, 132:2363-2369.
3. Andersson, U., Bird, A.G., Britton, S., and Palacios, R. (1981): Humoral and cellular immunity in human studies at the cell level from birth to two years of age. *Immunol. Rev.*, 57:5-38.
4. Andresson, U., Britton, S., De Ley, M., and Bird, G., (1983): Evidence for the ontogenic precedence of suppressor T cell functions in the human neonate. *Eur. J. Immunol.*, 13:6-13.
5. Bhan, A.K., Nadler, L.M., Stashenko, P., Clustey, R.T., and Schlossman, S.F. (1981): Stages of B cell differentiation in human lymphoid tissue. *J. Exp. Med.*, 154:737-749.
6. Bryson, Y.J., Winter, H.S., Gard, S.E., Fischer, T.J., and Stiehm, ER. (1980): Deficiency of immune interferon production by lymphocytes of normal newborns. *Cell. Immunol.*, 55:191-200.
7. Ceppellini, R., Bonnard, G.D., Coppo, F., Miggiano, V.C., Popisil, M., Curtoni, F.S., and Pellegrino, M. (1971): Mixed lymphocyte cultures and HLA. Reactivity of young fetuses, newborns and mothers at delivery. *Transpl. Proc.*, 3:58-66.
8. Debray-Sachs J., Bachs, M., Bach, J.F., and Dormont, J. (1971): Culture mixtes des lymphocytes du nouveau-né avec les lymphocytes de la mère. *Pathol. Biol.*, 19:171-175.
9. Foa, R., Giubellino, M.C., Fierro, M.T., Lusso, P., and Ferrando, M.L. (1984): Immature T lymphocytes in human cord blood identified by monoclonal antibodies: a model for the study of the differentiation pathway of T cells in humans. *Cell. Immunol.*, 89:194-201.
10. Handzel, Z.T., Levin, S., Dolphin, Z., Schlesinger, M., Hahn, T., Altman, Y., Schechter, B., Shneyour, A., and Trainin, N. (1980): Immune competence of newborn lymphocytes. *Pediatrics*, 65:491-496.
11. Hayward, A.R., and Kurnick, J. (1981): Newborn T cell suppession: early appearance, maintenance in culture, and lack of growth factor suppression. *J. Immunol.*, 126:50-53.
12. Hayward, A.R., and Malmberg, S. (1984): Response to human newborn lymphocytes to alloantigen: lack of evidence for suppression induction. *Ped. Res.*, 18:414-419.
13. Hercend, T., Reinherz, E.L., Menez, S., Schlossman, S.F., and Ritz, J. (1983): Phenotypic and functional heterogeneity of human cloned natural killer cell lines. *Nature*, 301:158-160.
14. Jacoby, D.R., Olding, L.B., and Oldstone, M.B.A. (1984): Immunologic regulation of fetal-maternal balance. *Adv. Immunol.*, 35:157-208.
15. Ko, H.S., Fu, S.M., Winchester, R.J., Yu, D.T.Y., and Kunkel, H.G. (1979): Ia determinants on stimulated human T lymphocytes. Occurrence on mitogen- and antigen-activated T cells. *J. Exp. Med.*, 150:246-255.
16. Leino, A., Ruuskanen, O., Kezo, P., Eskola, J., and Toivanen, P. (1981): Depressed phytohemagglutinin and concanavalin A responses in premature infants. *Clin. Immunol. Immunopathol.*, 19:260-267.
17. London, J., Berrih, S., and Bach, J.F. (1978): Peanut agglutinin I. A new tool for studying T lymphocyte subpopulations. *J. Immunol.*, 121:438-443.
18. Maccario, R., Ferrari, F.A., Siena, S., Vitiello, A., Martini, A., Siccardi, A.G., and Ugazio, A.G. (1981): Receptors for Peanut agglutinin on a high percentage of human cord-blood lymphocytes: phenotype characterization of Peanut-positive cells. *Thymus*, 2:329-337.
19. Maccario, R., Nespoli, L., Mingrat, G., Vitiello, A., Ugazio, A.G., and Burgio, G.R. (1983): Lymphocyte subpopulations in the neonate: identification of an immature subset of OKT8-positive, OKT3-negative cells. *J. Immunol.* 130:1129-1131.
20. Miyawaki, T., Yachie, A., Nagaoki, T., Mukai, M., Yokoi, T., Uwadana, N., and Taniguchi, N. (1982): Expression ability of Ia antigens on T cell subsets defined by monoclonal antibodies on Pokeweed mitogen stimulation in early human life. *J. Immunol.*, 128:11-15.

21. Ortaldo, J.R., and Herberman, R.B. (1984): Heterogeneity of natural killer cells. *Ann. Rev. Immunol.*, 2:359-394.
22. Porta, F.A., Maccario, R., Ferrari, F.A., Alberini, C.M., Montagna, D., De Amici, M., Giannetti, A., and Ugazio, A.G. (in press): Lymphocyte subpopulations in the neonate: high percentage of ANAE-positive cells with low avidity for sheep erythrocytes. *Thymus*.
23. Reinherz, E.L., Kung, P.C., Goldstein, G., Levey, R.H., and Schlossman, S.F. (1980): Discrete stages of human intrathymic differentiation: analysis of normal thymocytes and leukemic lymphoblasts of T-cell lineage. *Proc. Natl. Acad. Sci.*, 77, 1588-1592.
24. Reisner, Y., Linker-israeli, M., and Sharon, N. (1976): Separation of mouse thymocytes into two subpopulations by the use of peanut agglutinin. *Cell. Immunol.* 25:129-134.
25. Sheenhy, M.J., Quinteri, F.B., Leung, D.Y.M., Geha, R.S., Dubey, D.P., Limmer, C.E., and Yumis, E.J. (1983): A human large granular lymphocyte clone with natural killer-like activity and T cell-like surface. *J. Immunol.* 130, 542-526.
26. Toivanen, P., Uksila, J., Leino, A., Lassila, O., Hirvonen, T., and Ruuskanen O. (1981): Development of mitogen responding T cells and Natural Killer cells in the human fetus. *Immunol. Rev.*, 57:89-106.
27. Ugazio, A.G., Altamura, D., Giraudi, V., Mingrat, G., Belloni, C., and Burgio, G.R. (1976): Peripheral blood T lymphocyte subpopulations in newborns. *Boll. Ist. Sieroter. Milanese*, 55:451-459.
28. Vitiello, A., Maccario, R., Montagna, D., Porta, F.A., Alberini, C.M., Mingrat, G., Astaldi-Ricotti, G.C.B., Nespoli, L. and Ugazio, A.G. (1984): Lymphocyte subpopulations in the neonate: a subset of HNK-1⁻, OKT3⁻, OKT8⁺ lymphocytes displays natural killer activity. *Cell. Immunol.*, 85:252-257.
29. Yachie, A., Miyawaki, T., Nagaoki, T., Yokai, T., Uwadana, N., and Taniguchi, N. (1981): Regulation of B cell differentiation by T cell subsets defined with monoclonal OKT4 and OKT8 antibodies in human cord blood. *J. Immunol.*, 127, 1314-1317.

SECTION V
ACQUIRED IMMUNODEFICIENCY SYNDROME

Immune Deregulation
in the Lymphadenopathy Syndrome

Susanna Cunningham-Rundles[1], C. Metroka[1], J. Schneider[2],
H. Campbell[1], J. Gold[1], G. Hayward[3], and B. Safai[1]

[1] Memorial Sloan-Kettering Cancer Center, 1275 York Avenue, New York N.Y. 10021
[2] American Cyanamid, Pearl River, N.Y.
[3] Johns Hopkins Medical School, Baltimore, MD, USA

The Acquired Immunodeficiency Disease Syndrome (AIDS) is a recently described condition observed predominatly in male homosexuals characterized by opportunistic infections and/or the appearance of a rare tumor, Kaposi's Sarcoma (6, 8, 11, 12, 14, 16). The microbial agents and viruses found in AIDS are those pathogens which usually achieve life-threatening significance only in patients with underlying cellular immune deficiency and include *Pneumocystis carinii, Toxoplasma gondii, Entamoeba histolytica, Cryptococcus neoformans, Mycobacterium avium intracellular, Mycrobacterium tuberculosis, Candida albicans,* Cytomegalovirus, Herpes simplex virus and Epstein Barr virus.

AIDS has been described as essentially a disease of altered immunoregulation since profound cellular immune disfunction is observed in all patients and persists during period of clinical stability when a particular infection has been resolved (7). Within a short period of time, usually a few months, recurrence of infection or a new infection occurs.

Patients who present with Kaposi's Sarcoma, AIDS-KS, often develop or have had opportunistic infections. Those patients with AIDS-KS who are resistant to infection may possibly have a less severe form of AIDS. AIDS patients who survive opportunistic infections frequently develop KS. Since KS is known to develop in states of transient immunocompromise, such as prophylactic immuno-suppression in renal transplantation, and to resolve with return of immuno-competence, its appearance in AIDS has suggested a central role for immune deregulation in the pathogenesis.

Immunological assessment of patients with AIDS has revealed few differences between patients that can be easily related to presenting symptoms. Lymphopenia and leukopenia are usually observed in patients with AIDS related opportunistic infections, AIDS-OI and less commonly in AIDS-KS but immune response studied in culture systems using a standardized number of characterized cells may suggest that response deficiencies do not merely reflect relative number of cells in whole blood, even when relative proportions of helper/inducer to cytotoxic/suppressor cells are taken into account. AIDS patients as a whole have impaired *in vitro* response to T lymphocyte mitogens and antigens, to T independent B lymphocyte activators, and show poor effector cell activity either as specific primed killers or as natural, NK, killers. Some of these deficiencies appear related to lack of interleukin-2, IL-2 production, or to interferon synthesis that normally occurs as a part of specific activating processes. The relationship of aberrant and reduced response to the elevated serum immunoglobulins, bone marrow plasmocytosis, elevated serum interferon α, and immune complexes is not clear. Fauci (7) has suggested that spontaneous activation of peripheral blood B cells is the probable basis of hypergammaglobulinemia and is central to the refractoriness of these cells to further activation *in vitro*.

Evidence linking a T lymphotropic retrovirus to AIDS transmission (HTLV-III, LAV, ARV) has provided a probable common cause for the lethality of AIDS while raising many questions concerning the basis of differences in disease course in different clinical subgroups. Key issues include whether there may be "healthy" carriers, naturally occurring neutralizing antibody, and the related question of whether it is possible that natural host defense mechanisms might be potentially protective.

Among the populations of individuals considered at risk as a result of lifestyle factors, homosexual men with generalized lymphadenopathy syndrome constitute a relatively homogeneous group. Exposure to HTLV-III in this propulation in endemic regions is now known to exceed 80%, assuming that antibody detection reflects antigen presence. Analysis of immune function in this group may provide critical information concerning the etiology of AIDS. Increased incidence of generalized lymphadenopathy, LA, was first seen in large cities in 1981. We originally reported that 17% of our group of 90 patients developed AIDS during the 8 to 19 month follow-up period. The incidence of AIDS in this group is now about 22%. In this population we observed a subset of patient with markedly depressed lymphocyte response *in vitro* to phytohemagglutinin and pokeweed mitogen, and negative responses to *E. coli, C. albicans and S. aureus*. Of 17 patients identified, 12 or 70% developed AIDS during the observation period. In some cases these abnormalities were present 13 months before the onset of frank AIDS, suggesting that prognostic markers had been located.

The microbial activators were found to be the most sensitive pre-AIDS marker in this population. Since these agents activate B cells, this suggested that residual B cell function might prove a critical discriminator for the identification of patients with greater or lesser resistance to AIDS. Furthermore, we and others (2, 10, 13, 17) have found that approximately 10% of patients with LA develop B cell lymphomas, suggesting that this group of patients might provide a link between retroviral infection of T cells and B cell malignancies. In the studies presented here, the immunological characteristics of patients with LA are presented, and some preliminary indications suggesting that B cell deregulation is central to etiology are discussed.

Analysis of Lymphocyte Activation in AIDS and the Lymphadenopathy Syndrome

Characterization of immune response *in vitro* in AIDS has been undertaken by various groups using the methods that have proven fruitful in other diseases of the immune system. Initially, all studies tended to focus on the massive loss of immune function that is the hallmark of AIDS. Some cohesiveness could be obtained when sequential patients were studied according to initially presenting disease. We examined lymphocyte proliferative response *in vitro* to phytohemagglutinin, PHA, using a wide range of concentrations of mitogen in patients newly diagnosed as having AIDS and homosexual patients with LA without any discernible underlying immunodeficiency (3, 4). Some of these data are shown in Fig. 1. Patients with AIDS-KS showed a distribution of lymphocyte response to PHA from normal to negative; however, 75% of the responses were at least 2 SD below the mean of unselected normal controls. All but one patient with AIDS associated *Pneumocystis carinii* pneumonia had significantly reduced response. These cases have been previously described (11, 12).

The At Risk control group shown here were homosexual men not living in New York. Low responders within this group were those with greater promiscuity and drug use. Patients with LA included approximately 60% having an abnormal response to PHA. However, the remaining 40% were clearly within the normal range. Although it seemed possible that viral infection, possibly CMV or EBV might account for impaired T cell function in patients with LA, given the widespread nature of these viruses in the population being studied, there turned out to be no correlation between positive blood cultures and antibody titer and proliferative response. Study of patients not at risk for AIDS having these infections tended to suggest a much less impaired immune system and return to normal response was observed to coincide with clinical resolution. Since the LA patient population was defined to exclude drug abusers, drug abuse per se, known to affect immune response negatively, was not an issue. Since in other studies (1) we had found that response to microbial B cell activators was correlated with serum immunoglobulin level, we examined this response in AIDS.

Lymphocyte response to the B lymphocyte activator *E. Coli* was studied in the same patient populations and the results are shown in Figure 2. 80% of patients with AIDS-KS showed an abnormal response to *E. coli*. Among patients with abnormal response, it was possible to subgroup persons with absolutely no proliferative response (44%) from those who showed slight lymphocyte response. The potential significance of this observation will be discussed subsequently. 70% of patients with LA showed abnormally low

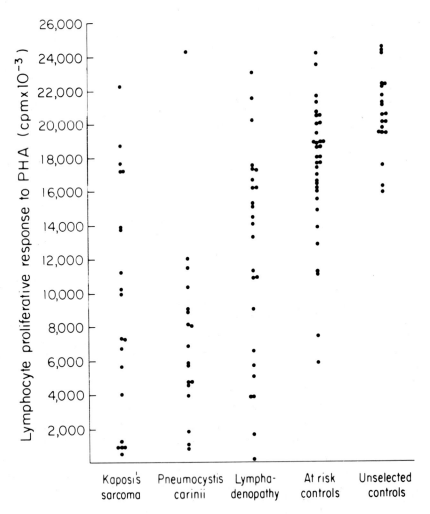

FIG. 1. Mean net maximum response to PHA following pulse labeling of 3-day cell cultures with ^{14}C thymidine is shown for defined AIDS patients, patients with LAS, a risk group of healthy homosexuals and laboratory controls.

response to *E. coli*. This was highly correlated with later development of frank AIDS (13). In contrast to all other groups, the At Risk control group contained a cluster of 10 persons with high lymphocyte proliferative response to *E. coli*. In addition, lymphocytes from the cluster group had unusually strong response to PWM with normal response to PHA. The low responders in this group were also those persons with longer and heavier use of drugs. These data suggested that lifestyle factors which allowed greater exposure to common viral pathogens in association with possible drug affected immune com-

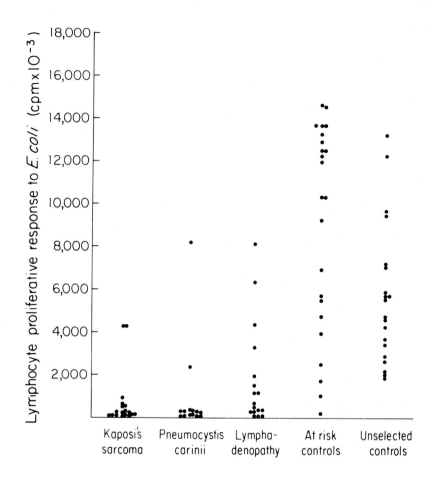

FIG. 2. Mean net maximum response to *E. coli* following pulse labeling of 3-day cell cultures with ^{14}C thymidine is shown for defined AIDS patients, patients with LAS, a risk group of healthy homosexuals and laboratory controls.

promise might lead to persistent viral infection. The immune system would therefore be especially vulnerable to infection with HTLV-III since the second signal required for retroviral replication would be in place.

Coculture Suppression of Normal Lymphocyte Response

We have observed that serum from AIDS patients suppresses lymphocyte response *in vitro* of control cell donors as previously published (2). However, the cellular response of AIDS patients cannot be corrected by a use of pooled normal human serum *in vitro* and the most likely explanation for this would appear to be lymphocyte subpopulation imbalance. All of the patients with AIDS-KS described here showed reduced percentage of helper/inducer T lymphocyte subset (OKT4$^+$) and increased percentage of suppressor/cytotoxic cells (OKT8$^+$). Of 19 patients with LA, all showed depression of helper/suppressor ratio with a range of 0.04 to 0.95 and a median of 0.29. We previously reported that suppressor cell function determined by means of the concanavalin A induction system was as strong as that of normal controls. Coculture experiments were carried out to evaluate cell-mediated suppression of response to PHA. Peripheral blood mononuclear cells, PBM from AIDS patients and LA patients were either added directly to control PBM prior to the addition of mitogen or cells were mixed and incubated for 12 hours before mitogen addition. As shown in Table 1, if third party cells were precultured

TABLE 1.   *Coculture Suppression of Normal Proliferative Response*

Third Party PBM	Preculture Period	Culture Addition	Response to PHA[1]
1. None	none	None	28,680
2. LA	None	None	24,624
3. LA	18 hr	None	14,924
4. LA	18 hr	Indomethacin	21,765
5. None	None	None	24,658
6. AIDS-KS	None	None	16,569
7. AIDS-KS	18 hr	None	12,104

[1] Net median cpm of maximum response following pulse labeling with ^{14}C thymidine.

with responder cells, suppression occurred. Furthermore, addition of indomethacin blocked suppression as shown in line 4.

Related results were obtained with PBM from the same AIDS and LA patients when filtered over G10 Sephadex columns to remove adherent cells. This method as carried out removes monocytes and does not affect helper/suppressor ratio although a small population of adherent T cells also remains attached to the column. As shown in Table 2, preincubation following filtration enabled cells to respond better to PHA than when PHA was added directly following filtration. This was particularly evident in LA patients.

TABLE 2.   *G-10 Filtration of PBM: Effect on Response to PHA in AIDS and LA Syndrome*

PBM Donor	Filtration	Preincubation	Response[1]
1. LA Syndrome	None	None	3,913
2. LA Syndrome	G-10	None	3,558
3. LA Syndrome	G-10	18 hr	6,969
4. AIDS-KS	None	None	7,896
5. AIDS-KS	G-10	None	11,953
6. AIDS-KS	G-10	18 hr	13,872

[1] Net median cpm of maximum response following labeling with ^{14}C thymidine.

Taken as a whole, these data suggested a possible role for prostaglandin in mediating suppression in AIDS. We have recently confirmed this indication (Tarter and Cunningham-Rundles, in preparation).

Restoration of Immune Response *in Vitro* by Immunomodulation

As described, lymphocyte activation *in vivo* in AIDS is characteristically reduced or negative *in vitro*. Among patients with LA, it is possible to distinguish persons having persistently and very significantly reduced response and in our population of 90 men, 70% of this group, which constituted 19% of the initial group, did develop AIDS. In part, this reduced lymphocyte activation *in vitro* could have been related to elevated acid labile serum interferon since we have found a correlation between presence of this lymphokine and subsequent evolution into AIDS. A number of workers have reported loss of Interleukin-2, IL-2, production in AIDS and have found partial restoration of proliferative response when IL-2 was added to the culture medium. We have recently investigated the effect of CL 246, 738, 3, 6-bis (2-piperidinoethoxy) acridine trihydrochloride previously shown to modulate cellular and humoral immunity in a murine model. When PBM from LA patients were primed with CL 246 and then stimulated with IL-2 PHA or PHA + IL-2, enhancement of the PHA response was significantly greater than that observed with IL-2 alone, PHA alone, or IL-2 + PHA, when cells from LA patients were primed with CL 246 first. In contrast, no effect was seen when the same treatments were applied to normal controls. This effect was observed only when patients had poor response to PHA and not in all cases, suggesting that modulation of the IL-2 receptor might be involved. In the data shown in Table 3, it appears that following priming with CL 246, response to PHA in the absence of

TABLE 3.   *Effect of CL 246[1] on Lymphocyte Activation* In Vitro *in LAS*

Cell Source	Primary Culture Addition	Secondary Culture Activator	Rsponse[2]
Control	None	IL-2	4,814
Control	CL 246	IL-2	4,138
Control	None	PHA	15,735
Control	CL 246	PHA	16,146
Control	None	PHA + IL-2	13,810
Control	CL 246	PHA + IL-2	17,284
LA	None	IL-2	1.598
LA	CL 246	IL-2	3,707
LA	None	PHA	2,164
LA	CL 246	PI IA	12,191
LA	None	PHA + IL-2	1,983
LA	CL 246	PHA + IL-2	13,204

[1] 2×10^{-4} µg/ml culture.
[2] Median net cpm following pulse labeling with ^{14}C thymidine.

exogenous IL-2 was observed. These data, although preliminary, suggest that modulation of immune response is a viable possibility in patients infected with HTLV-III.

Cytotoxicity in AIDS and the Lymphadenopathy Syndrome

Natural killer cell activity has been found to be depressed in both AIDS and the lymphadenopathy syndrome. We have previously observed that endogenous NK activity as assayed using the K 567 erythroleukemia target cell and freshly isolated PBM may be in the normal range in individual patients. Interestingly, approximately 66% of AIDS-KS patients have normal NK at the time of presentation (and providing this is the first sign of the syndrome), this sharply declines within 2 to 3 months. Among LA patients, however, 60% have negative NK initially. This may reflect a longer period of gradual progression before these patients seek medical attention compared to AIDS-KS with discernible lesions. In both groups, activated NK activity induced with interferon α or γ may be totally absent, suggesting exhaustion of the recruitable pool of pre-NK cells.

The potential role of the NK system in AIDS might be to destroy cells altered by retroviral infection. Clearly, this might play either a negative or a positive role in disease pathogenesis. We had previously found peripheral blood lymphocytes from AIDS or LA patients could serve as targets for NK lysis by control of effector cells (5). We subsequently attempted to establish cell lines specifically from lymphadenopathy patients (known to be infected with HTLV-III) in order to secure a homogenous source of cells. The cell populations obtained from culturing PBM in the absence of IL-2 were principally B lymphocytes by surface marker criteria as shown in Table 4. The cell

TABLE 4.   *Cell Surface Marker Analysis of AIDS Cell Lines*

Line	T3	T9	T10	T26	Leu 7	M-5	B7	DR
SLA 1	0	0	ND	30.5	20.4	ND	89.7	94.0
SLA 3	0	0	17.4	ND	8.6	0	83.5	93.2
SLA 4	1.6	0	34.8	ND	11.5	1.7	89.7	97.5
SLA 7	0	0	31.6	11.8	10.4	1.6	79.2	97.2

lines expressed variable density of the IL-2 receptor according to cell cycle and the OKT-10 activation marker. The lines secrete large amounts of interferon α which appears to be mainly acid labile and to contain HTLV-III virions (Metroka *et al.*, in preparation). When the cell lines were used as targets for cytotoxicity, normal PBM did not lyse these targets endogenously, but could be induced to lyse these targets with interferon α at a low level (5% to 10%). In contrast, AIDS patients could lyse the targets endogenously and showed an interferon augmented lysis comparable to that with the K 562 target cell. The cell lines contained multiple copies of the EBV genome by DNA hybridization analysis. It seemed possible that the cells had undergone spontaneous malignant transformation with expression of the Epstein-Barr nuclear antigen which might be recognized by AIDS patients' PBM primed *in vivo* to EBV since 100% of this population had ongoing or very recent EBV infection.

Consequently, AIDS patients' cells were studied before and after priming *in vitro* to an AIDS cell line (heterologous to the effector) and Raji which also expresses the EBV genome. The two cell donors shown in Table 5 showed

TABLE 5.   *Effect of Priming on Target Cytotoxicity in LAS*

Cell Donor	Priming Cell	Target	Cytotoxicity[2]
LA-1[1]	None	SLA-2[1]	48
LA-1	Raji	SLA-2	30
LA-1	SLA-2	SLA-2	84
LA-2	None	SLA-2	46
LA-2	Raji	SLA-2	100
LA-2	SLA-2	SLA-2	100
LA-1	None	Raji	12
LA-1	Raji	Raji	46
LA-1	SLA-2	Raji	24
LA-2	None	Raji	17
LA-2	Raji	Raji	100
LA-2	SLA-2	Raji	80

[1] Cell line derived from AIDS patient.
[2] ^{51}Cr release at effector/target ratio 100:1 following 18 hr assay.

marked differences in response. Both showed significantly stronger endogenous lysis of the SLA line relative to Raji. One effector exhibited strong killing of the unprimed SLA target, while the other did not. The reciprocal experiment showed the same trend in specificity.

Our data suggest that B lymphocytes from HTLV-III infected patients can undergo malignant transformation *in vitro* and that this is accompanied by secretion of acid labile interferon. It is possible that the B lymphocyte is also the source of this production *in vivo*. If so, this may explain the observed correlation between elevated interferon and poor prognosis. Furthermore, if these same cells may harbor retrovirus as we have found, then B cells secreting interferon may be the marker of retroviral infection. Vadhan has recently developed a model for predicting survival and response to interferon α therapy in which response to *E. coli* and absence of serum interferon were significant positive factors. Thus, the effect of EBV in B lymphocyte transformation in AIDS may be a dual one acting both to harbor and protect HTLV-III since these cells are not lysed and to promote malignant transformation which *in vivo* would lead to the development of B cell lymphomas.

For reasons that are not yet known, patients with lymphadenopathy have the greatest tendency to develop B cell neoplasia. Clarification of the mechanisms involved may provide essential new information on the development of cancer as a consequence of altered immunoregulation.

Acknowledgements

The authors gratefully acknowledge the technical assistance of R. Bedfor, A. Hoppin, A. Waring, and J. Weil. These studies were supported by NCI CA 34995 and NY AO-163.

REFERENCES

1. Cunningham-Rundles, S., Cunningham-Rundles, C., Ma, D.I., Siegal, F.P., Kosloff, C., Gupta, S., Smithwick, F.M., and Good, R.A. (1981): Impaired proliferative response to B lymphocyte activators in common varied immunodeficiency disease, 15:279-282.
2. Cunningham-Rundles, S., Michelis, M.A., and Masur, H. (1983): Serum suppression of lymphocyte activation *in vitro* in acquired immunodeficiency disease. *J. Clin. Immunol.,* 3:156-165.
3. Cunningham-Rundles, S. (1984): Analyses of altered immune function in the Acquired Immunodeficiency Syndrome. In: The Acquired Immunodeficiency Syndrome and Infections of Homosexual Men, edited by P. Macleod and D. Armstrong, pp. 331-340. Herder, N. York, NY.
4. Cunningham-Rundles, S., Safai, B., Metroka, C., Krown, S.E., Rubin, B.Y., and Stahl, W.E. (1984): Lymphocyte effector function *in vitro* in the Acquired Immune Deficiency Syndrome. in: AIDS: The Epidemic of Kaposi's Sarcoma and Opportunistic Infections, edited by A.E. Friedman-Kien and L.J. Lauberstein, pp. 153-159. Masson, USA.
5. Cunningham-Rundles, S., Metroka, C.E., Safai, B., Krim, M., Rubin, B.Y., and Hayward, G. (In press): Cytotoxic effector mechanisms in AIDS. *Int. Conference on AIDS,* edited by S. Gupta.
6. Elliott, J.H., Hoppes, S.L., Platt, M.S., Thomas, J.G., Patel, I.P., and Gansar, A. (1983): The acquired immunodeficiency syndrome and *Mycobacterium avium* intracellular bacteremia in a patient with hemophilia. *Ann. Int. Med.,* 98:290-293.
7. Fauci, A.S. (1982): The syndrome of Kaposi's Sarcoma and opportunistic infections: an epidemiologically restricted disorder of immunoregulation. *Ann. Intern. Med.* 96:777-782.
8. Gottlieb, M.S., Schroff, R., Schanker, H.M., Weisman, J.D., Fan, P.T., Wolf, R.A., and Saxon, A. (1981): *Pneumocystis carinii* pneumonia and mucosal candidiasis in previously healthy homosexual men: Evidence of a new acquired cellular immunodeficiency. *N. Engl. J. Med.,* 305:1425-1431.
9. Lane, H.C., Masur, H., Edgard, L.C., Uhalen, G., Rook, A.H., and Fauci, A.S. (1983): Abnormalities of B-cell activation and immunoregulation in patients with the acquired immunodeficiency disorder. *N. Engl. J. Med.,* 309:453-458. Persistent, generalized lymphadenopathy among homosexual males (1982): MMWR 31:249-251.
10. Levine, A.M., Meyer, P.B., Begandy, M.K., Parker, J.W., Taylor, C.R., Irwin, L., and Lukes, R.J. (1984): Development of B cell lymphomas in homosexual men. *Ann. Int. Med.,* 100:7-13.
11. Masur, H., Michelis, M.A., Greene, J.B., Onorato, I., Vande Sfouve, R.A., Holzman, R.S., Wormser, G., Brettman, L., Lange, M., and Cunningham-Rundles, S., (1981): A community acquired outbreak of *Pneumocystis carinii* pneumonia: initial manifestation of cellular immune dysfunction. *N. Engl. J. Med.,* 305:1431-1438.
12. Masur, H., Michelis, M.A., Wormser, G.P., Lewin, S., Gold, J., Tapper, M.A., Giron, J., Lerner, C.W., Armstrong, D., Setia, U., Sender, J.A., Siebken, R.S., Nicholas, P., Siegal, F.P., and Cunningham-Rundles, S., (1983): Previously healthy women with opportunistic infection vs. the initial manifestation of a community acquired cellular immunodeficiency extension of an emerging syndrome. *Ann. Int. Med.* 97:533-539.
13. Metroka, C.E., Cunningham-Rundles, S., Pollack, M.S., Sonnabend, J.A., Davis, J.M., Gordon, B., Fernandes, R.D., and Mouradian, J. (1982): Generalized lymphadenopathy in homosexual men. *Ann. Int. Med.* 99:585-591.
14. Siegal, F.P., Lopez, C., Hammer, G.S., Brown, A.E., Kornfeld, S.J., Gold, J., Hassett, J., Hirschman, S.Z., Cunningham-Rundles, C., Adelsbert, B.R., Parham, D.M., Siegal, M., Cunningham-Rundles, S., and Armstrong, D. (1981): Severe acquired immunodeficiency in male homosexuals manifested by chronic perianal ulcerative herpes simplex lesions. *N. Engl. J. Med.,* 305:1439-1444.

15. Vadhan, S.G., Real, F.X., Cunningham-Rundles, S., Oettgen, H.F., and Krown, S.E. (1984): Lymphocyte proliferative response to phytohemagglutinin (PHA) in patients with Kaposi's sarcoma and acquired immunodeficiency. *Proc. Am. Assoc. Clin. Res.* (In press).
16. Vieira, J., Frank, E., Spira, R.J., and Landesman, S.H. (1983): Acquired immune deficiency in Haitians: opportunistic infections in previously healthy Haitians. *N. Engl. J. Med.* 308:125-129.
17. Ziegler, J.L., Beckslead, J.A., Volberding, P.A., Abrams, D.I., Levine, A.M., Lukes, R.J., Gill, P.S., Burkes, R.L., Meyer, P.R., Metroka, C.E., Mouradian, J., Moore, A., Riggs S.A., Butler, J.J., Cabanillas, F.C., Hersh, E., Newell, G.R., Laubanstein, L.J., Knowles, D., Odajnyk, C., Raphael, B., Koziner, B., Urmacher, C., and Clarkson, B.D., (1984): Non-Hodgkin's lymphoma in 90 homosexual men. Relation to generalized lymphadenopathy and the Acquired Immunodeficiency Syndrome. *N. Engl. J. Med.,* 311:565-570.

Immunological Abnormalities in the Acquired Immunodeficiency Syndrome

J.B. Margolick, D.L. Bowen, H.C. Lane and A.S. Fauci

Laboratory of Immunoregulation
National Institute of Allergy and Infectious Disease
National Institutes of Health Bethesda, Maryland 20205, USA

The acquired immunodeficiency syndrome (AIDS) was first recognized in 1981 when the Centers for Disease Control reported 5 cases of *Pneumocystis carinii* pneumonia (8) and 26 cases of Kaposi's sarcoma (9) in previously healthy homosexual men. Because of the frequent occurrence of viral, fungal, parasitic, and neoplastic diseases known to be "opportunistic" in their predilection for patients with impaired or suppressed cellular immunity, AIDS was almost immediately recognized as due to a profound impairment of cellular immunity, with humoral immunity thought to be relatively spare (22, 35, 49). Although it is now known that B cell function in AIDS is also profoundly abnormal, patients with AIDS are not unusually susceptible to the bacterial diseases associated with humoral immunodeficiency and defective cellular immunity has remained the hallmark of the disease. This chapter will summarize what has been learned about the mechanisms underlying the collapse of cellular immunity in this devastating disease, and will outline how these mechanisms are intimately related to the properties of the retrovirus, known variously as human T-cell leukemia/lymphoma virus-III (HTLV-III), lymphadenopathy associated virus (LAV), and AIDS-related virus (ARV), which has recently been shown to be the causative agent of AIDS (19).

Immunologic Abnormalities in AIDS

The cellular immune system, i.e., T. cell function, is primarily affected, but functional abnormalities of B cells, mononuclear phagocytes, and natural killer cells have also been described.

Quantitative abnormalities of T cells

One of the first abnormalities to be described in AIDS was a decrease in the peripheral lymphocyte count in most patients (9, 22, 35, 49). When

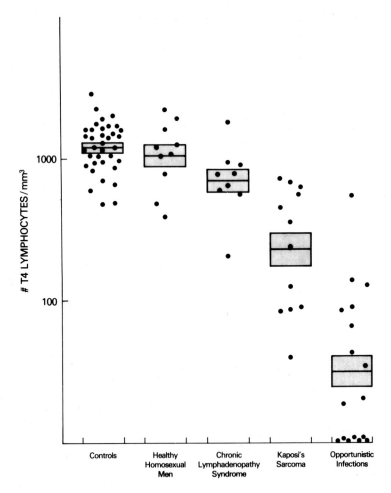

FIG. 1. Total number of peripheral blood T4$^+$ lymphocytes for the clinical subpopulations of patients with AIDS, patients with chronic lymphadenopathy syndrome, and control subjects. Those patients presenting with opportunistic infections have the lowest number of T4$^+$ cells (reprinted with permission from reference 28).

functional T lymphocyte subsets where quantitated using monoclonal antibodies, it became apparent that virtually all patients with AIDS had decreased numbers of circulating helper-inducer (OKT4$^+$ or Leu 3$^+$) T cells (49, 22, 36, 18) (Figure 1). This helper-inducer lymphopenia largely accounted for the overall lymphopenia, since these cells normally constitute about two-thirds of circulating lymphocytes. This defect was also responsible for the decreased T4/T8 ratios in patients with AIDS, who often had normal or elevated numbers of T8$^+$ (suppressor-cytotoxic) T lymphocytes (1, 49, 52, 17, 30). Therefore, the abnormally low T4/T8 ratio in AIDS was due to a different mechanism than that seen in non-AIDS patients with common viral infections such as cytomegalovirus and Epstein-Barr virus (7, 15, 16, 44) or in healthy male homosexuals, who generally had normal numbers of $T4^+$ cells but elevated numbers of $T8^+$ cells, usually due to a high frequency of infections with these latter viruses (1, 16, 30, 49, 52).

Functional abnormalities of T cells

Since the $T4^+$ lymphocyte plays an important role in the induction of many immune response (11, 17, 18, 43) (See below), and since patients with AIDS exhibit a marked variation in the extent of T4 cell depletion it is not surprising that multiple immunologic abnormalities have been observed in patients with AIDS, and that the degree of abnormality varies widely. Defective T cell responses observed in AIDS include in vivo defects such as impaired or absent delayed cutaneous hypersensitivity response (3-5, 8, 22, 35, 36, 48), as well as numerous in vitro defects such as decreased mitogen- and antigen-induced blastogenesis (10, 18, 24), decreased mitogen- and antigen-induced lymphokine production (10, 39), decreased cytotoxicity (46), decreased allogeneic (1, 12, 35) and autologous (24) mixed lymphocyte responses, and decreased T cell help for B cell immunoglobulin production (5, 29).

These in vitro parameters have generally been studied using unfractionated peripheral blood mononuclear cells (PBMC) from patients with AIDS. When correction is made for the wide variation in numbers and proportions of $T4^+$ cells present in the PBMC by studying purified $T4^+$ cells from the patients, certain of these abnormalities are no longer noted, indicating that they represent quantitative rather than qualitative defects. For example, the response of purified $T4^+$ cells from AIDS patients to pokeweed mitogen was normal (Figure 2a), as were the production of interleukin 2 and γ-IFN and the expression of IL 2 receptors (28). Purified $T4^+$ and $T8^+$ cells from patients with AIDS exhibited variable help and normal suppression, respectively, for B cell immunoglobulin synthesis in a pokeweed mitogen-driven system (29). However, the lack of T cell response to soluble antigens was not corrected by the use of purified $T4^+$ cells; in fact, the purified $T4^+$ cells from most patients failed to respond at all to soluble antigen (Figure 2b). This result, coupled with the consistent numerical decrease in $T4^+$ cells in AIDS, strongly supports the hypothesis that the lack of antigen-induced $T4^+$ cell responses is a fundamental defect in AIDS (28). The most likely mechanism for this defect is the physical absence or scarcity of the antigen-reactive $T4^+$ cell population. However, viable T4 cells, particularly the antigen-reactive subset of T4 cells, may also be functionally impaired as demonstrated by the variable help provided to B cells, as mentioned above, and their relative inability to be clonally expanded, as discussed below. The number of antigen-specific $T4^+$ cells present in AIDS patients has been analyzed using monoclonal antibodies such as Leu 8/TQ1 that have been reported to identify the suppressor-inducer subpopulation of $T4^+$ cells (40). In patients with AIDS-related complex man-

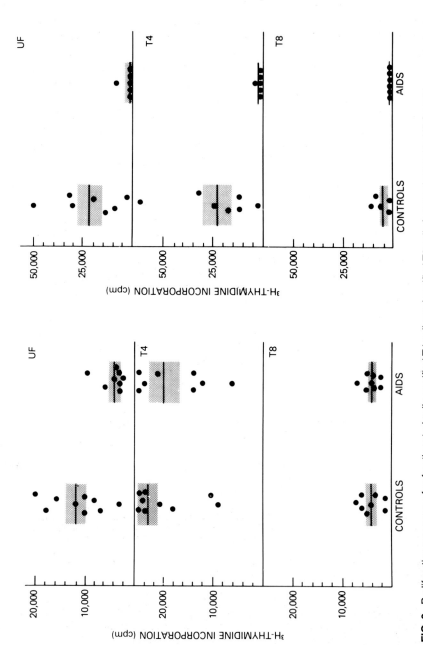

FIG. 2. Proliferative response of unfractionated cells, purified T4 cells and purified T8 cells from patients with AIDS and from controls. Lines and shaded areas represent the means φ SEM for each group. Proliferative response to pokeweed mitogen (A) and tetanus toxoid (B) are shown. The AIDS patients have normal responses to pokeweed mitogen, but responses to tetanus toxoid are greatly diminished in both the unfractionated cells and the purified T4 cells. (Reprinted with permission from reference 30).

ifested by chronic lymphadenopathy, the subpopulation of T4$^+$ Leu8$^+$ cells has been reported to be relatively depleted compared to the T4$^+$ Leu8$^-$ subpopulation (40). Monoclonal antibodies have recently been described which more precisely define the antigen-reactive subset of T4$^+$ cells (37). Current studies using these antibodies are underway aimed at determining whether this subset is selectively depleted early in the course of infection with the AIDS retrovirus (H.C. Lane and A.S. Fauci, unpublished observations).

When purified T4$^+$ and T8$^+$ cells form patients with AIDS were cultured under cloning conditions (i.e., limiting dilution in the presence of mitogen, feeder cells, and interleukin 2), both T4$^+$ and T8$^+$ cells from the AIDS patients had greatly reduced cloning efficiencies compared to cells from healthy heterosexual control donors (Figure 3) (34). Thus, it appears that the T

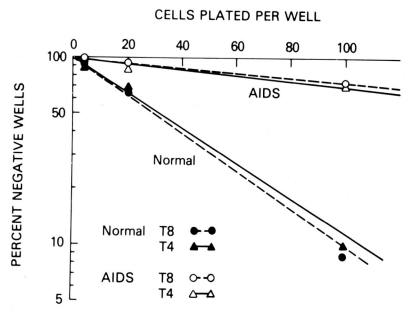

FIG. 3. Limiting dilution cloning analysis of purified T4 and T8 cells from a patient with the AIDS and from a normal donor. The straight lines indicate that the data conform to a one-hit Poisson distribution. There is a marked decrease in cloning efficiences of both T4 and T8 cells in patients with AIDS. The precursor frequencies are: normal T4 = 1/46, acquired immunodeficiency syndrome T4 = 1/276; normal T8 = 1/40, acquired immunodeficiency syndrome T8 = 1/368. (Reprinted with permission from reference 34).

cell defect in AIDS may extend to the level of the individual viable T cell, which exhibits and intrinsic defect in the ability to expand clonally. Of note, T4$^+$ and T8$^+$ cells appear to be affected approximately equally. In this study, the clones that ultimately were obtained from the AIDS T cells demonstrated normal proliferative responses to phytohemagglutinin and provided normal help (T4$^+$ clones) or suppression (T8$^+$ clones) to pokeweed mitogen-stimu-lated B cells.

Other abnormalities of T8$^+$ (suppressor-cytotoxic) cell function in AIDS have been described. There is generally an increased proportion of circulating T cells that express activation markers such as HLA-DR or T10 (22, 47). However, T8$^+$ cell function is decreased rather than increased. Thus, specific killing of cytomegalovirus-infected target cells by AIDS T8$^+$ cells was pro-foundly impaired compared to controls (46). This impairment was partially reversed by the addition of IL 2 to the cultures, demonstrating that the cytotoxic T8$^+$ cells were present and could be induced. These results strongly suggest that defective killing by T8$^+$ cells in AIDS may be secondary to a lack of an appropriate inductive signal delivered to the cytotoxic T8$^+$ cell by a normally functioning T4$^+$ cell. Similarly, lysis of K562 target cells by natural killer (NK) cells was abnormally low in AIDS patients but was improved by the addition of IL 2 to the cultures (46).

In summary, patients with AIDS manifest profound disturbances of T cell function that are most likely due to both 1) a marked decrease in the number of T4$^+$ cells and the amount of helper-inducer function available to stimulate other immunocompetent cells, and 2) intrinsic abnormalities of T cells that do not depend directly on abnormalities of other types of cells.

B Cell Abnormalities in AIDS

In contrast to the early recognition of a profound T cell defect in AIDS, B cell function was initially felt to be intact, since serum immunoglobulins were not decreased (20, 22, 35, 48, 51). In fact, serum immunoglobulins, especially IgG and IgA, are generally elevated, and patients with AIDS frequently have circulating immune complexes (32) and exhibit autoimmune phenome-na (53). The explanation for these observations is an intense polyclonal activa-tion of B cells similar to that seen in systemic lupus erythematosus and characterized by 1) greatly elevated numbers of circulating spontaneous im-munoglobulin-secreting cells (i.e., plaque-forming cells) and 2) greatly di-minished numbers of resting B cells that can be activated in vitro by standard B cell mitogens such as *Staphylococcus aureus* Cowan strain I and antibodies to surface IgM (29).

The mechanism for this generalized B cell activation in AIDS is not known. Possible mechanisms include viral infction and/or transformation of B cells with a B-lymphotropic virus such as Epstein-Barr virus (EBV) or with other viruses such as cytomegalovirus (CMV) that can induce B cell activation; infection with the AIDS retrovirus, which can infect EBV-transformed B cells (38); absence of the appropriate regulation of B cell activation by nor-mally functioning T cells; hypersecretion of B cell activating factors by virally transformed T cells, as has been reported for HTLV-I transformed T cells (47); or some combination of these mechanisms. Of note is the fact that CMV and EBV infections are present in virtually all patients with AIDS (42).

The high level of activated B cells in AIDS, as well as the increased responses of B cells to B cell growth factors in vitro, bear a striking resemblance to in vitro infection of B cells with EBV.

Patients with AIDS are unable to mount appropriate specific antibody responses either to new antigens such as keyhole limpet hemocyanin or recall antigens such as tetanus toxoid (2, 29). This lack of specific antibody response to antigen exposure or immunization may be due to the fact that most or all of the B cells are already activated and cannot be stimulated further, or to the above-mentioned defect in the antigen-specific T4$^+$ cell responsiveness required to initiate specific antibody responses. Whatever the mechanism, the fact remains that both the cellular and humoral arms of the immune system in patients with AIDS are unable to respond appropriately to antigen exposure. In particular, the use of standard antibody criteria for diagnosis of infections is unreliable in these patients (16, 33, 45).

Abnormalities of Mononuclear Phagocyte Function in AIDS

Although the number of circulating monocytes is generally normal in patients with AIDS, these cells have been reported to exhibit defective chemotaxis in response to a variety of stimuli (51) as well as defective killing of the parasitic organisms *Giardia lamblia and Toxoplasma gondii* in vitro (39). Extracellular killing of T. gondii was enhanced by the addition of γ-IFN to the cultures, suggesting that this defect may be related to defective helper-inducer cell function. Consistent with this interpretation is the report that AIDS monocytes respond to γ-IFN with normal increases in H_2O_2 release and cytotoxicity (23). Also, AIDS monocytes have been reported to have a defect in expression of surface Ia molecules (4), another effect which could be mediated by diminished γ-IFN levels. However, there is also evidence of monocyte pre-activation similar to that seen with B cells. Thus, AIDS monocytes spontaneously secrete interleukin 1 (IL 1) and prostaglandin E_2 (51) and have a diminished response to inducers of IL 1 release. At present it is unclear whether these abnormalities of monocyte function are related to direct infection of these cells with the AIDS retrovirus, lack of appropriate regulatory signals from T4$^+$ cells, or to secondary effects arising from the presence of multiple opportunistic infections in these patients.

Circulating Suppressor Factors in AIDS

Sera from patients with AIDS have been reported to contain factors that can suppress in vitro immune functions. One suppressive factor can inhibit a-IFN induced NK activity of normal PBMC as well as MLC- and phytohemagglutinin-stimulated proliferation of normal lymphocytes (12, 50). A different suppressor factor which did not affect NK activity has been detected in supernatants from a T-T hybridoma derived from T cells from a patient with AIDS (31). This factor suppressed B cell responses to mitogens as measured by proliferation and immunoglobulin synthesis, and resembles previously reported suppressor factors derived from T cells (23).

The exact nature and significance of these factors in the immunologic deficits seen in AIDS is not known and is still under investigation.

Other Serologic Abnormalities in AIDS

Also of unclear importance are a number of immune-related serological abnormalities that occur in AIDS. Anti-lymphocyte antibodies directed against both T4$^+$ and T8$^+$ lymphocytes have been reported in patients with AIDS (53). Patients with AIDS have been reported to have elevated circulating levels of β-2 microglobulin (6), a-1-thymosin (25), and an acid-labile α-interferon (15) similar to that observed in systemic lupus erythematosus. Serum levels of thymulin have been abnormally low in most patients with AIDS (14).

The AIDS Retrovirus and the Immunopathogenesis of AIDS

As has been emphasized several times in the preceeding sections, the constellation of immunologic deficits that occurs in AIDS is almost entirely compatible with an underlying defect in the T4$^+$ helper-inducer population, especially the antigen-specific subset of these cells (Figure 4). This observation, along with the decrease in T4$^+$ cells seen in virtually all patients with AIDS, strongly suggested that AIDS would prove to be caused by an agent selectively destructive to T4$^+$ lymphocytes. In addition, epidemiologic studies strongly suggested that AIDS was caused by an infectious agent, most likely a virus. Thus, a relationship of the putative AIDS agent to the newly identified class of human retroviruses called human T lymphotropic viruses (HTLV) was suspected early on. Viruses first isolated from patients with AIDS or related syndrome and strongly suspected of being causal for AIDS were originally designated lymphadenopathy-associated virus (LAV) (3) and HTLV-III (21). It is now clear that the underlying etiologic agent in AIDS is a previously undescribed human retrovirus with a selective tropism for T4 lymphocytes (19). For the sake of convenience, one can refer to the virus as HTLV-III/LAV until a more precise nomenclature is established.

HTLV-III/LAV is extremely cytopathic fro T4$^+$ lymphocytes, a fact which greatly complicated initial attempts to isolate and characterize it. However, permissive cell lines have been found and the virus has now been fully purified and its genome cloned. HTLV-III/LAV infection of T4$^+$ cells in vitro results in the production of infectious virus and the death of infected lymphocytes within 10-14 days. HTLV-III/LAV does not infect T8$^+$ lymphocytes (26), and in fact it appears that the T4 molecule may be necessary for the virus to enter a target cell, i.e., the T4 molecule itself may be the receptor for the virus (13, 27, 44). This conclusion is based on the observations that anti-T4 (CD4) antibodies, but not other antibodies, can block infection of cells with HTLV-III/LAV (13, 27) and that only cells that expressed T4 could be infected in

HYPOTHETICAL SCHEME FOR THE MODULATION OF THE HUMAN IMMUNE
SYSTEM IN AIDS BY HTLV

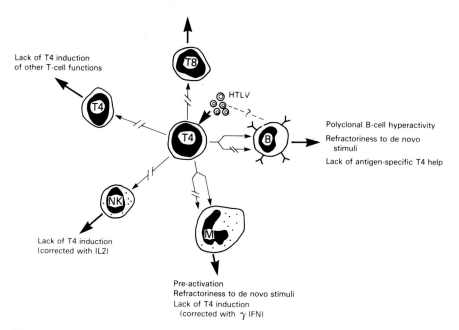

FIG. 4. Modulation of the human immune system by direct HTLV-III infection of the T4 helper/in-ducer lymphocyte subset. Infection of the helper/inducer cell with HTLV-III results in diverse functional defects due to a lack of inductive function for other T cells, cytotoxic cells (natural killer and T8), and monocytes, as well as a lack of helper function for the B cell. Reprinted with permission from *Clin. Res.* 32:491-9, 1985).

vitro (13, 44). Thus, the characteristics of HTLV-III/LAV coincide remarka-bly with those that were predicted for the causative agent of AIDS.

In addition to its well-documented cytopathic effect on $T4^+$ cells, it is possible that HTLV-III/LAV may cause loss of $T4^+$ cell function in other ways. For example, the virus could infect cells nonproductively or nonlytically, so that they are not killed directly but contain proviral nucleic acid sequences that interfere with cell replication or function. Alternatively, the virus could interfere with the function of the T4 molecule, either indirectly by inhibiting its expression in infected cells (13) or directly by binding to the molecule on the cell surface.

Finally, it should be kept in mind that the full spectrum of HTLV-III/LAV infectivity has not been defined and that direct effects on other immunocompe-tent cells, such as monocytes, natural killer cells, and B lymphocytes, may exist. In this regard, as previously mentioned, B cells that have been trans-formed with EBV may be susceptible to HTLV-III/LAV infection in vitro (38).

In conclusion, much has been learned in a very short time about both the immunologic defects in AIDS and the biology of HTLV-III/LAV the causative agent of AIDS. However, the mechanisms responsible for clinical infection with HTLV-III/LAV and for host resistance to this devastating infectious agent remain unknown. In addition, the mechanism for the preferential depletion of the antigen-specific subset of T4 cells in AIDS patients has not been fully determined. One hypothesis is that activated T4$^+$ cells are more susceptible to infection with HTLV-III/LAV than are resting T4^1 cells, as appears to be the case with HTLV-I. If this is the case, repeated antigenic exposure, for example by infections or transfusions with blood or blood products, could result in propagation and maintenance of HTLV-III/LAV infection and thus more rapid and extensive T4$^+$ cell depletion. The discovery of HTLV-III/LAV and its causative role in AIDS will facilitate progress toward the understanding, treatment, and prevention of the profound immune dysfunction that is the hallmark of AIDS.

REFERENCES

1. Ammann, A.J., Abrams, D., Conant, M., Chudwin, D., Cowan, M., Volberding, P., Lewis, B., Casavant, C. (1983): Acquired immune dysfunction in homosexual men: immunologic profiles. *Clin. Immunol. Immunopathol.* 27:315-325.
2. Ammann, A.J., Schiffman, G., Abrams, D., Volberding, P., Ziegler, J., Conant, M. (1984): B-cell immunodeficiency in acquired immune deficiency syndrome. *J.A.M.A.* 251:144-1449.
3. Barrè-Sinoussi, F., Chermann, J.-C., Rey, F., Nugeyre, M.T., Chamaret, S., Gruest, J., Dauguest, C., Axler-Blin, C., Brun-Vezinet, F., Rouzioux, C., Rozenbaum, W., Montagnier, L. (1983): Isolation of a T lymphotropic retrovirus from a patient at risk for acquired immune deficiency syndrome (AIDS). *Science* 220:868-871.
4. Belisto, D.V., Sanchez, M.R., Baer, R.L., Valentine, R., Thorbecke, G.J. (1984): Reduced Langerhans' cell Ia antigen and ATPase activity in patients with the acquired immunodeficiency syndrome *N. Engl. J. Med.* 310:1279-1281.
5. Benveniste E., Schroff, R., Stevens, R.H., Gottlieb, M.S. (1983): Immunoregulatory T cells in men with a new acquired immunodeficiency syndrome. *J. Clin. Immunol.* 3::359-367.
6. Bhalla, R.B. (1983): Abnormally high concentrations of beta 2 microglobulin in acquired immunodeficiency syndrome (AIDS) patients. *Clin. Chem.* 19:1560.
7. Carney, W.P., Rubin, R.H., Hoffman, R.A., Hansen, W.P., Healey, K., Hirsch, M.S. (1981): Analysis of T lymphocytes subsets in cytomegalovirus mononucleosis. *J. Immunol.* 126:2114-2116.
8. Centers for Disease Control. (1981): *Pneumocystis* pneumonia-Los Angeles. *Morbid. Mortal. Weekly Rep.* 30:250-252.
9. Centers for Disease Control. (1981): Kaposi's sarcoma and *Pneumocystis* pneumonia among homosexual men-New York City and California. *Morbid. Mortal. Weekly Rep.* 25:305-308.
10. Ciobanu, N., Welk, K., Kruger, G., Venuta, S., Gold, J., Feldman, S., Wang, C.Y., Koziner, B., Moore, M.A.S., Safai, B., Mertelsmann, R. (1983): Defective T-cell responses to PHA and mitogenic monoclonal antibodies in male homosexuals with acquired immune deficiency syndrome and its in vitro correction by interleukin-2. *J. Clin. Invest.* 3:332-342.
11. Corte, G., Mingari, M.C., Moretta, A., Damiani, G., Moretta, L., Bargellesi, A. (1982): Human T cell subpopulations defined by a monoclonal antibody. I. A small subset is responsible for proliferation to allogeneic cells or to soluble antigens and to helper activity for B cell differentiation. *J. Immunol.* 128:16-19.
12. Cunningham-Rundles, S., Michelis, M.A., Masur, H. (1983): Serum suppression of lymphocyte activation in vitro in acquired immunodeficiency disease. *J. Clin. Immunol.* 3:56-165.
13. Dalgleish, A.G., Beverley, P.C.L., Clapham, P.R., Crawford, D.H., Greaves, M.F., Weiss, R.A. (1984): The CD4 (T4) antigen is an essential component of the receptor for the acquired immunodeficiency syndrome retrovirus. *Nature* 312:763-767.

14. Dardenne, M., Bach, J.-F., Safai, B. (1983): Low serum thymic hormone levels in patients with acquired immunodeficiency syndrome. *N. Engl. J. Med.* 309:48-49.
15. DeStefano, E., Friedman, R.M., Friedman-Kien, A.E., Goedert, J.J., Henriksen, D., Preble, O.T., Sonnabend, J.A., Vilcek, J. (1982): Acid-labile human leukocyte interferon in homosexual men with Kaposi's sarcoma and lymphadenopathy. *J. Infect. Dis* 145:451-455.
16. Dylewski, J., Chou, S., Merigan, T.C. (1983): Absence of detectable IgM antibody during cytomegalovirus disease in patients with AIDS. *N. Engl. J. Med.* 309:493.
17. Fahey, J.L., Prince, H., Weaver, M.M., Groopman, J., Bisscher, B., Schwartz, K., Detel, R. (1983): Quantitative changes in the Th or Ts lymphocyte subsets that distinguish AIDS syndromes from other immune subset disorders. *Am. J. Med.* 76:95-100.
18. Fauci, A.S., Macher, A.M., Longo, D.L., Lane, H.C., Rook A.H., Masur, H., Gelmann, E.P. (1984): Acquired immunodeficiency syndrome: epidemiologic, clinical, immunologic, and therapeutic considerations. *Ann. Intern. Med.* 100:92-106.
19. Fauci, A.S., Masur, H., Markham, P.D., Hahn, B.H., Lane, H.C. The acquired immunodeficiency syndrome: an update. *Ann. Intern. Med.* (in press).
20. Friedman-Kien, A.E., Laubenstein, L., Dubin, R., Marmor, M., Zolla-Pazner, S. (1982): Disseminated Kaposi's sarcoma in homosexual men. *Ann. Intern. Med.* 96:693-700.
21. Gallo, R.C., Salahuddin, S.Z., Popovic, M., Sheared, G.M., Kaplan, M., Haynes, B.F., Palker, T.F., Redfield, R., Oleske, J., Safai, B., White, G. Foster, P., Markham, P.D. (1984): Frequent detection and isolation of cytopathic retroviruses (HTLV-III) from patients with AIDS and at risk for AIDS. *Science* 224:500-503.
22. Gottlieb, M.S., Schroff, R., Schander, H.M., Weisman, D.O., Fan, P.T., Wolf, R.A., Saxon, A. (1981): *Pneumocystis carinii* pneumonia and mucosal candidiasis in previously healthy homosexual men: evidence for a new acquired cellular immunodeficiency. *N. Engl. J. Med.* 305:1421-1430.
23. Greene, W.C., Fleisher, T.A., Nelson, D.L., Waldmann, T.A. (1982): Production of human suppressor T cell hybridomas. *J. Immunol.* 129:1986-1992.
24. Gupta, S., Safai, B. (1983): Deficient autologous mixed lymphocyte reaction in Kaposi's sarcoma associated with deficiency of Leu-3 positive responder cells. *J. Clin. Invest.* 71:296-300.
25. Hersh, E.M., Reuben, J.M., Rios, A., Mansell, P.W., Newell, G.R., McClure, J.E., Goldstein, A.L., (1983): Elevated serum thymosin alpha-1 levels associated with evidence of immune dysregulation in male homosexuals with a history of infectious diseases or Kaposi's sarcoma *N. Engl. J. Med.* 308:45-46.
26. Klatzmann, D., Barrè-Sinoussi, F., Nugeyre, M.T., Dauguet, C., Vilmer, E., Griscelli, C., Brun-Vezinet, F., Rouzioux, C., Gluckman, J.C., Chermann, J.-C., Montagnier, L. (1984): Selective tropism of lymphadenopathy associated virus (LAV) for helper-inducer T lymphocytes. *Science* 225:59-63.
27. Klatzmann, D., Champagne, E., Chamanet, E., Gruest, J., Guètard, D., Hercend, T., Gluckman, J.C., Montagnier, L. (1984): The T4 molecule behaves as the receptor for human retrovirus LAV. *Nature* 312:767-768.
28. Lane, H.C., Depper, J.M., Greene, W.S., Whalen, G., Waldmann, T.A., Fauci, A.S. Qualitative analysis of immune function in patients with the acquired immunodeficiency syndrome: evidence for a selective defect in soluble antigen recognition. *N. Engl. J. Med.* (in press).
29. Lane, H.C., Masur, H., Edgar, L.C., Whalen, G., Rook, A.H., Fauci, A.S. (1983): Abnormalities of B lymphocyte activation and immunoregulation in patients with the acquired immunodeficiency syndrome. *N. Engl. J. Med.* 309:453-458.
30. Lane, H.C., Masur, H., Gelmann, E.P., Longo, D.L., Steis, R.G., Chused, T., Whalen, G., Edgar, L.C., Fauci, A.S. (1985): Immunologic profiles define clinical subpopulations of patients with the acquired immunodeficiency syndrome. *Am. J. Med.* 78:417-422.
31. Laurence, J., Mayer, L. (1984): Immunoregulatory lymhokines of T hybridomas from AIDS patients: constitutive and inducible suppressor factor. *Science* 225:66-69.
32. Lightfoote, M.M., Folks, T.M., Sell, K.W. (1984): Analysis of immune complex components isolated from serum of AIDS patients. *Fed. Proc.* 43:1921.
33. Luft, D.J., Conley, F., Remington, J.S., Laverdiere, M., Levine, J.F., (1983): Outbreak of central-nervous system toxoplasmosis in Western Europe and North America. *Lancet* 1:781-783.
34. Margolick, J.B., Volkman, D.J., Lane, H.C., Fauci, A.S. Clonal analysis of T lymphocytes in the acquired immunodeficiency syndrome; evidence for an abnormality affecting individual helper and suppressor T cells. *J. Clin. Invest.* (in press).

35. Masur, H., Michelis, M.A., Greene, J.B., Onorato, I., Vande Stouwe, R.A., Holzman, R.S., Wormser, G., Brettman, L., Lange, M., Murray, H.W., Cunningham-Rundles, S., (1981): An outbreak of community-acquired *P. carinii* pneumonia: initial manifestation of cellular immune dysfunction. *N. Engl. J. Med.* 305:1431-1438.
36. Mildvan, D., Mathur, U., Enlow, R.W., Roman, P.L., Winchester, R.J., Cop., C., Singman, H., Alelsberg, B.R., Springland, I. (1982): Opportunistic infections and immunodeficiency in homosexual men. *Ann. Intern. Med.* 96:700-704.
37. Morimoto, C., Letvin, N.L., Boma, A.W., Hagan, M., Brown, H.M., Kornacki, M.M., and Schlossman, S.F. The Isolation and characterization of the human helper-inducer T cell subset. *J. Immunol.*, in press.
38. Montagnier, L., Gruest, J., Chamaret, S., Dauguet, C., Axler, C., Guètard, D., Nugeyre, M.T., Barrè-Sinoussi, F., Chermann, J.-C., Brunet, J.B., Klatzman, D., Gluckman, J.C. (1984): Adaptation of lymphadenopathy associated virus (LAV) to replication in EBV-transformed B lymphoblstoid cell lines. *Science* 225:63-66.
39. Murray, H.W., Rubin, B.Y., Masur, H., Roberts, R.B. (1984): Impaired production of lymphokines and immune (gamma) interferon in the acquired immunodeficiency syndrome. *N. Engl. J. Med.* 310:883-889.
40. Nicholson, J.K.A., McDougal, J.S., Spira, T.J., Cross, G.D., Jones, B.M., Reinherz, E.L. (1984): Immunomodulatory subsets of the T helper and T suppressor cell populations in homosexual men with chronic unexplained lymphadenopathy. *J. Clin. Invest.* 73:191-201.
41. Popovic, M., Read-Connole, E., Gallo, R.C. (1984): T4 positive human neoplastic cell lines susceptible for and permissive for HTLV-III. *Lancet* 2:1472-1473.
42. Quinnan, G.V., Masur, H., Rook, A.H., Armstrong, G., Frederick, W.R., Epstein, J. Manischewitz, J.F., Macher, A.M., Jackson, L., Ames, J., Straus, S.E. (1984): Herpesvirus infections in the acquired immune deficiency syndrome. *J.A.M.A.* 252:72-77.
43. Reinherz, E.L., Morimoto, C., Fitzgerald, K.A., Hussey, R.E., Daley, F.J., Schlossman, S.F. (1982): Heterogeneity of human T4 inducer T cells defined by a monoclonal antibody that delineated two functional subpopulations. *J. Immunol.* 128:463-468.
44. Reinherz, E.L., O'Brien, C., Rosenthal, P., Schlossman, S.F. (1980): The cellular basis of viral-induced immunodeficiency: analysis by monoclonal antibodies. *J. Immunol.* 125:1269-1276.
45. Roberts, C.J., Coccidioidomycosis in acquired immune deficiency syndrome. Depressed humoral as well as cellular immunity. *Am. J. Med.* 76:734-736.
46. Rook, A.H., Masur, H., Lane, H.C., Frederick, W., Kasahara, T., Macher, A.M., Djeu, J.Y., Manischewitz, J.F., Jackson, L., Fauci, A.S., Quinnan, G.V., Jr. (1983): Interleukin-2 enhances the depressed natural killer and cytomegalovirus-specific cytotoxic activities of lymphocytes from patients with the acquired immune deficiency syndrome. *J. Clin. Invest.* 72:398-403.
47. Salahuddin, S.Z., Markham, P.D., Lindner, S.G., Gootenberg, J., Popovic, M., Hemmi, H., Sarin, P.W., Gallo, R.C. (1984): Lymphokine production by cultered human T cells transformed by human T cell leukemia lymphoma virus I. *Science* 223:703-707.
48. Schroff, R.W., Gottlieb, M.D., Prince, H.E., Chai, L.L., Fahey, J.L. (1983): Immunological studies of homosexual men with immunodeficiency and Kaposi's sarcoma. *Clin. Immunol. Immunopathol.* 27:300-314.
49. Siegal, F.P., Lopez, E., Hammer, G.S., Brown, A.E., Kornfeld, S.J., Gold, J. Haset, J., Hirschman, S.Z., Cunningham-Rundles, C., Adelsberg, B.R., Parham, D.M., Siegal, M., Cunningham-Rundles, S., Armostrong, D. (1981): Severe acquired immunodeficiency in male homosexuals, manifested by chronic perianal ulcerative herpes simplex lesions. *N. Engl. J. Med.* 305:1439-1444.
50. Siegel, J.P., Djeu, J.Y., Stocks, N.I., Masur, H., Fauci, A.S., Lane, H.C., Gelmann, E.P., Quinnan, G.V. (1984): Serum from patients with the acquired immunodeficiency syndrome suppresses production of interleukin-2 by normal peripheral blood lymphocytes. *Clin. Res.* 32:358A.
51. Smith, P.S., Ohura, K., Masur, H., Lane, H.C., Fauci, A.S., Wahl, S.M. (1984): Monocyte function in the acquired immune deficiency syndrome: defective chemotaxis. *J. Clin. Invest.* 71:2121-2128.
52. Stahl, R.E., Friedman-Kien, A.E., Dubin, R., Marmor, M. Zolla-Pazner, S. (1982): Immunologic abnormalities in homosexual men: relationship to Kaposi's sarcoma. *Am. J. Med.* 73:171-178.
53. Williams, R.C., Masur, H., Spira, T.J. (1984): Lymphocyte-reactive antibodies in acquired immune deficiency syndrome. *J. Clin. Immunol.* 4:118-123.

Biology and Seroepidemiology
of HTLV-III

D. Markham, M.G. Sarngadharan, S. Zaki Salahuddin
and C. Gallo

Laboratory of Tumor Cell Biology National Cancer Institute
National Institutes of Health Bethesda, MD 20205, USA

INTRODUCTION

Human T cell leukemia (lymphotropic) virus type III (HTLV-III) (18, 56, 64) belongs to a group of human retroviruses including HTLV-I, the cause of Adult T-cell leukemia/lymphoma (51, 52) and HTLV-II isolated from a cell line established from a patient with a variant of hairy cell leukemia (30). These viruses share certain morphological, biochemical, and biological properties including: (a) isolation from human tissues, (b) tropism for T-lymphocytes, especially the T4 cell, (c) *in vitro* induction of multinucleated giant cells, (d) a hish molecular weight reverse transcriptase preferring Mg^{++-}, (e) the presence of only 3 major core proteins including a relatively small protein (p24), (f) the major core protein (p24) juxtaposed to the NH_2 terminal *gag* protein like HTLV-I and -II and unlike other retroviruses which have a small phosphoprotein in between the two, (g) distant antienic and nucleic acid relatedness, (h) an extra gene, x/lor, (i) a unique double splice to the 3' region, giving rise to a 1.8-2.2 Kb mRNA, (j) the phenomenon of trans-acting transcriptional activation of the viral LTR and probably some cellular regulatory elements very likely due to the protein encoded by the 2 Kb mRNA, (k) a likely African origin, and (l) the presence of common antigenic epitopes. Based on these similarities, and because of the uniform nomenclature for human T-cell leukemia (lymphotropic) viruses adopted at the first Cold Spring Harbor Meeting on HTLV (76), and for other reasons discussed below the virus causing AIDS and related syndrome was named HTLV-III.

When the Acquired Immunodeficiency Syndrome (AIDS) was recognized as a distinct new disease entity (reviewed in ref. 4,14), several features of the disease suggested that it could be caused by a retrovirus. These included: A) Epideiological studies which were most consistent with the involvement of an infectious agent (10, 29, 49). B) Evidence that the etiological agent was filterable using techniques that should not have allowed passage of fungi or bacteria (21, 32, 53). C) Immunological studies demonstrated that lymphocytes with the helper/inducer phenotype (OKT4/leu3a+) were drastically affected and could be the primary target (14, 34). Other than the recently recognized human retroviruses, HTLV-I and -II, few, if any infectious agents, e.g., bacteria, fungi, or other viruses, were known to have such an apparent cell specificity. D) By analogy to well-characterized animal retroviruses, e.g., feline leukemia virus, which may cause an AIDS-like disease in animals (25, 73).

In addition because of their tropism for T cells of the helper/inducer subgroup (14, 33), probable African origin (17), immune suppressive activity *in vitro* (44, 45, 54) and possibly *in vivo* (13) (in addition to their transforming effects) a T lymphotropic retrovirus possibly related to the HTLV group was considered a major candidate for causing AIDS (19).

Here the evidence linking HTLV-III as the etiologic agent of AIDS and related syndromes, and a description of its biological characteristics are presented.

Seroepidemiology of AIDS

Serological evidence implicating a human T-lymphotropic retrovirus in the etiology of AIDS was first obtained using a live-cell immunofluorescence assay. It was reported that ~36% of AIDS patients had serum antibodies that reacted with antigens present on HTLV-I-infected cells (12, 59). Subsequently, an even greater proportion of AIDS and ARC patients had evidence of exposure to an HTLV-I-related virus (13). The protein (antigen) recognized by these AIDS sera was shown to be an epitope of the HTLV-I envelope protein (38, 69). In addition, others found that ~10% of AIDS and ARC patients possessed serum antibodies to disrupted HTLV-I virions (59).

The etiological association between HTLV-III and AIDS was conclusively established by more direct seroepidemiological procedures once viral proteins became available. Sera from patients and donors were analyzed by indirect live cell membrane immuno-fluorescence assays, enzyme-linked immunosorbent assays (ELISA), Western blot analysis using patient sera and infected cells or purified virus or viral proteins, and by competition radioimmunoprecipitation using purified HTLV-III structural proteins (60, 64, 69). As summarized in Table 1, more than 90% of all AIDS and ARC patients were seropositive for antibodies to HTLV-III structural proteins. In contrast, control sera, including those from randomly collected healthy donors and people with non-AIDS related illnesses, were negative. Others with antibodies to HTLV-III included promiscuous homosexual men and intravenous drug users. Other individuals with none of the originally recognized risk factors for AIDS were also found to have antibodies to HTLV-III. These were otherwise healthy individuals who developed AIDS as a result of receiving blood transfusion(s) from individuals belonging to a defined AIDS risk group (29), and heterosexual contacts of "at-risk" groups (57).

TABLE 1.   *Patients with AIDS and related diseases and at Risk Donors Seropositive for Antibodies to HTLV-III*

Patients/Donors	Number Positive/Tested (%)
Patients with AIDS	288/297 (97)
Patients with ARC	327/360 (91)
Asymptomatic Homosexual Men	96/235 (41)
Transfusion AIDS Blood Donors	19/19 (100)
High-Risk Transfusion AIDS Donors	31/35 (87)
Renal Transplant Recipient from	
High Risk Donor	1/1
Controls	
Normal Donors[1]	0/515
Patients with Leukemias and Other	
Malignancies from HTLV-I Endemic Areas	0/515
Schizophrenics	0/30
Hodgkins Patients and Siblings	0/160
Renal Transplant Recipients and Other	
Immunosuppressed Donors	0/58
Miscellaneous Patients[2]	0/82

[1] These include randomly collected samples, black women from Baltimore (1962 collection), healthy Japanese from HTLV-I Endemic regions, healthy surinamese (methodone-treatment group), and other healthy random controls.
[2] These include heavily transfused patients and those with: hepatitis B virus infection, primary stage syphilis, rheumatoid arthritis, systemic lupus erythematosus, acute mononucleosis, lymphatic leukemias, B- and T-cell lymphomas, alopecia areata, idiopathic splenomegaly.

Representative patterns of antibody reactions in the confirmatory Western blot assays with selected sera from AIDS and ARC patients and healthy homosexuals at risk are shown in Figure 1. The viral protein most consistently detected had a molecular weight of ~41,000 and has been shown to be a processed product from the 3 ferminal of the HTLV-III *env-lor* gene (our unpublished data). Less frequently, the major HTLV-III internal protein, p24, and a 120K molecular weight product of the amino terminal end of the *env-lor* gene were also detected Additional reactivities against antigens of 66K, 51K, 31K, and 17K were also seen with some sera. Although there appeared to be a wide variation in antibody titer, serum antibody to HTLV-III was usually detected in most patients even before clinical symptoms were recognized. Generally, titers of HTLV-III antibodies were significantly lower in advanced AIDS patients than in ARC patients, or healthy normal, at risk, donors suggesting that the low titers found in some AIDS sera may be a natural consequence of the normal disease process.

Use of serological assays to identify infected individuals has some limitations in that in rare instances virus positive, seronegative, healthy at-risk donors were identified (61). These were highly selected individuals, many of whom were sampled because of a specific connection with AIDS or ARC patients, or by reference from clinicians, etc., and certainly represent an overestimate of the number of individuals in this category. However since efforts are

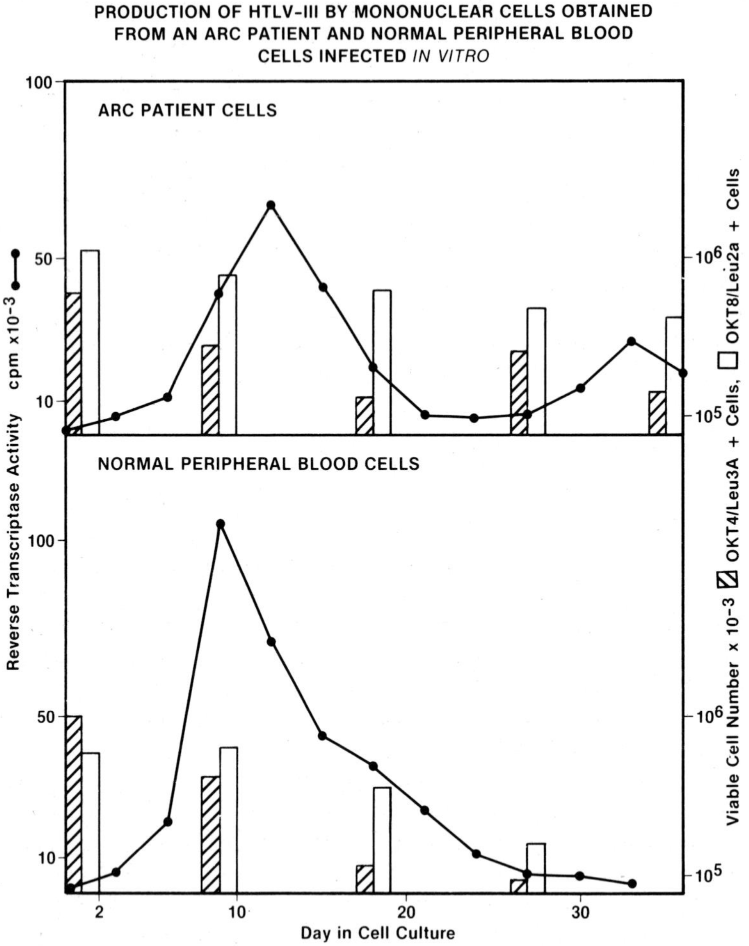

FIG. 1. Western Blot analysis of serum from AIDS (A) and ARC (B) patients and from healthy homosexual males at risk for AIDS (C). Proteins from disrupted HTLV-III were electrophoresed on polyacrylamide slab gels, transferred to nitrocellulose paper and incubated with serum from individual donors as described in *Materials and Methods*.

currently underway to screen blood donors as well as individuals in high risk groups for HTLV-III utilizing assays for antibody, the occurrence of seronegative but virus-positive persons without clinical symptoms suggests that other assays, possibly based on detection of viral antigens or proviral DNA, may be required in some instances.

Results of seroepidemiological studies now also demonstrate that, in addition to the U.S., Africa (6), and the Caribbean, HTLV-III is present in AIDS risk groups in Great Britain (7), Central and Southern (42, 67, 68) Europe, Scandinavia (35, 36), Australia (16), and South America (our unpublished observations). These observations are coincident with the emergence of AIDS and related diseases in these countries. Outside the U.S., the number of individuals with clinically recognized AIDS or its prodromes are so far relatively small and most were from homosexuals or recipients of blood or blood products, e.g., hemophiliacs. However, the number of exposed individuals, i.e., having antibodies to HTLV-III, is increasing rapidly.

In addition to the detection of antibody in patient sera which reacts with disrupted viral proteins, low titers of serum antibody able to neutralize infectious HTLV-III has been recently reported. This antibody co-purified with immunoglobulin fractions and was also found to react with HTLV-III envelope proteins, e.g., gp 120, gp 160, gp 41 (our personal observation with Dr. M. Robert-Guroff). The significance of these antibodies, e.g., whether or not they affect the disease process, remains to be determined.

Isolation of HTLV-III

The procedures used to isolate virus from AIDS and ARC patients and from other donors at risk for these diseases were patterned after those used for the isolation of other human T lymphotropic retroviruses, i.e., HTLV-I and II (30, 51, 52). The detection of virus positive cells and the characterization and comparison of the many viral isolates were conducted using HTLV-III-specific immunological reagents and nucleic acid probes which became available as a result of the ability to grow virus in large quantities. This occurred when HTLV-III was successfully transmitted for the first time to subclones of an estbalished human T-cell line (56).

After introduction into tissue culture, primary cells from patients usually produced virus within 2 to 3 weeks as illustrated in Fig. 2. Virus production then usually declined coincident with a loss of viable cells, especially those with the helper/inducer (OKT4/Leu3a+) phenotype. Often a second release of virus was observed, occuring several weeks after the initial detection of virus. An evaluation of the total cell count and the number of OKT4/Leu3a+ cells suggested that a minor population of cells susceptible to HTLV-III infection (possibly some OKT4/Leu3a+ lymphocytes) survived the initial release of virus and were either subsequently infected, or were otherwise induced to release virus.

More than 100 isolates from patients with AIDS or ARC and from healthy individuals at risk for AIDS have now been obtained in this laboratory (63). A summary of these HTLV-III isolates, some clinical information, and tissue sources are shown in Table 2. The frequency of HTLV-III isolation varied from ~50% for AIDS patients to ~85% for ARC patients and 30% for healthy individuals at risk for AIDS. HTLV-III was not found, however, in more than 150 samples from healthy heterosexual donors cultured in the same manner (data not shown).

Most HTLV-III isolates to date have been from peripheral blood leukocytes, however, in a smaller number of samples, infectious virus was also

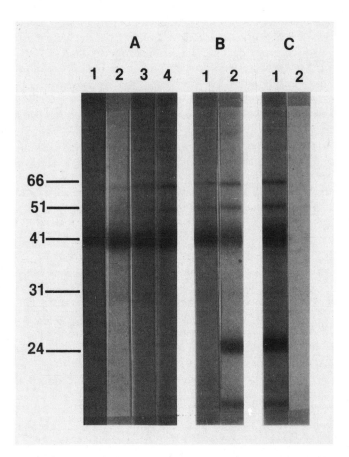

FIG. 2. HTLV-III produced by primary cells established in cell culture from an ARC patient (top) and by HTLV-III-infected normal peripheral blood cells (bottom). Top panel. Mononuclear cells were prepared from an ARC patients peripheral blood, as described in *Materials and Methods*. Virus release was monitored by reverse transcriptase activity in supernatant fluids and cell types were determined using cell specific monoclonal antibody as described in *Materials and Methods*. Bottom panel. Fresh mononuclear cells from normal donor were infected by cell-free HTLV-III and monitored as described above.

isolated from cells obtained from the bone marrow, ceriberal spinal fluid and lymph nodes. Relevant to the transmission of virus from positive carriers, HTLV-III was also isolated from cell-free plasma from AIDS and ARC patients. Epidemiological evidence suggesting that AIDS is linked to sexual practices was supported by the isolation of HTLV-III from cells found in the semen of an AIDS patients by D. Zagury and co-workers (79) and, simultaneously, by D. Ho and co-workers from a healthy homosexual male (28). HTLV-III was also isolated from cells found in the saliva of ARC patients and from several healthy homosexuals (22). Epidemiological studies indicate that

TABLE 2. *Summary of Donors and Tissue Sources of HTLV-III*

Tissue[1]	Donor/Patient[2]		
	Healthy	ARC (at Risk)	AIDS
Peripheral Blood	16/50	31/38	43/88
Bone Marrow	NT[3]	1/6	NT
Lymph Node	NT	4/4	NT
Brain	NT		2/3
CSF	NT	1/3	NT
Plasma	NT	3/6	NT
Saliva[4]	4/6	4/10	0/4
Semen[5]	1/1	NT	2/2

[1] Leukocytes from the indicated sources were introduced into cell cultures and monitored for infectious virus in all cases except plasma where cell free fluids were directly used to infect susceptable T-cells, CSF, cerebralspinal fluid.
[2] Healthy, clinical normal from AIDS risk group. ARC, AIDS-related complex, Number of isolates per number of donors tested.
[3] NT — Not tested.
[4] Collaborative studies with Dr. J. Groopman (22).
[5] Collaborative studies with Dr. D. Zagury (79) and Drs. D. Ho and M. Hirsch (28).

HTLV-III is not easily transmitted by casual contact (e.g., sneeze, cough, etc.) (27); however, it is possible that heavy salivary exchange may also be involved.

The virus isolated from infected leukocytes has a uniform morphological appearance with a diameter of 100 to 120 nm, and is frequently seen budding from the envelope of infected cells. A possibly unique feature of the virions is the cylindrically shaped core observed in many presumably mature virions. A careful morphological evaluation of the production of virus demonstrated many similarities between HTLV-III and some lentiviruses, e.g., visna virus (20).

A number of culture conditions and media additives were tested for their ability to improve virus expression and hydrocortisone was found to be of particular value (41). For example, in ~50% of virus positive samples tested the amount of virus was substantially increased when 5μg/ml hydrocortisone was used to supplement growth media. More importantly, in ~15% of AIDS specimens, the inclusion of hydrocortisone permitted the isolation of virus that would otherwise have gone undetected.

Some indication that fresh cells other than those with the OKT4/leu 3+ as their predominant phenotype could be infected by HTLV-III, e.g., some B-lymphocytic cells and monocytoid cells was seen (our personal observation). It is possible, however, that a small percentage of those cells may contain the OKT4/leu3a+ markers and are therefore infectable by HTLV-III. It is likely that these cells could be involved as a natural reservoir of virus *in vivo*, and thus contribute to persistent infection without the accompanying pathological consequences usually observed in AIDS. In addition other human T or pre-T cell lines (e.g., JM, CEM-CCRF, Molt 3, Molt 4) which have been found to be permissive for productive infection by HTLV-III (11, 56 and our personal observations) some B-lymphoblastic cell lines can also be productively infected by HTLV-III (48, and our personal observation). The cytopathic effect of HTLV-III described with fresh lymphocytes is also observed with T- and B-cell lines, although it is not as pronounced since many cells in the population survive and can, at least transiently, produce virus (our personal observations). These established cell lines not only serve as sources of large amounts of virus, but also as model systems to study the cytopathic effect of HTLV-III on stable populations of susceptible cells. In addition to T and B cell lines, preliminary results indicate that cells of the monocyte-macrophage lineage can also be infected (Salahuddin et al., *Science*, In Press).

Subhuman primates, e.g., chimpanzees, can also be infected by HTLV-III (1, 15). In addition to an immunological response, i.e., production of specific antibody, virus was isolated from lymphocytes collected at different intervals post-infection, and some clinical manifestations similar to the lymphadenopathy seen in humans were observed. These and other animal studies will not only help to further establish the cause-and-effect association between HTLV-III and AIDS, but will likely prove valuable in the development of model systems to study the disease process, and hopefully its prevention and/or cure.

The mechanisms responsible for the profound cytopathic effect of HTLV-III on infected cells, particularly those with the OKT4/leu 3a phenotype, are not known. Recent observations suggest that the tropism for T4 lymphocytes results from the similarity, or proximity of the virus receptor to the T4 antigens recognized on the surface of susceptible cells by specific antibodies, e.g., OKT4, leu3a, etc. (11, 34, 55). Fresh cells from patients and cells infected *in vitro* by HTLV-III contain both unintegrated as well as integrated proviral DNA (70-72). It is, therefore, possible that a latent form of virus could exist in resting cells. In other retrovirus systems, it was suggested that the accumulation of unintegrated proviral DNA was involved in the cytopathic effect (31, 77).

HTLV-III, like HTLV-I and -II, contains genes which encode a trans-acting transcriptional enhancing activity. Whereas for HTLV-I and -II, it has been suggested that this activity likely plays a primary role in the transformation process, it is not clear how, or whether, this activity is involved in the cytopathology of HTLV-III. It has been suggested that like HTLV-I (62), HTLV-III-infected cells liberate potent immunoregulatory factors which suppress the function of T- and other cells of the immune system (37) and, could therefore contribute to the generalized immunosuppressive effect observed. Our preliminary experience with T cells infected by HTLV-III *in vitro* supports this possibility. For example, supernatant fluids from fresh cultured human mononuclear leukocytes infected with HTLV-III contain activities able to suppress the activation of both T- and B-cells (Markham et al., in preparation). The significance of these observations and how, or if, these activities differ from those obtained from stimulated normal T cells remain to be elucidated.

Transmission of HTLV-III by Heterosexual Contact

Earlier epidemiological observations had suggested that AIDS could be contracted by female sexual partners of male members of high-risk groups. This was noted in a study of AIDS an ARC cases in the U.S. (23, 26) and in studies in Africa which demonstrated the almost equal occurrence of these syndromes in men and women (8, 9, 50, 74). Seroepidemiological tests of donor sera further demonstrated the elevated (36%) prevalence of antibodies to HTLV-III in female contacts of AIDS and ARC patients (our personal observations with M. Robert-Guroff), and similar studies revealed a very high prevalence (~60%) of HTLV-III serum antibodies in a prostitute population in parts of Africa (our personal observation with C. Saxinger). This male-to-female transmission of virus, and consequently disease, was directly shown in a case study of seven families where the husband had either AIDS or ARC (57). Five spouses with no other risk factor had evidence of HTLV-III infection documented by seropositivity and/or isolation of virus. Three of these 5 spouses had also developed ARC. Of 11 children belonging to these families, only one, a 14 month old child, was seropositive for HTLV-III. The antibody in this one infant was likely a result of congenital infection.

Female-to-male transmission of virus was also suggested in a carefully controlled study involving U.S. military personnal presenting with AIDS or ARC. Seven out of 19 men in this study gave no history linking them to a recognized AIDS risk group. All 19 were seropositive for antibody to HTLV-III and infectious virus was isolated from their peripheral blood lymphocytes. The only common factor among the 7 patients with no conventional risk factor was the frequent employment of prostitutes, or other frequent heterosexual contacts (more than 6 encounters with prostitutes per year for 2 consecutive years, or more than 10 different heterosexual partners per year for 2 years). These contacts occurred in various parts of the world, with New York and Germany being frequently mentioned (our personal observation with R. Redfield). The studies suggest that, in addition to concern for the rise of HTLV-III infection and the consequential disease in various parts of the world occurring in AIDS risk groups, at least certain heterosexually promiscuous groups should also be monitored.

Origin of HTLV-III

The geographical origin of HTLV-III, although not precisely defined, appears to be Africa. Earlier serological studies demonstrating a high prevalence of seropositivity to HTLV-I in parts of Africa (reviewed in ref. 66) were extended to include exposure to HTLV-III (8, 9, 66). Recently, C. Saxinger in this laboratory, collaborating with other investigators tested sera collected in Uganda in 1972-73 as part of a Burkitt lymphoma study, for antibodies to HTLV-III. Surprisingly, ~65% of rural, poor, Ugandan children from the West Nile Bank region had low levels of antibodies reacting with HTLV-III (66). Since the disease AIDS only was recognized some years later in Africa, it is not clear whether the disease previously existed but remained unrecognized (possibly responsible for many of the deaths occurring at an early age observed in parts of Africa), or that the preexisting virus has recently become more pathogenic. Alternatively, these children may represent a population of individuals resistant to the effects of the virus.

These observations, coupled with the detection of antibodies reacting with HTLV-I in the sera of many species of many Old World primates (24, 65), and the occasional detection or isolation of virus closely related to HTLV-I from some animals (24, 78), are consistent with the suggestion that AIDS began in Africa and probably Central Africa. But the apparent spread of AIDS to other parts of Africa and other parts of the world, i.e., Caribbean, U.S., Europe, etc., remains to be determined.

Control of HTLV-III

The number of individuals suffering from disease caused by HTLV-III has increased at an alarming rate since its initial reports. Individuals infected by the virus are no longer limited to a restricted population in the U.S., but now include people with any one of several risk factors throughout the world. Two aspects of the control of HTLV-III (and its diseases) that need careful investigation are treatment of already infected individuals, and prevention of the further spread of the virus. Possibly the most likely approaches for the treatment of infected people will be to find ways to: 1) inhibit virus infection, and/or replication, 2) remove infected cells, including those possibly serving as a virus reservoir, and 3) replace lost T-lymphocytes.

Procedures for the replacement of T-lymphocytes are now well tested, e.g., by transplantation or by treatment with TCGF. However, those for the control HTLV-III infection or replication, and for the identification and removal of infected cells, remain to be develope. In this regard, certain drugs which were found to inhibit viral reverse transcriptase activity, e.g., Suramin, are promising candidates since they inhibit virus infection *in vitro* (46, 58). Clinical trials using this drug are currently in progress and preliminary results of testing the peripheral blood mononuclear cells from treated patients are encouraging. Using release of virus is one criteria, the ability to isolate virus was inversely related with the level of suramin achieved. (5, 419. Other inhibitors of retroviral reverse transcriptase activity, e.g., antimoniotungstate (J.C. Chermann et al., personal communication) and Ribavirin (43) are also being tested.

Use of vaccines to prevent infection and/or moderate the disease process is being actively pursued by different approaches in several laboratories. It is important, however, to determine if the genomic diversity noted among may

HTLV-III isolates (discussed previously) yield antigenically different viruses. If so, neutralization of virus might not have broad application. It is encouraging that low titers of neutralizing antibodies to HTLV-III have been detected in the serum of many different infected individuals suggesting that many individuals have mounted an immune response able to neutralize at least one HTLV-III isolate (M. Robert-Guroff *et al.*, submitted: D.D. Ho *et al.*, submitted; R. Weiss *et al.*, personal communication).

DISCUSSION

The frequent isolation of HTLV-III from patients with AIDS and ARC, and the detection of antibodies specific for HTLV-III in nearly all patients with these diseases, leaves little doubt that HTLV-III is etiologically involved. This etiologic association is further strengthened by the detection of HTLV-III infection in hemophiliacs and children with AIDS, and in HTLV-III infected blood donors and the otherwise healthy recipients of this blood who subsequently develop AIDS. Furthermore, a comparison of the ability of HTLV-III to selectively infect OKT4/leu3a cells with a resulting cytopathic effect, is consistent with clinical observations in ARC/AIDS patients.

Several groups of investigators have also detected retroviral infections in patients with AIDS and in individuals at risk for AIDS. They designated these viral isolates variously as LAV (lymphadenopathy-associated virus) (2, 48) $IDAV_1$, $IADV_2$ (immune deficiency-associated virus) (75). In the initial studies these viruses were not characterized and their relationship to each other, and prevalence in disease was not clear. Subsequent studies have now clearly demonstrated that these and other virus isolates (3, 18, 22, 39, 63) are very similar to HTLV-III. For all the reasons mentioned, and because lymphadenopathy can have numerous causes, it does not seem appropriate to name this virus after one clinical manifestation of the AIDS spectrum of diseases.

Although the basic characterization of HTLV-III as a new retrovirus is well advanced, there are many questions concerning its biological and biochemical properties which remain to be answered. This includes the fundamental question concerning the mechanism by which a virus exerts its cytopathic effects and causes AIDS. The nucleotide sequence analysis of HTLV-III is now completed and its analysis should provide crucial information concerning the structural-functional relationships of the viral genome.

Information, along with expression studies and analyses of viral-specific proteins, will be important to ongoing efforts to control viral infection and expression. The development of specific neutralizing antisera, and drugs inhibiting viral infection or replication, will undoubtedly be important. Of crucial importance to the development of effective vaccines will be the definition of the degree of genomic diversity which is present in HTLV-III and the determination whether these differences have biological significance. The growth of HTLV-III in large quantities, the availability of many isolates from patients and donors with various disease manifestations and from different parts of the world, and the cloning of its genome will provide the needed biological and immunologic reagents and molecular probes to address these questions. Such studies involving patients with AIDS and ARC, as well as apparently healthy carriers, will undoubtedly lead in the near future to a fuller understanding of HTLV-III and the disease(s) it produces.

REFERENCES

1. Alter, H.J., Eichberg, J.W., Masur, H., Saxinger, W.C., Macher, A.M., Lane, H.C., Fauci, A.S.: Transmission of HTLV-III Infection from human plasma to chimpanzees: An animal model for AIDS. *Sciences* 226:549-552, 1984.
2. Barré-Sinoussi, F., Chermann, J.C., Rey, F., Nugeyne, M.T., Chamaret, S., Gruest, J., Dauguet, C., Axler-Blin, C., Vezinet-Brun, F., Rouzioux, C., Rozenbaum, W., and Montagnier, L.: Isolation of a T-lymphotropic retrovirus from a patient at risk for acquired immune deficiency syndrome (AIDS). *Science,* 220:868-871, 1983.
3. Bieberfeld, G., Bredberg-Ruden, U., Bottiger, B., Bieberfeld, P., Morfeldt-Mansson, L., Suni, J., Valeri, A., Saxinger, C., Gallo, R.C.: Antibodies to human T-lymphotropic virus (HTLV) type III demonstrated by a dot immuno-binding assay. *Scand. J. Immunol.,* in press.
4. Broder, S., Gallo, R.C.: A pathogenic retrovirus (HTLV-III) linked to AIDS. *N. Engl. J. Med.* 311-1292-1297, 1984.
5. Broder, S., Vanchan, R., Collins, J.M., Lane, H.G., Markham, P.D., et al.: Effects of Suramin in patients with AIDS or AIDS-related complex: Clinical pharmacology and suppression of HTLV-III replication. The Lancet, submitted.
6. Brun-Vezinet, F., Rouzioux, C., Montagnier, L., Chamaret, S., Gruest, J., Barré-Sinoussi, F., Geroldi, D., Chermann, J.C., McCormick, J., Mitchell, S., Plat, P., Taelman, H., Mirlanga, K.B., Wobin, D., Mbendi, N., Mazebo, P., Kayembo, K., Bredts, C., Desmyter, J., Fernard, F.M., Quem, T.C.: Prevalence of antibodies to lymphoadenopathy-associated retrovirus in African patients with AIDS. *Science,* 226:453-456, 1984.
7. Cheingsong-Popov, R., Weiss, R.A., Dalgleish, A., Tedder, R.S., Shanson, D.C., Jeffries, D.J., Ferns, R.B., Briggs, E.M., Weller, I.V.D., Mitton, S., Adler, M.W., Farthing, C., Lawrence, A.G., Gazzard, B.G., Weber, J., Harris, J.R.W., Pinchng, A.J., Craske, J., Barbara, J.A.J.: Prevalence of antibody to HTLV-III in AIDS and AIDS-risk patients in Britian *The Lancet,* Sept. 1:477-480, 1984.
8. Clumeck, N., Sonnett, J., Taelman, H.: Acquired Immunodeficiency Syndrome in African Patients. *N. Engl. J. Med.,* 310:492-497, 1984.
9. Clumeck, N., Robert-Guroff, M., Von De Preer, P., Jennings, A., Demol, P., Gallo, R.C.: Seriepidemiological studies of HTLV-III antibody prevalence among selected groups of heterosexual Africans. Submitted for publication.
10. Curran, J.W., Lawrence, D.W., Jaffe, H., *et al.:* Acquired immunodeficiency syndrome (AIDS) associated with transfusions. *N. Engl. J. Med.* 310:69-75, 1984.
11. Delgleish, A.G., Beverly, P.C.L., Clapham, P.R., Crawford, D.H., Greaves, M.F., Weiss, R.A.: The CD4(T4) antigen is an essential component of the receeptor for the AIDS retrovirus. *Nature* 312:763-767, 1984.
12. Essex, M., McLane, M.F., Lee, T.H., Falk, L., Howe, C.W.S., Mullins, J.I., Cabradilla, C., and Francis, D.P.: Antibodies to cell membrane antigens associated with human T-cell leukemia virus in patientis with AIDS. *Science,* 220:859-862, 1983.
13. Essex, M.E., McLane, M.F., Tachibana, N., Francis, D.P., and Lee, T.-H.: Seroepidemiology of human T-cell leukemia virus in relation to immunosuppression and the acquired immunodeficiency syndrome. In: *Human T-Cell Leukemia/Lymphoma Virus,* R.C. Gallo, M. Essex and L. Gross (eds.), Cold Sring Harbor Laboratory, New York, pp. 355-362, 1984.
14. Fauci, A.S., Macher, A.M., Longo, D.L., Lane, H.C., Rook, A.H., Masur, H., Gelmann, E.P.: Acquired immunodeficiency syndrome: epidemiological, clinical, immunologic, and therapeutic considerations. *Ann. Int. Med.* 100:92-106, 1984.
15. Francis, D.P., Feorino, P.M., Broderson, J.R., McClure, H.M., Getchell, J.P., McGrath, C.R., Swenson, B., McDougal, J.S., Palmer, E.L., Harrison, A.K., Barré-Sinoussi, F., Chermann, J.C., Montagnier, L., Curran, J.W., Cabradilla, C.D., Layanaraman, V.S.: Infection of chimpanzees with lymphadenopathy associated virus. *Lancet* ii: 1276-1277, 1984.

16. Frazer, I.H., Sarngadharan, M.G., Mackay, I.R., Gallo, R.C.: Antibody to human T cell leukemia virus type III in Australian homosexual men with lymphadenopathy. *The Medical J. of Australia,* 141:247-276, 1984.

17. Gallo, R.C.: Human T-cell leukemia-lymphoma virus and T-cell malignancies in adults. In: L.M. Franks, J. Wyke, and R.A. Weiss (eds.), *Cancer Surveys,* Vol. 3, Oxford University Press, Oxford, pp. 113-159, 1984.

18. Gallo, R.C., Salahuddin, S.Z., Popovic, M., Shearer, G.M., Kaplan, M., Haynes, B.F., Palker, T.J., Redfield, R., Oleske, J., Safai, B., White, F., Foster, P., and Markham, P.D.: Frequent Detection and Isolation of Cytopathic Retroviruses (HTLV-III) from Patients with AIDS and a risk for AIDS. *Science,* 224:500-503, 1984.

19. Gallo, R.C., Essex, M., Gross, L., (eds.) *Human T-Cell Leukemia/Lymphoma Virus.* Cold Spring Harbor Press, New York, 1984.

20. Gonda, M.A., Wong-Staal, F., Gallo, R.C., Clements, J., Narayan, D., Gilden, R.V.; Sequence homology and morphologic similarity of HTLV-III and Visna Virus, a pathogenic lentivirus. *Science* 227:173-177, 1984.

21. Garther, L.G., Wernicke, D., Eberle, J., Zoulek, G., Deinhardt, F., Schranm, W.: Increase in prevalence of anti-HTLV-III in haemophiliacs. *Lancet* i: 1275-1276, 1984.

22. Groopman, J.E., Salahuddin, S.Z., Sarngadharan, M.G., Markham, P.D., Gonda, M., Sliski, A., Gallo, R.C.: Isolation of HTLV-III from saliva of pre-AIDS, AIDS and healthy homosexual men at risk for AIDS. *Science,* 226:447-449, 1984.

23. Guinan, M.E., Thomas, D.A., Pinksy, Goodrich, J.T., Selik, R.M., Jaffe, H.W., Haverkos, H.W., Noble, G., Curran, J.W.: Heterosexual and homosexual patients with the acquired immunodeficiency syndrome. *Ann. Intern. Med.* 100-213-218, 1984.

24. Guo, H.G., Wong-Staal, F., Gallo, R.C.: Novel viral sequences related to a human T-cell leukemia virus in T-cells of a seropositive baboon. *Science* 223:1195-1197, 1984.

25. Hardy, W.D., Jr., Hess, P.W., MacEwen, E.G., McClelland, A.J., Zuckermann, E.E., Essex, M., Cotter, S.M., Jarrett, O.: Biology of feline leukemia virus in natural environment. *Cancer Res.* 36:582-588, 1976.

26. Harris, C., Small, C.B., Klein, R.E., Friedland, G.A., Moll, B., Emeson, E.F., Spigland, I., Steigbiglel, N.H.: Immunodeficiency in female sexual partners of men with the acquired immunodeficiency syndrome. *N. Engl. J. Med.* 308:1180-1184, 1983.

27. Hirsch, M.W., Wormser, C.P., Schooley, R.T., Ho, D.D., Hopkins, C.C., Joline, C., Danconsur, F., Sarngadharan, M.G., Saxinger, C., Gallo, R.C.: Risk of nosocomial infection with human T-cell lymphotropic virus III (HTLV-III). *N. Engl. J. Med.* 312:1-4, 1985.

28. Ho, D.B., Schooling, R.T., Rota, T.R., Kaplan, J.C., Flyn, T., Salahuddin, Z., Gonda, M., and Hirsch, M.S.: HTLV-III in the semen and blood of a healthy homosexual man. *Science* 226:451-453, 1984.

29. Jaffe, H.N., Sarngadharan, M.G., Devico, A., Bruch, L., Getchell, J.P., Kalyanaraman, V.S., Kilbourne, B.W., Peterman, T.A., Haverkos, H.W., McDougal, J.S., Stoneburner, R.L., Gallo, R.C., Francis, D.P., Curren, J.W.: Serologic evidence of an etiologic role for a human T-lymphotropic retrovirus in transfusion-associated AIDS. In Press.

30. Kalyanaraman, V.S., Sarngadharan, M.G., Robert-Gufoff, M., Miyoshi I., Blayney, D., Golde, D., and Gallo, R.C.: A new subtype of human T-cell leukemia. *Science,* 218:571-573, 1982.

31. Keshet, E. and Temin, H.M.: Cell killing by spleen necrosis virus is correlated with a transcient accumulation of spleen necrosis virus DNA. *J. Virol.* 31:376-388, 1979.

32. Kitchen, L.W., Barin, F., Sullivan, J.L., McLane, M.F., Brettler, D.B., Levene, P.H., Essex, M.: Aetiology of AIDS antibdies to human T cell leukemia virus (type III)in haemophiliacs. *Nature,* 312:3367-3369, 1984.

33. Klatzmann, D., Barré-Sinoussi, F., Nugeyre, M.T., Dauguet, C., Vilmer, F., Griscelli, C., Brun-Vezinet, F., Rousioux, C., Gluckman, J.C., Chermann, J.C., Montagnier, L.: Selective tropism of lymphadenopathy associated virus (LAV) for the helper/inducer T lymphocytes. *Science,* 225:59-63, 1984.

34. Klatzmann, D., Champagne, E., Chamaret, S., Gruest, J., Gaetard, D., Hercent, T., Cluckman, J.C., Montagnier, L.: T lymphocyte T4 molecule behaves as the receptor for human retrovirus LAV. *Nature* 312:767-765, 1984.

35. Krohn, K., Ranki, A., Antonev, J., Valle, S.L., Suni, J., Vaheri, A. Saxinger, C., Gallo, R.C.: Immune functions in homosexual men with antibodies to HTLV-III in Finland. *Clin. Exp. Immunol.,* in press.

36. Lange-Wantzin, C., Saxigenr, W.C., Gallo, R.C.: Prevalence of HTLV-III antibodies in Danish homosexuals with venereal disease. *ACTA Dermatovenerealogica,* (Stockholm), in Press.

37. Lawrence, J., and Mayer, S.: Immunoregulatory lymphokines of T-hybridomas from AIDS patients: constitutive and inducible suppressor factors. *Science*, 225:66-69, 1984.
38. Lee, T.H., Coligan, J.E., Homma, T., McLane, M.F., Tachibana, N., and Essex, M.: Human T-cell leukemia virus-associated cell membrane antigens: Identity of the major antigens recognized by the virus infection. *Proc. Natl. Acad. Sci. USA*, 81:3856-3860.
39. Levy, J.A., Hoffman A.D., Kramer, S.M., Landin, J.A., Shimabukuro, J.M., and Oshiro, L.S.: Isolation of lymphocytopathic retroviruses from San Francisco patients with AIDS. *Science* 225:890-892, 1984.
40. Markham, P.D., Resnick, L., Yarchoan, R., Redfield, R., Mitsuya, H., Lane, C., Fauci, A, Broden, S., and Gallo, R.C.: Suppression of HTLV-III production by cultured lymphocytes from AIDS and ARC patients treated *in vitro and in vivo*. Submitted.
41. Markham, P.D., Salahuddin, S.Z., Veren, K., Orndorff, S., Gallo, R.C.: Enhanced expression and isolation of HTLV-III using hydrocortisone and other hormones. *Int. J. Cancer*, Submitted, 1985.
42. Matherz, D., Leibwitch, J., Mathern, S., Salmot, A.G., Catalen, P., Zagury, D.: Antibodies to HTLV-III associated antigens in populations exposed to AIDS virus in France. *Lancet* ii:460, 1984.
43. McCormick, J.B., Mitchell, S.W., Getchell, J.P., Hicks, DR.: Ribavirin suppresses replication of lymphadenopathy associated virus in cultures of human adult T-lymphocytes. *Lancet* ii:1367-1369, 1984.
44. Mitsuya, H., Guo, H.G., Megson, M.E., Trainer, C., Reitz, M.S., Broder, S.: Transformation and cytopathogenic effect in an immune human T-cell clone infected by HTLV-I *Science*, 223:1293-1296, 1984.
45. Mitsuya, H., Matis, L.A., Megson, M., Bunn, P.A., Murray, C., Mann, D.L., Gallo, R.C., and Broder, S.: Generation of an HLA-restricted cytotoxic T-cell line reactive against cultured tumor cells from a patient infected with human T-cell leukemia/lymphoma virus. *J. Exp. Med.*, 158:994-999, 1983.
46. Mitsuya, H., Popovic, M., Yarchoor, R., Matusushita, S., Gallo, R.C., Broder, S.: Suramin protection of T cells *in vitro* against infectivity and cytopathic effect of HTLV-III. *Science*, 226:172-174, 1984.
47. Montagnier, L., Grust, J., Chamaret, S., Daugnet, C., Axler, C., Guetard, D., Nugeyere, M.T., Barré-Sinoussi, F., Cherman, J.C., Brunet, J.B., Klatzmann, D., Glockman, J.C.: Adaptation of lymphadenopathy-associated virus (LAV) to replication in EBV-transformed, B-lymphoblastoid cells lines *Science* 225:63-66, 1984.
48. Montagnier, L., Chermann, J.C., Barré-Sinoussi, F., Chamaret, S., Gruest, J., Nugeyre, M.T., Rey, F., Dauguet, C., Axler-BLin, C., Vezinet-Brux, F., Rouzioux, C., Saimot, G.A., Rozenbaum, W., Gluckman, J.C., Klatzmann, D., Vilmer, E., Griscelli, C., Foyer-Gazengel, C., and Brunet, J.B.: A new human T-lymphotropic retrovirus: characterization and possible role in lymphadenopathy and acquired immune deficiency syndrome. In: *Human T-cell leukemia (Lympoma Virus)*, R.C. Gallo, M.E. Enox, and L. Gross (eds.). Cold Spring Harbor Laboratories, pp. 363-379, 1984.
49. O'Duffy, A.F., Isles, A.F.: Transfusion-induced AIDS in four premature babies. *Lancet* ii;1346, 1984.
50. Piot, P., Quinn, T.C., Taelman, H., Feinsod, F.M., Minlanger, K.B., Wobin, O., Mbendi, N., Mazebo, P., Ndanji, K., Stevens, W., Kalambayi, K., Mitchell, S., Bridts, C., McCormick, J.B.: Acquired immunodeficiency syndrome in a heterosexual population in Zaire. *Lancet* II:65-69, 1984.
51. Poiesz, B.J., Ruscetti, F.W., Gazdar, A.F., Bunn, P.A., Minna, J.D., and Gallo, R.C.: Detection and isolation of type-C retrovirus particles from fresh and cultured lymphocytes of a patient with cutaneous T-cell lymphoma. *Proc. natl. Acad. Sci. USA*, 77:7415-7419, 1980.
52. Poiesz, B.J., Ruscetti, F.W., Reitz, M.S., Kalyanaraman, V.S., and Gallo, R.C.: Isolation of a new type-C retrovirus (HTLV) in primary uncultured cells of a patient with Sézary T-cell leukemia. *Nature*, 294:268-271, 1981.
53. Poon, M.C., Landey, A., Prasthofer, E.F., Stagno, S.: Acquired immunodeficiency syndrome with *Pneumocystis carinii* pneumonia, and Mycobacterium avium intracellulare infection in a previously healthy patient with classic hemophilia: clinical, immunologica, and virologic finding. *Am. Inst. Med.* 98:287-290, 1983.
54. Popovic, M., Flomenberg, N., Volkman, D.J., Mann, D., Fauci, A.S., Dupont, B., and Gallo, R.C.: Alteration of T-cell functions by infection with HTLV-I or HTLV-II. *Science*, 226:459-462, 1984.
55. Popovic, M., Read-Connole, E., Gallo, R.C.: T4 positive human neoplastic cell lines susceptible to and permissive for HTLV-III. The *Lancet* II:1472-1473, 1984.

56. Popovic, M., Sarngadharan, M.G., Reed, E., and Gallo, R.C.: Detection, isolation, and continuous production of cytopathic human T lyphotropic retrovirus (HTLV-III) from patients with AIDS and pre-AIDS. *Science,* 224:497-500, 1984.
57. Redfield, R.R., Markham, P.D., Salahuddin, S.Z., Sarngadharan, M.G., Bodner, A.J., Falk, T.M., Ballow, W.R, Wright, D.G., Gallo, R.C.: Frequent transmission of HTLV-III among spouses of patients with AIDS-related complex (ARC) and the acquired immunodeficiency syndrome (AIDS): A family study. *J. Am. Med. Assoc.,* In Press, 1985.
58. Resnick, L., Markham, P.D., Veren, K., Salahuddin, S.Z., Gallo, R.C.: Combined acyclovir and suramin therapy synergistically suppresses the infection of human mononuclear leukocytes by HTLV-III. *The Lancet,* submitted.
59. Robert-Guroff, M., Safai, B., Gelmann, E., Mensell, P.W.A., Groopman, J.E., Sidhu, G.S., Friedman-Kien, A.E., Begley, A.C., Blayney, D.W., Lange, M., Gutterman, J.W., Goedert, J.L., Steigbigel, N.H., Johnson, J.M., Downing, R., Gallo, R.C.: HTLV-I specific antibody in AIDS patients and others at risk. *Lancet* ii:128-131, 1984.
60. Safai, B., Sarngadharan, M.G., Groopman, J.E., Popovic, M., Schüpbach, J. Sarngadharan, M.G., Arnett, K., Sliski, A., Gallo, R.C.: Seroepidemiological studies of HTLV-III in AIDS. *Lancet,* 1:1438-1440, 1984.
61. Salahuddin, S.Z., Groopman, J.E., Markham, P.D., Sarngadharan, M.G., Redfield, R.R., McLane, M.F., Essex, M., Sliski, A., Gallo, R.C.: HTLV-III symptom-free seronegative persons. *The Lancet* ii:1418-1420, 1984.
62. Salahuddin, S.Z., Markham, P.D., Lindner, S.G., Gootenberg, J., Popovic, M., Hemmi, H., Sarin, P.S., and Gallo, R.C.: Lymphokine production by cultured human T-cells transformed by human T-cell leukemia-lymphoma virus. *Science* 223:703-706, 1984.
63. Salahuddin, S.Z., Markham, P.D., Popovic, M., Patel, A., Orndorf, S., Gold, J., Fladager, A., Gallo, R.C.: Isolation of infectious HTLV-III from AIDS and ARC patients and healthy carriers: A study of risk factors and tissue sources *Proc. Natl. Acad. Sci. USA,* in press, 1985.
64. Sarngadharan, M.G., Popovic, M., Bruck, L., Shüpbach, J., and Gallo, R.C.: Antibodies reactive with a human T-lymphotropic retrovirus (HTLV-III) in the sera of patients with acquired immune deficiency syndrome. *Science,* 224:506-508, 1984.
65. Saxinger, W.C., Lange-Wentzin, G., Thomsen, K., Lapin, B., Yakovleva, L., Li, Y.W., Guo, H.C., Robert-Guroff, M., Blattner, W.A., Ito, Y., Gallo, R.C.: Human T-cell leukemia virus: A disease family of related exogenous retroviruses of humans and Old World primates. In: *Human T-cell Leukemia/Lymphoma Virus.* (Gallo, R.C., Essex, M., and Gross, L., eds.). Cold Spring Harbor Press. p. 232-330, New York, 1984.
66. Saxinger, C., Levine, R.H., Deen, A.G., De The, G., Sarngadharan, M.G., Gallo, R.C.: Evidence for exposure to HTLV-III in Uganda prior to 1973. *Science,* in press.
67. Schneider, J., Boyer, H., Biengle, U., Wernet, P., Hunsman, G.: Antibodies to HTLV-III in German blood donors. *Lancet* i:275-276, 1985.
68. Schüpbach, J., Haller, O., Vogt, M., Luthy, R., Jaller, H., Ralz, O., Popovic, M., Sarngadharan, M.G., Gallo, R.C.: Antibodies to HTLV-III in Swiss patients with AIDS and pre-AIDS and in groups at risk for AIDS. *N. Engl. J. Med.* 312:265-270, 1985.
69. Schüpbach, J., Sarngadharan, M.G. and Gallo, R.C.: Antigens on HTLV-infected cells recognized by leukemia and AIDS sera are related to HTLV viral glycoprotein. *Science,* 224:607-610, 1984.
70. Shaw, G.M., Gonda, M.A., Flickenger, G.H., Hahn, B.H., Gallo, R.C., Wong-Staal, F.: Genomes of evolutionarily divergent members of the HTLV family are highly conserved especially in pX. *Proc. Natl. Acad. Sci.* 81:4544-4548, 1984.
71. Shaw, G.M., Hahn, B.H., Arya, S.K., Groopman, J.E., Gallo, R.C., Wong-Staal, F.: Molecular characterization of HTLV-III in AIDS. *Science* 226:1165-1171, 1984.
72. Shaw, G.M., Harper, M.E., Hahn, B.H., Epstein, L.G., Gajdusek, D.C., Price, R.W., Navia, B.A., Petito, G.K., O'Hara, C.J., Groopman, J.E., Cho, E.S., Oleske, J.M., Wong-Staal, F., Gallo, R.C.: HTLV-III infection in brains of children and adults with AIDS encephalopathy. *Science,* 227:177-182, 1985.
73. Trainor, Z., Wernicke, D., Unger-Waron, H., Essex, M.: Suppression of the humoral antibody response in natural retroviral infection. *Science* 220:858-859, 1983.
74. Van de Perre, P., Rouvroy, D., Lepage, P., Bogaerts, J., Kestelyn, P., Kayihigi, J., Hekker, A.C., Butzler, O.B., Clumeck, N.: Acquired immuno-deficiency syndrome in Rwanda. *Lancet* ii: 62-65, 1984.
75. Vilmer, F., Barré-Sinoussi, F., Rouzioux, C., Gazengel, C., Brun-Vezinet, F., Dauguet, C., Fischer, A., Manigne, P., Chermann, J.C., Griscelli, C., Montagnier, L.: Isolation of new lymphotropic retrovirus from two siblings with hemophilia B, one with AIDS. *Lancet* i:753-757, 1984.

76. Watanabe, T., Seiki, M., and Yoshida M.: Retrovirus terminology. *Science* 222:1178, 1983.
77. Weller, S.K., Jay, A.E., and Temin, H.M.: Correlation between cell killing and massive second-round reproduction by members of some groups of avian leukemia viruses. *J. Virol.* 33:494-506, 1980.
78. Yamamoto, N., Koubayashi, N., Takeuchi, K., Koyanagi, Y., Hatanaka, M., Hinuma, Y., Chosa, T., Schneider, J., Hunsmann, G.: Characterization of African green monkey B-cell lines releasing an adult T-cell leukemia virus-related agent. *Int. J. Cancer* 34:77-82, 1984.
79. Zagury, D., Bernard, J., Leibowitch, J., Safai, B., Groopman, J.E., Veldman, M., Sarngadharan, Gallo, R.C.: HTLV-III in cells cultured from semen of two patients with AIDS. *Science* 226:449-451, 1984.

Seropositivity to HTLV-III/LAV in Danish Subpopulations

P. Ebbesen*, M. Melbye*, and R.J. Biggar**

* The Institute of Cancer Research
Danish Cancer Society
Radiumstationen DK-8000 Aarhus C, Denmark
** Environmental Epidemiology Branch
National Cancer Institute
Landow Building 3C19
Bethesda, Maryland 20205, USA

Danes have the highest incidence of AIDS among the indigenous populations of Europe (14). In the following I shall discuss aspects of a series of previously published studies on Danes which may have some general relevance.

The only large-scale European study giving quantitative data on the various aspects of gay sexuality has been carried out in Aarhus and Copenhagen (9). The data conform with those of Bell and Weinberg on the sex behaviour of gays in the San Francisco Bay area in the 70th (2). Most notable is a mean of 28 new partners a year in Copenhagen for men 20-40-year old, and only moderately less in the much smaller provincial town. Furthermore, half the men also had sex with women. The major difference in behaviour between the metropolis and the provincial town was the frequency of sex with foreigners, in particular US citizens, with the Copenhageners leading. This is also the place where the Danish AIDS cases have occurred. In this respect it now appears natural that in 1982 we found a very strong statistical correlation between sex contact with an American and low T-helper value. Relative risk ratios (odds ratios) with 95% confidence intervals calculated by the exact method compared T-helper/suppressor ratios in groups exposed and not exposed. The relative risk of a low (more than 50% reduction) T-helper/suppressor ratio was 7.7 for those Danish gays visiting the US in 1980-81 (4). Later sera stored from that study revealed a similar very strong correlation between seropositivity to HTLV-III/LAV and contact with US citizens (relative risk 3.59 (13). Clearly, Europe received part of the epidemic from the US while at the same time especially France and Belgium had virus brought from Central Africa. In this connection it should be mentioned that Dr. Gigase's

Belgian group, the people of Gallo's and Fraumeni's laboratories, and our group are presently participating in studies of the East-Zairian population. The results so far indicate that in a rural population of Eastern Zaire both men and women have at least 12% seropositive and that 1/3 of the children have antibodies reacting with the ELISA and Western blot (6) although no AIDS cases have been observed in this area. Kaposi's sarcoma is frequent in that part of Zaire but was found to occur independently of antibodies to HTLV-III/LAV (5). The African connection clearly is not yet as well understood as the US-European transfer of virus.

The percentage of seropositives in Danish homosexuals has since December 1981 gone up by nearly 1 percent a month. Western blot analysis showed the person's reactivity against the various HTLV-III epitopes including P15, P24 and P41 to wax and wane in parallel. A team of European colleagues are presently soliciting information about the rise in seropositivity in the different West and East European countries over the years. If the increase in percentage of seropositive Europeans roughly follows the Danish curve, and if the present level of seropositivity in Western-Europe gays is about 30% and the mean latency period is about 2 years, the peak of new cases in European homosexuals might well be as far away as 5 years in future.

A particular route for HTLV-III/LAV into Denmark has been factor VIII preparations produced in the US. In collaboration with Scottish and US colleagues the serology of Danish and Scottish haemophiliacs was comapred (15). 22 Danish haemophiliacs (mean age, 22.8 yr, range 12-46) and 77 Scottish haemophiliacs (mean 34.9 yr, range 13-72) were enrolled. 12 (57%) of 21 Danish haemophilia A patients had antibodies against HTLV-III, as did a single haemophilia B patient (total, 59% positive; table I). Between 1979 and 1984 antibody-positive subjects with haemophilia A had received significantly ($p < 0.05$) larger quantities of factor VIII concentrate made from US donor material (mean 498.800 units) than antibody-negative subjects (mean 83.800 units). There was no statistical difference between the amounts of locally manufactured concentrate used in the two groups. The 2 subjects who

TABLE 1.   *HTLV-III seropositivity in healthy Scottish and Danish*

	Total tested	HTLV-III antibody positive (%)
Scotland		
No treatment	11	0 (0.0)
Local	28	2 (7.1)
Commercial	4	1 (25.0)
Both	34	9 (26.5)
Total	77	12 (15.6)
Denmark		
Local	2	0 (0.0)
Commercial	1	1 (100.0)
Both	19	12 (63.2)
Total	22	13 (59.1)

had not received factor concentrate made from US donor material in the period 1979-84 were both seronegative, whereas the seropositive haemophilia B patient had used only US manufactured factor IX concentrate.

In Scotland, 11 (18%) of 62 haemophilia A patients and 1 (78%) of 15 haemophilia B patients were HTLV-III positive. All but 2 of the seropositive subjects were known to have received commercial factor concentrate in the period 1979-84. Seropositive haemophilia patients had received more commercial clotting factor concentrate than had seronegative subjects (p < 0.001), whereas there was no statistical difference between the two groups in use of local products. As shown in table 1, 40% of subjects receiving commercial factor concentrate either alone or in combination with local products had antibodies against HTLV-III, compared with 7% of those recorded as receiving only local products. HTLV-III seropositivity was more common in persons more exposed to commercially produced factor VIII. The proportion with antibody rose from 11.8% among subjects in the bottom third of commercial product use to 29.4% in the middle third and 77.8% in the top third (trend analysis, p < 0.001). In contrast, no significant difference in seropositivity was observed between groups classified according to their use of locally produced factor VIII concentrate.

Since 1982, almost all treatment in Glasgow has been with locally produced factor concentrate. Therefore exposure to the HTLV-III antigen is likely to have taken place among Scottish patients before then. In line with this observation are data from another study showing that some American haemophiliacs were infected as far back as in 1979 (10). In terms of prevalence of HTLV-III antibodies and incidence of AIDS, European homosexuals area 1-2 years behind those in the United States (14). However, the prevalence rates of HTLV-III antibodies in Danish haemophiliacs are similar to those in American haemophiliacs, probably because of the use of US plasma products. Furthermore, the estimated incidence of AIDS among American haemophiliacs, 1-2 per thousand, is very close to that in European haemophiliacs (1 per thousand) (7). Plasma collected from the Scottish haemophiliacs between 1974 and 1984 showed antibodies to HTLV-III/LAV appearing after 1980 (12). The virus seems to be new to the haemophiliac environment having entered at about the time when the AIDS epidemic started.

There are only a few reports on heterosexual transmission of AIDS (11), including one report of AIDS in both a haemophiliac and his spouse (16). The high prevalence rate of HTLV-III antibodies in patients with haemophilia prompted us to evaluate the risk of transmission of HTLV-III to household members.

In September-October, 1984, we examined 26 Danish haemophiliacs (mean age 22.0 yr; range 4-71 yr) and their household members (9 female spouses or regular female sexual partners, 15 fathers, 17 mothers, 12 siblings and 11 children). Serum were assayed for antibodies against HTLV-III using the Western blot analysis.

None of 29 household members of 12 seronegative subjects were seropositive. However, 1 of 35 household members of 14 seropositive haemophiliacs was positive. She was a 17-year-old who had lived together with her haemophiliac friend for one year and had practiced vaginal, oral and anal sex with him. The seropositive partner did not belong to any known risk group and never participated in the preparation or administration of her partner's factor VIII concentrate. Analysis of sera from both the patient and his partner showed identical profiles on Western blots, including P15, P24, P41-P45, P61-64. Among the other 8 couples in this study, all had practiced vaginal and oral sex but only one other couple had practiced anal intercourse. Neither member of that couple was seropositive.

This study shows that heterosexual transmission of HTLV-III as detected by HTLV-III antibody positivity can occur between haemophiliacs and their sexual partners. Furthermore, it suggests that, as in homosexual men, HTLV-III infection might be facilitated by the practice of anal intercourse. In contrast, we found no serologic evidence that other household members had been infected by their HTLV-III seropositive haemophiliac housemate.

A multitude of infections are of course known to florish in the immune deficient in particular we found more cytomegalovirus to be excreted in the sperm of gay men with low T-helper/suppressor ratio (3) and recently we found the frequency of oral *candida albicans* isolation on primary plates to vary inversely with the H/S ratio (18). Both cytomegalovirus and candida (17) may have immunosupressive effects, something which makes interpretations difficult. The battered immune system of many gays, independent of infection with HTLV-III/LAV is, however, an important reality. I will use this as a pretext for presenting another Danish subpopulation, our mice.

Danish male mice grouped solely with males do mount each other and often fight. It is, however, possible to find sublines where biting does not take place. If crowded in the boxes these apparently docile mice develop chronic lesions — amyloidosis, sometimes anaemia, weight loss and loss of fur. All males in the group are affected to about the same degree and the lesions also develop in specific pathogen-free mice (8, Table II). The immune capacity of these fellows is impaired as measured by skin graft rejection and rejection of Moloney sarcoma virus-induced tumor (1). Other immune parameters are presently being studied along with the beta-adrenergic receptor density of the brain. What we know at present is that the all male crowding causes an acceleration of certain organic lesions, immune defects and a significant shortening of the mean survival time as compared to breeder males. Its possible relevance to acquired immune deficiency in humans is probably as a model for chronic physical and psychologic stress which may also be important for the main group at risk for AIDS. We are presently following this line of thought by entering a prospective study of 20,000 human adults with the purpose of determining the pattern of non-infectious diseases in relation to sex habits.

TABLE 2.   Influence of grouping and various treatments on mean survival time of three strains of mice. The animals were segregated at weaning

	Mean survival time in months						
	Sex segregated 10 per box	One of one sex 9 of opposite sex	Half and half (5/5)	Only one per box	Sex segregated 10 per box reserpine tranquillizer	One male 9 castrated males	Castrates
Males							
DBA	12	19	9	21	17	18	20
BALB/c	13	21		22			21
CBA	14	19					
Females							
DBA	19	17	16				
BALB/c	21	21	20	20			18
CBA	17	16					

REFERENCES

1. Amkraut, A., and Solomon, G.F. (1972): Stress and murine sarcoma virus (Moloney)-induced tumors. *Cancer Res.,* 32:1428-1433.
2. Bell, A., and Weinberg., M. (1978): *Homosexualities.* Mitchell Beazley, London.
3. Biggar, R.J., Andersen, H.K., Ebbesen, P., Melbye, M., Goedert, J.J., Mann, D.L., and Strong, D.M. (1983): Seminal fluid excretion of cytomegalovirus related to immunosuppression in homosexual men. *Brit. Med. J.,* 286:2010-2012.
4. Biggar, R.J., Melbye, M., Ebbesen, P., Mann, D.L., Goedert, J.J., Weinstock, R., Strong, D.M., and Blattner, W.A. (1984): Low T-lymphocyte ratios in homosexual men. Epidemiologic evidence for a transmissible agent. *JAMA,* 251:1441-1446.
5. Biggar, R.J., Melbye, M., Kestens, L., Sarngadharan, M.G., de Feyter, M., Blattner, W.A., Gallo, R.C., and Gigase, P.L. (1984): Kaposi's sarcoma in Zaire is not associated with HTLV-III infection. *N. Engl. J. Med.* 311:1051-1052.
6. Biggar, R.J., Melbye, M., Kestens, L., de Feyter, M., Saxinger, C., Bodner, A.J., Paluko, L., Blattner, W.A., and Gigase, P.L. (1985): Seroepidemiology of HTLV-III antibodies in a remote population of eastern Zaire. *Br. Med. J.,* (in press).
7. Bloom, A.L. (1984): Acquired immunodeficiency syndrome and other possible immunological disorders in European haemophiliacs. *Lancet,* i:1452-1455.
8. Ebbesen, P. (1984): Grouping stress as a way of obtaining permanent changes in the lymphoid organs of mice. In: *Lymphoid Cell Functions in Aging,* edited by A.L. de Weck, Vol. 3, pp. 47-52. EURAGE Series Topics in Aging Research in Europe.
9. Ebbesen, P., Melbye, M., and Biggar, R.J. (1984): Sex habits, recent disease, and drug use in two groups of Danish male homosexuals. *Arch. Sex. Behavior,* 13:291-300.
10. Goedert, J.J., Sarngadharan, M.G., Eyster, M.E., et al. (1985): Antibodies reactive with human T cell leukemia viruses in the serum of hemophiliacs receiving factor VIII concentrate. *Blood,* 65: (in press).
11. Harris, C., Small, C.B., Klein, R.S., et al. (1983): Immunodeficiency in female sexual partners of men with the acquired immunodeficiency syndrome. *N. Engl. J. Med.,* 308:1181-1184.
12. Madhok, R., Melbye, M., Lowe, G.D.O., Forbes, C.D., Froebel, K.S., Bodner, A.J., and Biggar, R.J. (1985): HTLV-III antibody in sequential plasma samples: From haemophiliacs 1974-84. *Lancet,* i:524-525.
13. Melbye, M., Biggar, R.J., Ebbesen, P. et al. (1984): Seroepidemiology of HTLV-III in Danish homosexual men: Prevalence, transmission, and disease outcome. *Br. Med. J.,* 289:573-575.
14. Melbye, M., Biggar, R.J., and Ebbesen, P. (1984): Epidemiology. Europe and Africa. In: *AIDS: A Basic Guide for Clinicians,* edited by P. Ebbesen, R.J. Biggar, and M. Melbye, pp. 29-41. Munksgaard/Saunders, Copenhagen/Philadelphia.

15. Melbye, M., Froebel, K.S., Madhok, R., Biggar, R.J., Sarin, P.S., Stenbjerg, S., Lowe, G.D.O., Forbes, C.D., Goedert, J.J., Gallo, R.C., and Ebbesen, P. (1984): HTLV-III seropositivity in European haemophiliacs exposed to factor VIII concentrate imported from the USA. *Lancet,* ii:1444-1446.
16. Pitchenik, A.E., Shafron, R.D., Glasserm, and Spira, T.J. (1984): The acquired immunodeficiency syndrome in the wife of a hemophiliac. *Ann. Intern. Med.,* 100:62-65.
17. Rogers, M.F., Morens, D.M., Stewart, J.A., Kaminski, R.M., Spira, T.J., Feorino, P.M., Larsen, S.A., Francis, D.P., Wilson, M., Kaufman, L., and Task Force for AIDS, Atlanta, Ge. (1983): National case-control study of Kaposi's sarcoma and Pneumocystis carinii pneumonia in homosexual men: part 2, laboratory results. *Ann. Intern. Med.,* 99:151-158.
18. Schonheyder, H., Melbye, M., Biggar, R.J., Ebbesen, P., Neuland, C.Y., and Stenderup, A. (1984): Oral yeast flora and antibodies to candida albicans in homosexual men. *Mykosen,* 27:539-544.

A Two-years Immunological Survey of Hemophiliacs from Apulia, Italy

G. Lucivero, T. Ripa, A. Dell'Osso, A.M. Sonnante,
A. Iacobelli and L. Bonomo[1]

Institute of Medical Clinics II, Clinical Immunology
University of Bari, Policlinico, 70124 Bari, Italy
[1]Institute of Medical Clinics VI, University of Rome "La Sapienza"
Policlinico Umberto I, 00161, Rome, Italy

Since cases of Pneumocystis carinii pneumonia have been reported in patients with hemophilia A treated with commercial purified factor VIII concentrates (2), the hemophiliacs' community has became progressively aware that the substitutive therapy with preparations of antihemophilic factor represents a risk for developing the acquired immunodeficiency syndrome (AIDS) or its prodromes such as a persistent systemic lymphadenopathy (3, 5, 22). Early in 1983, immunological studies carried out in otherwise healthy hemophiliacs revealed that the distribution of circulating T-lymphocyte subsets as well as the assays for cell-mediated immunity (responses to mitogens, natural killer activity) were significantly abnormal in the hemophiliacs treated with commercial purified preparations of antihemophilic factor, but not in those patients treated with cryoprecipitated from single or a few donors (14, 17, 20, 25, 34).

Recently a new human T-cell lymphotropic retrovirus, baptized lymphadenopathy-associated virus (LAV) by Montagnier's group (32) or human T-lymphotropic retrovirus III by Gallo's group (27) has been isolated from patients with AIDS, from hemophiliacs or from persons at risk for this syndrome. Moreover antibodies specific for LAV/HTLV-III have been detected in patients with AIDS or in at risk populations (8, 24, 28) and a coincidental appearance of LAV/HTLV-III antibodies in hemophiliacs and the onset of the AIDS epidemics has also been reported (6). Therefore the hypothesis has been put forwards that the LAV/HTLV-III retrovirus is a marker for AIDS and probably represents the etiological agent in this syndrome (4).

Up today Italy has not been hit severely by the AIDS epidemic; however recent evidences from several major cities suggest that the incidence of this syndrome and its prodromes has been progressively increasing in homosexuals, intravenous-drug abusers, hemophiliacs and other populations at risk during the last two years (1). In this regard, in February 1983 we began a clinical and immunological survey of hemophiliacs from Apulia, a region in the South of Italy, in order to detect early symptoms or immune clinical or laboratory alteration suggestive for AIDS. Beside clinical examinations, we looked at the main immunological abnormalities observed in AIDS, such as lymphopenia, selective depletion of T-cells with helper-inducer phenotype (T lymphocytes bearing the Leu 3a/T4 surface antigen) and polyclonal activation of B lymphocytes with elevated serum immunoglobulins (29).

MATERIALS AND METHODS

Study Groups

We have examined 62 patients (mean age 21.1 years; range 7-64 years) with severe hemophilia A (Factor VIII:C < 1%) and 12 patients (mean age 22.0 years; range 15-33 years) with hemophilia B (Factor IX < 1%). No clinical symptom suggestive of immunodeficiency was present at the time of the first examination and in the two following years of survey in the subjects with hemophilia A. On the other hand one patient with hemophilia B was affected by Hodgkin's lymphoma since December 1981 and had been treated with chemotherapy and radiotherapy for induction of remission. One additional B hemophiliac developed systemic lymphadenopathy without other symptoms in May 1984. The other 10 patients with hemophilia B were healthy at the time of examination and thereafter. Twenty three healthy relatives (15 parent, 4 siblings and 4 spouses) of hemophiliacs were also examined for immunological abnormalities.

Sixthy-two age-matched normal donors without history of omosexuality or drug-abuse represented the control population.

Since 1983 the patients were examined at least twice, with six-twelve months intervals.

Differential Treatment of Patients with hemophilia A.

Since 1978 one group of A hemophiliacs (N = 33) has been treated exclusively with commercial cryoprecipitated and lyophilized factor VIII concentrates prepared from a limited pool of plasma (approximately 500 donors). Moreover since 1981 the plasma for these lyophilized cryoprecipitates was obtained from Italian blood banks. The remaining patients (N = 29) were treated with commercial high and intermediate purity Factor VIII concentrates prepared from a large pool of plasma (more than 3,000 donors).

The patients with hemophilia B were treated with commercial prothrombin complex concentrates.

White Cell Counts and Lymphocyte Surface-Marker Analysis

Peripheral blood samples were drawn by venipuncture from the study groups after informed consent. The patients were untreated for at least one week, before sampling of blood. The blood samples were collected in EDTA for blood counts and white cell differential counts and in heparin for surface-marker analysis.

Peripheral blood mononuclear cells were fractionated from diluted (1:4) heparinized blood by centrifugation on Ficoll-Hypaque density gradient. The percentages of T lymphocytes were assessed by rosette formation with neuraminidase-treated sheep erythrocytes (E rosettes) (33). B lymphocytes positive for surface immunoglobulins were detected by direct immunofluorescence with FITC-conjugated goat antibodies to human immunoglobulins.

A panel of four murine monoclonal antibodies specific for surface antigens expressed by T lymphocytes (anti-Leu4), T-cell subsets with helper-inducer (anti-Leu3a) or suppressor-cytotoxic (anti-Leu2a) phenotypes and by lymphoid cells with natural killer activity (anti-Leu7) was used by indirect immunofluorescence.

Briefly 1 x 10^6 mononuclear cells were first incubated with 10 µl of each monoclonal antibody for 30 minutes at 4°C, then washed twice with cold PBS supplemented with 0.2 g % sodium azide and incubated with 10 µl of FITC-conjugated goat antibodies to mouse IgG or IgM. Monoclonal murine IgG or IgM unrelated to human lymphocyte antigens were used as negative controls in the experiments. Finally the cells were washed twice with cold PBS + 0.2% sodium azide, resuspendend at the concentration of 1 x 10^6 ml in the same solution and spun onto glass slides by cytocentrifugation (Shandon Cytospin). The cytologic preparations were fixed in ethanol (95%) - acetic acid (5%) solution at -20°C for 20 minutes, rehydrated in PBS, mounted in Elvanol under coversplips and examined with a Leitz-Dialux 20 microscope equipped for epi-illumination fluorescence and phase contrast. The percentages of positive cells were calculated by examining at least 300 cells.

Serum IgG, IgA and IgM Assays

The levels of serum IgG, IgA and IgM were assayed in the patients and in the control group by laser nephelometry (Laser Nephelometer, Behring Institute).

Anti-HTLV III Antibodies

The assay for anti-HTLV III antibodies in the serum of patients with hemophilia and their healthy relatives was kindly performed by Prof. F. Aiuti (Clinical Immunology, University of Rome «La Sapienza», Rome, Italy). The anti-HTLV III antibodies were detected by indirect immunofluorescence method using HTLV-III-infected HT-9 cells and fluorochrome-conjugated goat antiserum specific for human immunoglobulins (1).

Student's t test and variance analysis were used for statistical evaluation of the diffrences observed within the study groups. The correlations between age or dosage of substitutive therapy and lymphocyte subsets or serum immunoglobulins in patients with hemophilia A were esthablished by linear regression analysis.

RESULTS AND DISCUSSION

Lymphocyte Subsets in Patients with Hemophilia A and B

The absolute values of white cells and lymphocytes as well as the percentages and absolute numbers of T and B lymphocytes and Leu7-positive lymphoid cells did not differ significantly in the patients with hemophilia A or B and in the control group (Table 1). However the analysis of T-lymphocyte subsets with helper-inducer or suppressor-cytotoxic phenotypes demonstrated a significant reduction of the helper cells (Leu 3a$^+$) and a significant increase of the suppressor cells (Leu 2a$^+$) in patients with hemophilia A and B

TABLE 1.   *Analyses of blood cells in hemophiliacs and controls*

	Controls (N = 60)	Hemophilia A (N + 62)	Hemophilia B (N + 12)
White cells/μl	5180 ±600[a]	5123 ±340	4307 ±658
Lymphocytes/μl	1490 ±172	1439 ±95	4307 ±210
E-rosettes			
per cent	68.9 ±2.1	70.0 ±1.2	67.9 ±2.9
cells/μl	1026 ±32	1007 ±18	934 ±40
Leu4/T3			
per cent	63.7 ±3.2	65.3 ±2.0	59.5 ±3.1
cells/μl	949 ±48	939 ±29	818 ±42
Leu 7			
per cent	24.9 ±2.8	21.5 ±1.4	25.4 ±1.8
cells/μl	371 ±42	309 ±20	349 ±25
B cells			
per cent	12.7 ±0.8	10.2 ±1.2	9.8 ±1.1
cells/μl	189 ±12	147 ±17	134 ±15

[a] Values are expressed as means ± S.E.M.

TABLE 2.   *Analyses of T-Lymphocyte subsets in Hemophiliacs and controls*

	Controls (N = 60)	Hemophilia A (N + 62)	Hemophilia B (N + 12)
Leu 3a/T4			
per cent	41.2 ±1.6	36.1 ±1.1[a]	30.1 ±2.9[b]
cells/μl	614 ±24	519 ±16[a]	414 ±40[b]
Leu 2a/T8			
per cent	27.7 ±1.4	35.0 ±1.2[c]	33.8 ±3.0[d]
cells/μl	413 ±21	503 ±17[c]	465 ±41[d]
Leu 3a/Leu 2a			
RATIO	1.63 ±0.17	1.09 ±0.05[e]	1.02 ±0.16[e]
Patients with			
ratio < 1 (%)	13	45	50

[a] Significantly different from controls (P < 0.01)
[b] Significantly different from controls (P < 0.005)
[c] Significantly different from controls (P < 0.001)
[d] Significantly different from controls (P < 0.05)
[e] Significantly different from controls (P < 0.001)

(Table 2). These data are in good agreement with previous studies performed in healthy hemophiliacs (14, 17, 20, 31, 34).

Even if the role of the substitutive therapy in the induction of the imbalance in the lymphocyte subsets has been pointed out by several reports, the actual mechanisms responsible for these alterations have not been identified (7, 18, 19, 25, 30). Rasi et al (25) reported normal ratios of helper/suppressor T cells in patients with hemophilia A treated with cryoprecipitates from small pool of plasma. Moreover Lee et al. suggested that T-cell subset abnormalities in hemophiliacs might be related to HLA proteins in plasma products (16) or to different plasma fractionation methods (15).

Lymphocyte subsets and differential treatment in Hemophilia A.

We have examined patients with severe hemophilia A that have been treated since 1978 with high or intermediate purity factor VIII concentrates prepared from a large (> 10,000 donors) pool of plasma or, alternatively, with commercial lyophilized factor VIII concentrates prepared by cryoprecipitation from a pool of plasma from approximately 500 donors. As shown in Table 3 the patients treated with purified F-VIII concentrates presented sig-

TABLE 3. *Lymphocyte subsets in hemophiliacs according to type of product used patients treated with F-VIII concentrates*

	Purified (N = 29)	Cryoprecip. (N − 33)	Significance
Lymphocytes/μl	1935 ±105	1819 ±80	N.S.
E rosettes (%)	70.5 ±1.5	69.4 ±2.0	N.S.
Leu 4/T3 (%)	65.9 ±3.2	64.5 ±1.7	N.S.
Leu 3a/ T4 (%)	33.3 ±1.7[a]	38.5 ±1.4[b]	P < 0.02
Leu 2a/ T8 (%)	36.9 ±2.2[a]	33.3 ±3.0[a]	N.S.
Leu3a/Leu2a ratio	0.98 ±0.08[a]	1.19 ±0.06[a]	P < 0.05
Leu 7 (%)	25.9 ±2.4[b]	19.0 ±1.6[a]	P < 0.02
B cells (%)	10.9 ±1.1	9.4 ±0.8	N.S.

[a] Significantly different from controls
[b] Non significantly different from controls.

nificantly lower percentages of helper (Leu 3a$^+$) cells and lower helper/suppressor ratios compared to the hemophiliacs treated with commercial cryoprecipitates. It is noteworthy that the values of helper cells in the latter group did not differ from the controls. On the opposite the hemophiliacs treated with cryoprecipitates presented levels of Leu 7 positive cells significantly lower than the controls. The percentages and the absolute numbers of suppressor T cells (Leu 2a$^+$) were uniformly higher than the control values in both groups of hemophiliacs.

Correlations between age, dose of therapy and lymphocyte subsets

No correlation was observed between age of patients and the percentages of Leu 3a$^+$, Leu 2a$^+$ or Leu 7$^+$ cells and between dosage of substitutive therapy (Factor VIII units/year) and Leu 3a[+] or Leu 7[+] cells. A significant positive correlation was observed between dosage of Factor VIII used and percentages (and absolute numbers) of Leu 2a[+] lymphocytes in the whole population of A hemophiliacs. However when the analysis was performed in the two groups of patients according to the type of treatment, the positive correlation between expansion of the Leu 2a[+] cell population and dose of Factor VIII transfused was confirmed only in the group of patients treated with purified Factor VIII concentrates (Fig. 1). These data confirm previous reports on the influence of treatment in the imbalance of T-cell subsets (7, 10, 14, 19, 25, 31) and indicate that type of treatment and dosage might alter selectively different subpopulations of T lymphocytes or Leu 7[+] cells.

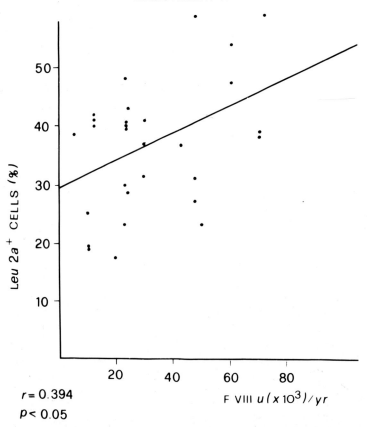

CORRELATION BETWEEN DOSAGE OF PURIFIED F-VIII CONCENTRATES AND Leu 2a[+] CELLS IN HEMOPHILIA A

$r = 0.394$

$p < 0.05$

F VIII $u(\times 10^3)/yr$

FIG. 1. Correlation (by linear regression analysis) between dosage of purified factor VIII concentrates transfused (expressed as Factor VIII units/year) and percentages of Leu 2a[+] cells in individual patients. Correlation coefficient r − 0.394; significance p < 0.05.

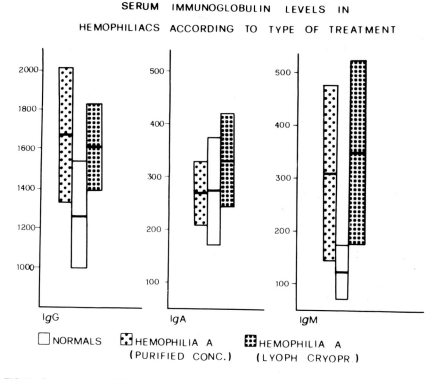

SERUM IMMUNOGLOBULIN LEVELS IN
HEMOPHILIACS ACCORDING TO TYPE OF TREATMENT

IgG   IgA   IgM

☐ NORMALS   ⊞ HEMOPHILIA A (PURIFIED CONC.)   ⊞ HEMOPHILIA A (LYOPH CRYOPR.)

FIG. 2. Serum immunoglobulins levels in patients with hemophilia A, according to treatment with high and intermediate purity Factor VIII concentrates (purified conc.) or with commercial lyophilized cryoprecipitates (lyoph. cryopr.). Mean values ± S.D. are indicated in the figure.

Serum Immunoglobulins levels in patients with hemophilia A

Serum IgG and IgM levels were significantly higher in hemophiliacs than in controls (Fig. 2). On the other hand serum IgA were significantly elevated in the group of patients treated with commercial cryoprecipitates. The increase of IgA correlated with the age of patients but not with the dosage of the substitutive therapy (data not shown). Moreover 70% of patients treated with cryoprecipitates and 32% of patients on therapy with purified concentrates presented levels of one or more classes of serum immunoglobulins beyond the upper limit of the normal range. Abnormalities of B-cell activation with hypergammaglobulinemia have been reported in patients with acquired immunodeficiency syndrome (12). However in our patients, the increased levels of serum immunoglobulins seem to be related to the substitutive therapy. The commercial cryoprecipitates, that determine a higher antigenic load of proteins (21) might induce a stronger stimulation of the B lymphoid system with increased secretion of IgA.

Anti-HTLV III antibodies in Hemophiliacs

It has been hypothesised that the recently identified T-cell lymphotropic retrovirus HTLV-III/LAV represents the etiologic agent of AIDS. This hypothesis is also supported by the finding of anti-HTLV-III IgG antibodies in the populations at risk for AIDS but not in normal subjects. It has been reported that up to 74% of hemophiliacs without signs of immunodeficiency have antibodies to this retrovirus (3, 11, 13, 24) and that the prevalence of anti-HTLV-III antibodies in hemophiliacs increased progressively in the last two-three years and correlated with the onset of the AIDS epidemic (6, 8).

In our study groups, 13% of patients with hemophilia A and 50% of B hemophiliacs presented antibodies to HTLV-III (Table 4). The lowest inci-

TABLE 4. *Anti-HTLV III antibodies in Hemophiliacs from Apulia (Italy)*

PATIENTS	N. Positive for anti-HTLV III Ab.	% Positive
Hemophilia A	4/31	13
A. Treatment with purified FVIII conc.	3/14	21
B. Treatment with lyophilized cryopr.	1/17	6
Hemophilia B	4[a]/8	50

[a] One patient affected by Hodgkin's lymphoma; one additional patient with persistent systemic lymphadenopathy.

dence (6%) was observed in the group treated with commercial cryoprecipitated. It is noteworthy that two patients with hemophilia B and antibodies to HTLV-III were respectively affected by Hodgkin's disease in homosexual men with generalized lymphadenopathy have been reported recently (26). However, in spite of chemo- and radiotherapy, our patient with Hodgkin's disease have not developed opportunistic infections and is currently in clinical remission. The other hemophiliacs positive for anti-HTLV-III antibodies were in good health and did not differ significantly from the negative ones as regard to lymphocyte subsets and serum IgG (data not shown). A longer follow-up is required to understand whether the hemophiliacs positive for HTLV-III antibodies are at greater risk for AIDS or have to be considered healthy carriers (13).

Immunological findings in healthy relatives of Hemophiliacs

No immunological alteration has been observed in healthy relatives of hemophiliacs. These results are in good agreement with previous reports (23); moreover none of the examined relatives was positive for anti-HTLV-III antibodies and this finding confirms that the immunological changes observed in healthy hemophiliacs are not linked to an easily transmissible infectious agent (9).

Immunological Survey (1983-85) in Hemophiliacs

The immunological status of hemophiliacs, evaluated by surface-marker analysis, remained stable in 68% of patients during the period of this survey. The remaining 32% of patients presented changes in the distribution of lymphocyte subset with increase (64%) or decrease (40%) of the helper/suppressor ratio. Until now no patient (except one) has developed lymphopenia or severe depletion of helper lymphocytes or has shown symptoms suggestive of AIDS or the AIDS-related complex.

CONCLUSIONS

The presented results indicate that the immunological abnormalities observed in hemophiliacs are secondary to therapy with blood products. However dose and type of therapy and the lenght of treatment have selective influences on different lymphocyte subsets. More precisely, the dose of factor VIII transfused is related to the expansion of the suppressor cell population. On the other hand the use of purified factor VIII concentrates induces a more profound reduction of helper lymphocytes while the commercial cryoprecipitates seem to alter the Leu 7^+ cells and to induce more frequently polyclonal secretion of immunoglobulins. The different proteic content of blood products (i.e. cryoprecipitates vs. high or intermediate purity factor VIII concentrates) (21), the method differences in plasma fractionation and the presence of infectious agents in these blood products are likely to act with different mechanism in the induction of the quantitative or qualitative derangement of individual players of the immunological orchestra. In the context of chronic antigenic stimulation of the immune system, retrovirus infection might represent the last ring of a chain of immunological alterations towards the development of AIDS. However further studies are needed to clarify the role of LAV/HTLV-III infection in development of immune changes and clinical symptoms in hemophiliacs.

Aknowledgments

This work was supported by Grant N. 8400786.44 of the C.N.R., Finalized Project "Oncologia" and by Grant M.P.I. 40%, N. 91020/080. The authorss thank Dr. M. Grande and V. De Mitrio for referring the patient with hemophilia B and Hodgkin's disease.

REFERENCES

1. Aiuti, F. (1984): Sindrome da immunodeficienza acquisita (AIDS). Stato dell'arte, 1984. *Immunol. Clin. Sper.*, III:221-249.
2. Anonymous (1982): Pneumocystis carinii pneumonia among persons with hemophilia A. *Morbid. Mortal. Weekly Rep.*, 31:365-367.
3. Anonymous (1984): Update Acquired immunodeficiency syndrome (AIDS) in persons with hemophilia. *Morbid. Mortal. Weekly Rep.*, 33:589-591.

4. Broder, S. and Gallo, R.C. (1984): A pathogenic retrovirus (HTLV-III) linked to AIDS. *N. Engl. J. Med.*, 311:1292-1297.
5. Daly, H.M. and Scott, G.L. (1983): Fatal AIDS in A hemophiliacs in the UK. *Lancet*, II:1190.
6. Evatt, B.L., Gomperts, E.D., McDouglas, J.S. and Ramsey, R.B. (1985): Coincidental appearance of LAV/HTLV-III antibodies in hemophiliacs and the onset of the AIDS epidemics. *N. Engl. J. Med.*, 312:483-486.
7. Froebel, K.S., Madhok, R., Forbes, C.D., Lennies, S.E., Lowe, G.D. and Sturrock, R.D. (1983): Immunological abnormalities in haemophilia: are they caused by American factor VIII concentrate? *Br. Med. J.*, 287: 1091-1093.
8. Gurtler, L.G., Wernicke, D., Eberle, J., Zoulek, G., Deinhardt, F. and Schramm, W. (1984): Increase in prevalence of anti-HTLV III in haemophiliacs. *Lancet*, II: 1275-1276.
9. Hirsh, M.S., Wormser, G.P., Schooley, R.T., Ho, D.D., Felsenstein, D., Hopkins, C.C., Joline, C., Duncanson, F., Sangadharan, M.G., Saxinger, C. and Gallo, R.C. (1985): Risk of nosocomial infection with human T-cell lymphotropic virus III (HTLV-III). *N. Engl. J. Med.*, 312:1-4.
10. Kessler, C.M., Schulof, R.S., Alabaster, O., Goldstein, A.L., Naylor, P.H., Phillips, T.M., Luban, N.L.C., Kelleher J.F. and Reaman, G.H. (1984): Inverse correlation between age related abnormalities of T-cell immunity and circulating thymosin α-l levels in haemophilia A. *Br. J. Haematol.*, 58:325-336.
11. Kitchen, L.W., Barin, F., Sullivan, J.L., McLane, M.F., Brettler, D.B., Levine, P.H. and Essex, M. (1984): Aetiology of AIDS-antibodies to human T-cell leukaemia virus (type III) in haemophliacs. *Nature*, 312: 367-369.
12. Lane, H.C., Masur, H., Edgar, L.C., Whalen, G., Rook, A.H. and Fauci, A.S. (1983): Abnormalities of B-cell activation and immunoregulation in patients with the acquired immunodeficiency syndrome. *N. Engl. J. Med.*, 309: 453-458.
13. Laurence, J., Brun-Vezinet, F., Schutzer, S.E., Rouzioux, C., Klatzmann, D., Barré-Sinoussi, F., Chermann, J.-C. and Montagnier, L. (1984): Lymphadenopathy-associated viral antibody in AIDS. Immune correlations and definition of a carrier state. *N. Engl. J. Med.*, 311:1269-1273.
14. Lederman, M.M., Ratnoff, O.D., Scillian, J.J., Jones, P.K. and Schacter, B. (1983): Impaired cell-mediated immunity in patients with classical hemophilia. *N. Engl. J. Med.*, 308:79-83.
15. Lee, C.A., Janossy, G., Ashley, J. and Kernoff, P.B.A. (1983): Plasma fractionation methods and T-cell subsets in haemophilia. *Lancet*, II:158-159.
16. Lee, C.A., Kernoff, P.B.A., Karayiannis, P., Waters, J. and Thomas, H.C. (1984): Abnormal T-lymphocyte subsets in hemophilia: relation to HLA proteins in plasma products. *N. Engl. J. Med.*, 310:1058.
17. Luban, N.L.C., Kelleher, J.F. and Reaman, G.H. (1983): Altered distribution of T lymphocyte subpopulations in children and adolescents with haemophilia. *Lancet*, II: 503:505.
18. Lucivero, G., Ripa, T., Dell'Osso, A. and Bonomo, L. (1985): Lymphocyte subpopulations in patients with hemophilia A and healthy relatives. The role of the therapy in the induction of immunological abnormalities in hemophiliacs. *Immunol. Clin. Sper.*, in press.
19. Mannucci, P.M., Gringeri, A., Ammassari, M. and Mari, D. (1984): Abnormalities of lymphocyte subsets are correlated with concentrate consumption in asymptomatic italian hemophiliacs treated with concentrated made from american plasma. *Americ. J. Hematol.*, 17:167-176.
20. Menitove, J.E., Aster, R.H., Casper, J.T., Lauer, S.J., Gottschall, J.T., Williams, J.E., Gill, J.C., Wheeler, D.V., Piaskowski, V., Kirchner, P. and Montgomery, R.R. (1983): T-lymphocytes subpopulations in patients with classic hemophilia treated with cryoprecipitate and lyophilized concentrates. *N. Engl. J. Med.*, 308:83-86.
21. Morfini, M., Longo, G., Matucci, M., Vannini, S., Messori, A., Filimberti, E., Duminuco, M., Avanzi, G. and Rossi-Ferrini, P. (1984): Cryoprecipitates and Factor VIII commercial concentrates: in vitro characteristics and in vivo compartmental analysis. *La Ricerca Clin. Lab.*, 14: 681-691.
22. Ragni, M.V., Lewis, J.H., Spero, J.A. and Bontempo, F.A. (1983): Acquired-immunodeficiency-like syndrome in two haemophiliacs. *Lancet*, I: 213-214.
23. Ragni, M.V., Bontempo, F.A., Lewis, J.H., Spero, J.A. and Rabin, B.S. (1983): An immunological study of spouses and siblings of asymptomatic hemophiliacs. *Blood*, 62: 1297-1299.
24. Ramsey, R.B., Palmer, E.L., McDouglas, J.S., Kalyanaraman, V.S., Jackson, D.W.,

Chorba, T.L., Holman, R.C. and Evatt, B.L. (1984): Antibody to lymphadenopathy-associated virus in haemophiliacs with and without AIDS. *Lancet*, II: 1297-1299.
25. Rasi, V.P.O., Koistinen, J.L.K., Lohman, C.M. and Silvennoinen, O.J. (1984): Normal T-cell subsets ratios in patients with severe haemophilia A treated with cryoprecipitate. *Lancet*, I:461.
26. Schoeppel, S.L., Hoppe, R.T. and Dorfman, R.F. (1985): Hodgkin's disease in homosexual men with generalized lymphadenopathy. *Ann. Intern. Med.*, 102: 68-70.
27. Schüpbach, J., Popovic, M., Gilden, R.V., Gonda, M.A., Sarngadharan, M.G. and Gallo, R.C. (1984): Serological analysis of a subgroup of human T-lymphotropic retroviruses (HTLV-III) associated with AIDS. *Science*, 224:503-505.
28. Schüpbach, J., Haller, O., Vogt, M., Luthy, R., Joller, H., Oelz, O, Popovic, M., Sarngadharan, M.G. and Gallo, R.C. (1985): Antibodies to HTLV-III in Swiss patients with AIDS and pre-AIDS and in groups at risk for AIDS. *N. Engl. J. Med.*, 312: 2665-270.
29. Seligmann, M., Chess, L., Fahey, J.L., Fauci, A.S., Lachmann, P.J., L'Age-Stehr, J., Ngu, J., Pinching, A.J., Rosen, F.S., Spira, T.J., and Wybran, J. (1984): AIDS- An immunological reevaluation. *N. Engl. J. Med.*, 311: 1286-1292.
30. Tsoukas, C., Gervais, F., Shuster, J., Gold, P., O'Shaughnessy, M. and Robert-Guroff, M. (1984): Association of HTLV-III antibodies and cellular immune status of hemophiliacs. *N. Engl. J. Med.*, 311: 1514-1515.
31. Unzeitig, J.C., Church, J.A., Gomperts, E.D., Nye, C.A., Pasquale, S., and Richards, W. (1984): Abnormal T-cell subsets and mitogen responses in hemophiliacs exposed to factor concentrate. *Amer. J. Dis. Children*, 138: 645-648.
32. Vilner, E., Barrè-Sinoussi, F., Fouzioux, C., Gazengel, C., Vezinet Brun, F., Dauquet, C., Fischer, A., Manigne, P., Chermann, J.C., Griscelli, C. and Montagnier, L. (1984): Isolation of new lymphotropic retrovirus from two siblings with haemophilia B, one with AIDS. *Lancet*, I: 753-757.
33. Weiner, M.S., Bianco, C. and Nussenzweig, V. (1973): Enhanced binding of neuraminidase-treated sheep erythrocytes to human T lymphocytes. *Blood*, 42: 939-946.
34. Weintrub, P.S., Koerper, M.A., Addiego, J.E., Drew, W.L., Lennette, E.T., Miner, R., Cowan M.J. and Amman, A.J. (1983): Immunological abnormalities in patients with hemophilia A. *J. Pediat.*, 103: 692-695.

Epidemiological Survey on HTLV-III Infection in Italy: 1981-1985

M. Carbonari, B. Scarpati, G. Scano, G. Turbessi,
C. Lanzalone, G. Luzi, R. Bonomo, F. Giordano and F. Aiuti

*Dept. of Allergy and Clinical Immunology University of Rome "La Sapienza"
and Italian Red Cross "Centro Trasfusionale", Rome, Italy*

ABSTRACT

An extensive epidemiological survey on the distribution of serum antibodies to human T lymphotropic retrovirus III (HTLV III) in patients and normal donors is reported. ELISA and IFA have been performed to evaluate all the sera. This study was carried out in people living in large as well as small cities in different regions in Italy. Serum samples of 29 patients with Acquired Immunodeficiency Syndrome (AIDS), 520 with AIDS Related Complex (ARC) and 2059 from individuals at risk for these diseases were analized. Percentage of positive sera was from 87.5% in AIDS, and varied from 100% to 45% in ARC. Positive sera in individuals at risk for AIDS or ARC ranged from 20.7% in homosexuals to 26.6% in drug abusers and 27.4% in haemophiliacs. No positive sera were observed, in 1984, by IFA, among 660 normal individuals, relatives of patients with AIDS, ARC or among people at risk living in small cities. On the contrary, in 1985, using ELISA method, we found 7 positive sera among 8979 blood donors and 9 seropositive among relatives of seropositive individuals at risk for AIDS and ARC. These data confirm that HTLV-III infection is mainly diffused in the categories at risk for AIDS, but at the present time it seems to spread through heterosexual transmission in subjects not considered at risk for AIDS.

INTRODUCTION

The Acquired Immune Deficiency Syndrome (AIDS), a new epidemic form of acquired cellular immunodeficiency, appeared in USA in 1979 and spread to Western European Countries over the last six years. Increasing literature on AIDS expresses the exponential diffusion of the disease as also confirmed by a recent CDC meeting in Atlanta. Acquired Immunodeficiency Syndrome (AIDS) is a disease caused by a family of retroviruses recently identified: the human T lymphotropic virus (HTLV III) (9) or Lymphoadenopathy-Associated or Immunodeficiency-Associated Virus (LAV/IDAV) (4). Up to now, more than 10.000 cases have been reported in U.S.A. (12), approximately 500 in Northern Europe (13), and 50 patients have been reported in Italy (June 1985). In addition, in the last two years a large group of patients with a syndrome characterized by generalized lymphoadenopathy has been identified in USA and in Italy (1) (mainly in homosexuals, drug addicts and haemophiliacs). In the present study we report an update of the prevalence of specific antibodies to HTLV III/LAV in patients with AIDS, with AIDS-Related Complex (ARC), in subjects at risk for AIDS and in individuals having sexual intercourse with those subjects.

PATIENTS

Serum samples were obtained from patients and normal individuals from 14 Italian cities: Rome, Milan, Florence, Cagliari, Verona, Turin, Genoa, Viterbo, Catanzaro, Bari, Brescia, Pisa, Naples and Trento.

AIDS

Sera were collected from 29 patients with AIDS, 5 of them were children from seropositive mothers, born after 19 82; 21 had opportunistic infection (OI), 4 had OI and Kaposi's Sarcoma (KS) and 4 had only KS. Some of the sera were collected at an early stage of the disease, while the majority were obtained at a later phase.

ARC Patients

Criteria for selection of ARC patients were those established by the CDC-NIH Working Group (2). All the patients had unexplained lymphoadenopathy involving two or more extrainguinal sites, showed two or more additional symptoms such as fatigue, muscle pain, night sweats, weight loss and moderate fever. They also had three or more of the following immunological abnormalities: cutaneous anergy, lymphopenia, inversion of the T4/T8 ratio, increased Ig levels, elevated antibody titers to CMV and/or EBV. The overall population consisted of 520 patients, 352 of whom were drug addicts, 151 were homosexuals, 15 haemophiliacs and 2 children whose mothers were drug addicts (Table 1). In some patients (30 drug abusers and 5 homosexuals)

TABLE 1.   *HTLV-III antibodies detected in AIDS/ARC by IFA and ELISA systems*

PATIENTS		IFA+/Total	%(+)	ELISA+/Total	%(+)
AIDS		15/25	60	25/29	86.2
ARC:	Drug addicts	40/79	50.6	247/352	70.1
	Homosexuals	7/12	58.3	105/151	69.5
	Haemophiliacs	15/15	100	15/15	100
	Children	0/2		2/2	

serum samples had also been collected one or two years before when the subjects were symptom-free.

Individuals at risk for AIDS and ARC

Homosexuals. Samples were collected from 333 high promiscuity apparently healthy homosexuals or bisexuals. Some of them had recurrent venereal infections and a high incidence of hepatitis B (27%). All cases were symptom-free at the time of the blood collection and after a periods of 8-10 month none had developed AIDS. *Drug addicts.* 1179 intravenous heroin addicts without ARC were studied. Approximately 35% of them showed immunological abnormalities. None developed AIDS in the last 8-10 months of observation. *Haemophiliacs.* 522 haemophiliacs without ARC were also selected. The majority of them had immunological abnormalities as previously described by us (11) and others (6, 7). *Multiply Transfused Patients:* 25 patients affected by Cooley, which periodically undergo blood transfusion, were also selected (Table 2).

TABLE 2. *Individuals at Risk for AIDS and ARC*

	IFA+/TOT	ELISA +/TOTAL		
		A	B	C
Homosexuals	16/134	70/133	—	28/66
Drug Abusers	119/564	241/410	—	112/205
Haemophiliacs	46/199	60/215	—	27/108
Multiply transf. subjects	0/23	2/2	—	—

Controls and other categories

Five hundred and fifty sera were collected, in 1984, from various categories. As normal controls we tested a healthy population homogeneous for sex and age including: 80 females and 50 males whose age varied from 18 to 65 years, 280 blood donors from five different blood banks and 140 military servicemen. Other categories were constituited by: 55 laboratory and hospital personnel and 30 normal relatives of AIDS and ARC patients. In 1985, we have examined the specimens of 8979 blood donors of both sexes, aged 18-65 years, negative for risk factors of AIDS. Finally, we have checked 73 sera of normal partners and/or relatives of patients with AIDS or ARC.
In order to assess the prevalence of antibodies against HTLV III in Africa, we have also examined some African sera, affected by various infectious diseases and Kaposi's sarcoma, collected during 1975 (Somalia), 1980 (Tanzania) and 1984 (Camerun). Partners and/or children of bisexuals and drug additcs, relatives of patients with AIDS or ARC and people working in hospitals with patients with AIDS or ARC were also included in our analysis. Some individuals were studied as members of families.

METHODS

Cell lines

The neoplastic aneuploid T cell line HT, derived from an adult with lymphoid leukemia of T4 cells was infected with HTLV III and produced HTLV III virus in sufficient quantities to be visualized by indirect immunofluorescence (IFA) using both a rabbit antiserum to HTLV III and patient serum (9). The percentage of positive cells of cell clone H9 derived from the parenteral cell HT line varies from 5 to 80%, according to different cell preparation as evaluated by IFA. Non infected H9 clone was negative with all the positive sera.

Immunofluorescence assay (IFA)

The assay was performed as described elsewhere (3). In order to evaluate the presence of IgM antibodies we used as a second reagent a fluorescein conjugated monoclonal anti-mu antibody as well as an anti-IgM heteroantiserum in 148 cases positive for HTLV III antibodies (37 ARC patients, 14 AIDS patients and 97 at risk subjects). Fluorescent positive cells were evaluated by means of a Leitz Orthoplan Microscope. Results have been considered as positive only when more than 5% of the cell displayed a linear and/or spotted membrane fluorescence. Controls included: non infected H9 clone normal sera, as well as sera positive for antinuclear antibodies (ANA) and rheumatoid factor (RF). Each positive sera was tested at various dilutions ranging from 1:8 to 1:128. The majority of the positive sera showed intense fluorescence at least up to the 1:64 dilution.

ELISA assay

ELISA assay was performed with test kits developed by three different companies. HTLV III antigen used in the test was derived from HTLV III virus propagated in T-lymphocyte culture. After mass propagation of the virus by cell culture techniques, the virus was purified by ultracentrifugation and inactivated by disruption. The antigen further purified was used to sensitize the plastic coated iron metal beads (A = Litton) or plastic beads (B = Abbott) or the test well (C = Electronucleonics), according with the various kits. Sera were allowed to react with the antigen. Solid phase, after washing several times was incubated with peroxidase-labeled goat anti-human IgG. The solid phase was again washed extensively and allowed to react for 30 minutes with 200 μl of substrate; this was o-phenylendiamine (OPD) in B and C kits and was 2,2'azino-di-ethyl-benzothiazoline- sulfonate in A kit. Reactions were blocked with a stop solution and the colour yeld was measured with a Dynatech ELISA plate reader on a selected wavelenght of 492 nm and/or 690 nm. An absorbance reading greater than or equal to the cut-off was given as positive.

RESULTS

AIDS patients

Fifteen out of 25 patients were positive with indirect immunofluorescence test (60%), while 25/29 were positive using the ELISA techniques (86.2%). In 1 case with OI and KS the antibody titer against HTLV III, declined during the follow-up of 11 months from 1/128 to 1/8 (IFA); in 4 cases it remained unchanged. All the cases were positive for antibodies against EBV and/or CMV and 3 were HBsAg positive.

ARC patients

The results are summarized in Table 1. Antibodies against HTLV III were positive in 369 out of 520 sera of patients with ARC obtained from different Italian cities. The highest percentage of positive sera was found among haemophiliacs (100%). IFA positive sera were positive with ELISA as well. No significant differences were found among the kits used. In the group of drug addicts significant difference in prevalence of seropositive patients occurred selecting different geographical areas. The percentage of positive sera was 82.8% in those patients who had been affected by ARC for a period of more than six months. Among the drug addicts with ARC, 20 were females including two prostitutes (14 positive for HTLV III antibodies). One of the two prostitutes had delivered a child who died 5 months later of repeated infections and severe T cell deficiency. The serum of the child collected in the second month of life showed a positive titer of IgG antibodies to HTLV III, probably of maternal origin. Two more children, born from drug addicts females, showed an ARC syndrome and a positivity for HTLV III antibody. An interesting finding was the absence of antibodies against HTLV III in 15 cases (10 drug abusers from Milan and 5 homosexuals from Rome) that were collected 1-2 years before (when they were symptoms-free). None of the patients with ARC observed for a period ranging from 1 to 2 years developed AIDS. During the last 6 months only one haemophilic child showed weight loss and opportunistic infections (two episodes).

Individuals at risk for AIDS and ARC

The results are summarized in Table 2. 134 sera of homosexuals, 564 of drug abusers, 199 of haemophiliacs and 23 of polytransfused were examined with IFA. The overall positivity was 19.6% ranging from 23.1% in haemophiliacs to 11.9% in homosexuals. ELISA was used to study 760 sera with kit A and 379 sera with C. We found 52.4% positive homosexuals, 58.8% drug abusers and 27.9% haemophiliacs with A; 42.4% positive in homosexuals, 54.6% drug abusers and 25% haemophiliacs with C.

Controls and other categories

No positives were found among 550 healthy donors in 1984 (IFA). The same results have been obtained among the relatives of the patients with AIDS and/or ARC checked. In 1985 (ELISA techniques) the specimens of 8979 blood donors of both sexes, negative for risk factors of AIDS were examined (kit B) 8910 donor samples were negative in the first run and were not tested further. 60 were initially reactive (0.67%) and 18 (0.19%) were in the grey-zone. 42 out of these 60 reactive samples were negative after the second test and 18 were confirmed positive. On reinvestigation, with the same kit, 17 out of the 18 grey-zone specimens confirmed in grey-zon and 1 was found positive. All 61 reactive samples have been investigated in other confirmatory tests (A, C). Only one has been confirmed with test C and six with the other one (Table 3). Furthermore, we have also revealed the seropositivity in 9 out of others

TABLE 3. *ELISA techniques. Results in blood donors, relatives of at AIDS Risk patients and African individuals*

	ELISA+		
	A	B	C
Blood donors	6/61	18/8979	1/61
Relatives	9/79	—	—
African	2/18	—	1/18

79 relatives tested. None of them was at risk for AIDS and/or ARC. Among African sera, 15/120 were positive using IFA (15.8%). The highest percentage of positivity (70%) was found among Somalian subjects suffering from leprosy. We have then tested the same sera with the uninfected line and obtained the same pattern of florescence. 18 out these sera were also examined with ELISA techniques and all but two were negative with kit A (11%). Only one serum was reactive with C (5.5%).

Heterosexual transmission of HTLV III

In Table 4 the prevalence of HTLV-III antibodies among contacts or relatives of seropositive individuals is shown. Two findings seem to be particularly interesting: 11 out of 12 children born from HTLV-III positive mothers after 1982 developed seropositivity (5 AIDS, 2 ARC and 4 IgM positive) while none of 16 children born from HTLV-III positive mothers before 1980 was positive; in addition, 13 out of 22 females partners of bisexual men, drug abusers and hemlophiliacs became positive for anti HTLV-III antibodies (3 ARC, 10 seropositive healthy).

TABLE 4.   *HTLV III antibodies in relatives and sexual contact of seropositive individuals at Risk for AIDS*

	SERUM (+)			SERUM (−)
	AIDS	ARC	HEALTHY	
12 children from mothers positive born after 1982	5	2	4(IgM)	1
16 children from mothers positive born before 1980	0	0	0	16
22 females (not drug abus.) partners of bisexual men, drug abusers, haemophiliacs	0	3	10	9
6 males partners of drug abusers (females)	0	0	2	4
60 relatives of same house-hold of homosexuals, drug abusers, haemophiliacs	0	0	1	59

Presence of IgM antibodies

Twenty-one percent of subjects at risk for AIDS and ARC, which were positive for HTLV III antibodies, showed a detectable titer of IgM isotype. Among the seropositive ARC patients, 13.5% presented IgM antibodies. Conversely, no IgM to HTLV III could be demonstrated among the AIDS patients. In 5 cases the IgM antibody titer was significantly higher than the IgG one (Table 5).

TABLE 5.   *IgM antibodies in seropositive cases for HTLV III*

	Seropositive	IgM+	Percentage
Cases			
AIDS	15	0	0
ARC	37	5	13.5
AT RISK SUB.S	97	20	21

DISCUSSION

This investigation reports an epidemiological study on the prevalence of antibodies to HTLV III/LAV in AIDS, ARC patients and subjects at risk for AIDS in Italy. A pilot trial carried out by the Food and Drug Administration (FDA) within the past months indicates that the test kits developed by different contractors, all using the ELISA method, show a wide range of variations in their sensitivity and selectivity, and may be subject to significant false positive and false negative rates (5). Our results obtained in AIDS patients, confirm that antibodies to HTLV III/LAV are frequently found in this group. Sera wich were reactive by IFA were all positive with ELISA without any difference among the kits employed (A, B, C). A great number of ARC patients were also seropositive fo HTLV III/LAV. This finding confirms that HTLV III/LAV not only is the cause of AIDS but also of ARC in epidemiologically related risk group. Table 1 shows the concordance of IFA and ELISA; sera positive in any assay gave positive reactions in all kit tests. Moreover some sera displaying a doubtful interpretation (presence of positive cells lower than 5%, by IFA) were tested with ELISA. In all the cases we obtained a positive result with ELISA (evidence of a higher sensitivity of ELISA versus IFA). The presence of some seronegative ARC subjects may suggest that their lymphadenophaty was unrelated to HTLV III/LAV infection or perhaps that they did not produce a detectable antibody response. Heterogeneity was also found in different geographical areas. Drug abusers with ARC from Sardinia showed a significantly lower positivity of antibodies to HTLV III/LAV in comparison to those collected in Milan. It is particularly noteworthy that in AIDS and ARC patients, we were not able to demonstrate any significant difference among the ELISA kits used, probably on reason of the relative homogeneity of the population examined.

Surprisingly, we were able to demonstrate that the presence of HTLV III/LAV antibodies in categories at risk for AIDS is diffused more than we might suspecte by the low incidence of AIDS patients. However we believe that the prevalence of seropositivity among members of risk groups require careful interpretation. Even if HTLV III/LAV is etiologically related to AIDS and ARC, we should not assume that these disorders will develop in all patients infected with such a retrovirus. It is as important to stress that in this population we identified some discrepancies among the test kits employed. Several hypothesis may be put forward to explain the variation of the results: hetereogeneity of samples examined, different sensitivity and specificity of the ELISA tests that might be improved with a better calibration of them or difference for the antigen purification. The importance of this finding became greater when we examined specimens from controls and other categories. No positive sera were found among healthy people examined in 1984 by IFA, whereas, in 1985, were found 0.67% not reliable reactive among blood donors. The pilot trial mentioned above, reported that five companies obtained positive readings from a low of 5 to a high of about 100 out of 3000 blood donors samples examined. Each company then ran its own confirmatory tests on the positives obtained on the ELISA tests. These confirmatory tests, using the so-called Western Blot technique, suggests a false positive rate of one out of every ten that were scored positive by the ELISA test. In addition, some carriers of the retrovirus may show no antibody response whatsoever.

False positive tests recorded among African sera by IFA and perhaps by ELISA, could be explained by the high prevalence of autoantibodies and particularly of lymphocytotoxic autoantibodies found in leprosy (data not shown). The negativity of both tests in our Kaposi's sarcoma patients, confirms the finding that the KS endemic in Africa greatly differs from the form of disseminated tumor frequently observed in African patient with AIDS.

Finally, in this paper we report that a significant percentage of positive cases have IgM antibodies to HTLV III/LAV suggesting the possibility of an early infection (8). Furthermore, the prevalence of IgM antibodies was decreasing from individuals at risk to ARC patients and completely absent in AIDS patients. This appears to be evidence for a primary antibody response to a recently acquired infection.

REFERENCES

1. Aiuti, F., 1983: La sindrome da immunodeficienza acquisita (AIDS). *Immunol. Clin. Sper.* II: 67-74.
2. Aiuti, F., Allen J.R., Bijkerk, H., 1983: AIDS in Europe. Status quo 1983. *Eur. J. Cancer Clin. Oncol.* 20: 155-173.
3. Aiuti, F., Rossi, P., Sirianni, M.C., Carbonari, M., Popovic, M., Sarngadharan, M.G., Contu, L., Moroni, M., Romagnani, S., Gallo, R.C., IgM and IgG antibodies to human T-lymphotropic retrovirus HTLV-III in patients with lymphoadenopathy sindrome and in individuals at risk for AIDS in Italy. *Brit. Med. J.* (in press).
4. Barrè-Sinoussi, F., Chermann, J.C., Rey, F., Nugeyre, M.T., Chamaret, S., Gruest, J., Dauguet, C., Axler-Blin, C., Vezinet-Brun, F., Rouzioux, C., Rozenbaum, W., Montagnier, L., 1983: Isolation of a T-lymphotropic retrovirus from a patient at risk for Acquired Immune Deficiency Syndrome (AIDS). *Science* 220: 868-871.
5. Budiansky, S., 1984: AIDS screening. *Nature* 312: 583.
6. Centers for Disease Control. 1982: Pneumocystis Carinii pneumonia among persons with haemophilia A. *MMWR* 31: 365-367.
7. Cheingsong-Popov, R., Weiss, R.A., Dagleish, A., Tedder, R.S., Shanson, D.C., Jeffries, D.J., Ferns, R.B., Weller, I.V.D., Mitton, S., Adler, M.W., Fathing, C., Lawrence, A.B., Gazzard, B.G., Weber, J., Harris, J.R.W., Pinching, A.J., Craske, J., Barbara, J.A.J. 1984: Prevalence of antibody to human T-lymphotropic virus type III in AIDS and AIDS-risk patients in Britain. *Lancet* II: 477-480.
8. Fiorilli, M., Carbonari, M., Scarpati, B., Scano, G., Gaetano, C., Aiuti, F., 1985: Immunoglobulins in the Acquired Immunodeficiency Syndrome *Ann. Int. Med.,* 102(6): 862.
9. Gallo, R.C., Salahuddin, S.Z., Popovic, M., Shearer, G.M., Kaplan, M., Haynes, B.F., Palker, T.J., Redfield, R., Oleske, J., Safai, B., White, G., Foster, P., Markham, P.D., 1984: Frequent detection and isolation of cytopathic retroviruses (HTLV III) from patients with AIDS. *Science* 224: 500-502.
10. Mildvan, D., Mathur, U., Enlow, R.W., 1982: Persistent, generalized lymphadenopathy among homosexuals male, *MMWR* 31: 249-251.
11. Pandolfi, F., De Rossi, G., Mariani, G., Carbonari, M., Ensoli, B., Napolitano, M., Lopez, M., Mandelli, F., Aiuti, F., Impairment of cellular immunity and OKT4 lymphocytes in symptom-free haemophiliacs with antibodies to HTLV III. *Diag. Immunol.* (in press).
12. Renold, F.K., 1984: Le SIDA aux Etats-Unis. *Med. et Hyg.* 42: 1561-1566.
13. Siegal, F.P., Lopez, C., Hammer, G.S., 1981: Severe acquired immunodeficiency in male homosexuals manifested by chronic perianal ulcerative herpes simplex lesions. *N. Engl. J. Med.* 42: 1561-1566.

SECTION VI
IMMUNOTHERAPY
OF IMMUNODEFICIENCIES

Bone Marrow Transplantation in 1985

Neena Kapoor and Robert A. Good

*Original research was aided by grants from the National Institutes
of Health AI-19495, AG-03592, NS-18851 and the March
of Dimes Birth Defects Foundation grant #1-789*

Physicians and medical scientists have been intrigued from ancient times with the possibility of removing diseased parts of the body and replacing them with healthy organs (1). Real understanding of the obstacles to tissue transplantation, however, began to develop only about forty years ago with Medawar's linking of transplantation rejection to immunology. In this early work, Sir Peter Medawar (1-3) showed that skin grafts from an unrelated donor are rejected but autologous skin grafts were accepted and that a second skin graft from the same foreign donor is rejected with accelerated tempo. The fundamental earlier work by Gorer permitted these experiments to quickly be linked to the immunogenetics of the major histocompatibility systems (MHC) and also to tumor rejection (4-6). The operational possibility of bone marrow transplantation emerged in 1949 when Jacobson et al. demonstrated the protective effect of hematopoietic tissues upon irradiated subjects (7). He reported that protecting the spleen by lead shielding following high dose irradiation diminished mortality of rabbits and was accompanied by accelerated hematopoietic recovery. In 1951 these investigators showed that the implantation of an autologous or isogeneic spleen (8) or the intraperitoneal injection of a suspension of isogeneic spleen cells following lethal irradiation in mice also had a protective influence. In the same year, Lorenz and co-worker (9) obtained similar results in mice using isogeneic bone marrow. Some investigators thought this protective influence of hematopoietic cells or tissues was due to humoral factors (10). However, by 1956 several laboratories had demonstrated using a variety of genetic markers that the protective effect against lethal irradiation is attributable to colonization of hematopoietic sites by cells from the donor (11). Soon thereafter it was established for mice that hematopoietic reconstruction following lethal irradiation and bone marrow transplantation is attributable to donor cells (12,13). Thomas et al. (14) described occasionally successful allotransplantation of marrow in dogs following lethal irradiation.

Early Attempts at Marrow Transplantation

These successful allotransplantations in experimental animals stimulated attempts to apply this form of therapy to the patients with bone marrow failure or with leukemia. Mathe in 1959 (15) described his experience with leukemic patients who had been given marrow transplants following 200 to 400 rads of total body irradiation. These patients failed to achieve engraftment and probably died of their original disease. Mathe also reported his experience in treating five patients who were accidently exposed to the radiation with gamma rays and neutrons (16). The patients were given allogeneic bone marrow at various intervals. They all had transient engraftment with donor type cells but finally the autologous marrow recovered. A third report from the same group appeared in 1962. In this study 24 leukemic patients were irradiated with a dose of irradiation known to be 100% lethal and were given marrow from multiple donors at variable times. In this group, the marrow graft was accepted in 17 cases and one patient survived who had been given marrow from a monozygotic twin (17) (syngeneic transplant). Some of the deaths where myeloidrestoration had occurred after total body irradiation were attributed to graft-versus-host disease which had been described first by Barnes and co-workers in 1956 (13, 18) and later confirmed by many others (19-23).

Graft Vs Host Reactions

Cohen, Vos and van Bekkum (24) drew attention to severe weight loss and skin lesions which appeared in irradiation chimeras during the delayed mortality following marrow transplantation. Perhaps the most convincing evidence for a secondary disease (graft-versus-host disease) mechanism in radiation chimeras not directly attributable to the irradiation was the observation that, by altering the number of lymphoid cells injected together with the bone marrow, the severity of secondary disease could be increased or decreased (25). Later, it was well established in murine models that graft-versus-host disease is initiated by the thymus-derived "T" lymphocytes of donor origin (26-28). It was also suggested by the same group of investigators that it is immuno-incompetent recipients who are at risk for graft-versus-host disease when allogeneic hematopoietic cells are infused (26, 28), thus establishing immunogenetics as a key factor in successful marrow transplantation.

Major Histocompatibility Complex

A major break in transplant immunology was initially made by Gorer when he discovered and initiated the definition of the serology of the alloantigens determined by the major histocompatibility complex (MHC complex) of the mouse (5-7). The genetic system identified in the mouse by these alloantigens was implicated first in blood typing of mice and then by rejection of tumor grafts and finally for rejection of tissue grafts. This system responsible in a major way for histocompatibility or incompatibility of tissues in the mouse was named H-2 by Snell (29).

Dausset (30) in 1954 discovered the first HLA antigen in man and he and Van Rood independently generated evidence that this system is a crucial determinant of antigeneic specificity of humans. The relatively recent detailed understanding of the major histocompatibility system derived from extensive further investigations of Dausset (31), Van Rood (32), Ceppellini and Von Rood (33), Amos and co-workers (34), Terasaki (35), Festenstein and De-mant (36), and others. Application of this knowledge made possible improved tissue transplantation first in experimental animals (37-42) and then in man (43). It was this surging knowledge of the potentiality of transplantation usign H-2 matched donors which led us to the conclusion that HLA matched sibling donors might make possible bone marrow transplantation with no graft-versus-host disease (GVHD) or perhaps tolerable graft-versus-host reaction (44, 92).

These insights permitted Good and his colleagues in Minneapolis (44, 43) and Bach and his colleagues in Wisconsin (45) to carry out the initial transplantation to treat successfully severe combined immunodeficiency disease (SCID) and also aplastic anemia (44, 46) and Wiskott-Aldrich syndrome (45, 49) and to launch treatment of several forms of leukemia and lymphoma (47, 48) congenital hematopoietic disease and other forms of genetically determined disease by bone marrow transplantation (50, 52).

Effective Treatment for More than 40 Lethal Diseases

Since these beginnings, marrow transplantation has now emerged as the preferred treatment for some 50 otherwise lethal genetic, congenital, acquired or malignant disease that involve the hematopoietic and lymphoid systems.

The diseases listed by the international bone marrow transplantation registry that are treated preferentially at this juncture by methods which include bone marrow transplantation are listed in Table 1 (51).

At the present time, bone marrow transplantation is the treatment of choice for all forms of severe combined immunodeficiency, many forms of acute and chronic leukemia and all known forms of aplastic anemia if a histocompatible sibling or close relative donor is available. In addition, progress is being made to make marrow transplantation safer and more tolerable by over-coming the major complications and obstacles to marrow transplantation (50).

Overcoming the Obstacles

Over the past sixteen years since effective allogeneic marrow transplantation was introduced as a therapeutic modality (44), great progress has been made in overcoming or minimizing each of these complicating problems and marrow transplantation is consequently being rapidly extended to treatment of new disease and new patient groups in the diseases where it is the accepted modality of treatment. Further, individual marrow transplantation services are being rapidly expanded as is reflected in a description of the development of typical service. Further, new marrow transplantation services are being rapidly introduced in departments of Pediatrics or Medicine so that it now seems predictable that a great many major medical centers will be developing bone marrow transplantation centers within the next few years. Already more than 100 such bone marrow transplantation services are reporting marrow transplants to the International Bone Marrow Transplantation Registry a striking increase over the fewer than twelve or so which reported case to the Registry only five years ago.

Progress Permissive of Marrow Transplantation

Progress has been related to improvements in immunogenetics, irradiation, application and development of immunosuppressive regimens, safer, more effective myeloablation, improved chemotherapy of leukemias, new and better use of antibiotics, and chemotherapeutics both for treatment and prophylaxis of infection, improved protective isolation and improved decontamination of mouth, respiratory tract, skin and bowel. Further improvement in intensive support systems and improvements in use of blood and blood products - all have contributed significantly to the improvements in management of the patient undergoing bone marrow transplantation. Thus, marrow transplantation once relegated almost entirely to last ditch therapy can be considered as a primary treatment for many of the disease listed in Table 1.

Needed Improvements

Much needed and also very much to be anticipated in the near future are new and improved means to facilitate rapid hematopoietic recovery, means to facilitate more prompt immunologic reconstruction, to permit more complete ablation of malignant cells from the body, and to treat and prevent the major virus infections like Herpes simplex, E-B virus (EBV), and cytomegalovirus (CMV) infection. Better means are also needed to decontaminate the body of potential bacterial, fungal, parasitic and viral pathogens, to diagnose promptly and treat effectively opportunistic infection and to prevent complicating secondary malignancies. With the development of these measures which are surely to be anticipated, it can be certain that bone marrow transplantation will continue for the foreseeable future to develop rapidly as a means of treatment for: 1. genetic and acquired abnormalities of hematopoiesis; 2. abnormalities and deficiencies of immunologic cells and function; 3. hematopoietic and lymphoid malignancies and 4. genetically determined enzymatic and protein deficiencies and abnormalities. Only with time and as a reflection of the tempo of the new developments will we be able to measure the full potentiality of this therapeutic use of marrow transplantation as a form of cellular engineering.

TABLE 1.   *Diseases now treatable by bone marrow transplantation*

Leukemia, Lymphoma and Other Malignant Diseases:

M1, Acute undifferentiated leukemia
M2, Acute myelogenous leukemia
M3, Acute pregranulocytic leukemia
M4, Acute myelomonocytic leukemia
M5, Acute monocytic leukemia
M6, Acute erythroleukemia
ALL, T cell
ALL, B cell
ALL, Non-T, Non-B
ALL, cALLa
ALL, Pre-B cell
ALL, L1
ALL, L2
ALL, L3
Chronic myelogenous leukemia
Acute histiocytic leukemia (malignant histiocytosis)
Acute megakaryocytic leukemia
Acute (malignant) myelosclerosis
Myelodysplasia (Refractory Anemia with Excess of Blasts)
Myelodysplasia (Chronic Myelomonocytic Leukemia)
Myelodysplasia (Refractory Anemia with Excess of Blasts in Transformation)
Hodgkin's Disease
Lymphoma (including Burkitt's)
Lymphosarcoma
Ewings's sarcoma
Immunoblastic sarcoma
Cancer

Aplastic Anemia and Hemoglobinopathies:

Severe aplastic anemia
Fanconi's anemia
Pure red cell aplasia
Thalassemia major
Paroxysmal nocturnal hemoglobinuria
Osteopetrosis
Myelofibrosis

Immunodeficiency Diseases and Genetic Disorders:

SCID with adenosine deaminase deficiency
SCID with reticular dysgenesis
SCID with low T and B cell numbers
SCID with low T and normal B cell numbers (Swiss)
SCID with bare lymphocytes (absence of HLA antigen expression)
CID
Wiskott-Aldrich syndrome
Cartilage-hair syndrome
Nezelof syndrome
X-linked (Bruton-type) agammaglobulinemia
Ataxia telangiectasia
DiGeorge syndrome
Thymic aplasia
Thymic hypoplasia
T cell deficiency
Chronic Granulomatous disease
Hurler's disease

Marrow Transplantation Procedure

Marrow transplantation is achieved by providing stem cells that can repopulate hematopoietic and lymphoid cells in the marrow spaces and throughout the lymphoid tissues. Marrow transplantation may employ stem cells of autologous, syngeneic or allogeneic origin. The application of autologous marrow transplantation for treatment of malignancies is currently of great interest because a most limiting factor to the administration of aggressive irradiation and chemotherapy to destroy malignant cells widely disseminated in the body is the hematotoxicity of the anti-malignancy treatment. Cryopreservation of marrow and autologous marrow transplantation offers a potential alternative to allogenic marrow transplantation to correct the dire consequences of this toxicity. The rationale, technology and preliminary clinical results of autologous marrow transplantation have been extensively reviewed by Graze and Gale (52), Deisseroth and Abrams (53), Dicke et al. (54), Kaizer et al. (55), and Santos and Kaizer (56).

Whereas autologous marrow transplantation is promising for the rescue of the hematopoietic system following lethal radiation and/or chemotherapy, its role in the treatment of hematopoietic malignancy still remains conjectural. Studies of animal model system has suggested that it may be possible to eliminate tumor cells from tumor plus bone marrow cell suspensions using pharmacological, immunological, or plant-lectin separation methods (50, 61). Recent studies show that purging of the marrow may be best achieved by using cytotoxic antisera to a tumor-associated antigen in presence of complement (57, 58) or by use of monoclonal antibodies or lectins specific for tumor cells that have been coupled to toxic molecules such as ricin (59-61).

Syngeneic marrow transplantation is severely restricted for use in humans because of the relatively rare occurrence of identical twins. Syngeneic transplants are performed in the same way as allogeneic transplants and generally are accompanied by fewer complications than are allogeneic transplants due to the fact that engraftment is prompt and graft-versus-host disease absent. In the present chapter, we will devote most of our discussion to allogeneic marrow transplants, since it is this approach that constitutes the overwhelming majority of treatment procedures used in bone marrow transplantation today. At present, marrow transplantation is mostly restricted to patients who have histocompatible HLA-matched sibling donors.

The antigens determined by the major histocompatibility (HLA) complexes in man are coded for in genes located on the short arm of chromosome number six. Usually this component of the genome is inherited as a unit. From study of families with intra-HLA recombinant chromosomes, it has been shown that the HLA region is comprised of four major genetic loci which contain alleles which code for well defined polymorphic antigenic systems that are involved in tissue and marrow transplantation rejection.

HLA Matching

HLA A, B and C antigens are called Class I antigens. They are expressed on all nucleated cells and can be identified using serological testing. These antigen are also expressed on platelets. HLA D and Dr antigens are called Class II antigens and are selectively expressed on B lymphocytes. They can also be identified on activated T lymphocytes. Some of these antigen are also expressed on monocytes and on immature bone marrow hematopoietic cells. Since a single maternal and a single paternal haplotype are expressed in each offspring, each HLA complex is transmitted as a single Mendelian trait. Each of four genotypes may be represented in the offspring of two parents. This distribution yields a 25% chance that siblings will be identical to each other at both MHC (HLA) determinants. HLA typing can be established by serological testing for antigens coded on HLA A, B, C and DR loci. Demonstration of compatibility at the D locus on the other hand is achieved using bidirectional mixed leukocyte culture and genotypes at the D locus may be precisely defined using unidirectional mixed leukocyte cultures that employ cells homozygous for D locus determinants that have been irradiated and cannot themselves divide. An ideal donor for marrow transplantation is a sibling who is HLA A, B, C, Dr identical and has lymphocytes mutually unresponsive with those of the potential recipient in mixed leukocyte culture (MLC) and thus is also identical with the recipient at the D locus. Statistically, one sibling in four in a family will be matched at the MHC. Further, since American families average approximately 2.5 children to a family and taking into account linkage disequilibriums and genetic recombination, it has been calculated that a matched sibling donor will be available in approximately 40% of families. Thus, if marrow transplantation is needed for treatment, e.g., of malignant diseases, a donor is available 40% of the time. If one is considering treatment of genetically determined disease, however, the chances of having a sibling perfectly matched at the MHC is considerably smaller since, depending upon the mode of inheritance of the disease in question, a sibling may also have the disease with significant frequency. Thus, when one deals with correction of genetically determined disease by marrow transplantation, the chance of having a suitable matched sibling who does not share full expression of disease is approximately 25%.

Preparation of Marrow Recipient for Transplantation

Although approximately fifty otherwise lethal diseases have been treated successfully by bone marrow transplantation, they may be divided for purposed of this setion into: 1. many different hematopoietic malignancies; 2. the severe aplastic anemias; 3. congenital, generally genetic, hematopoietic disorders and 4. various forms of immunodeficiency with the forms of severe combined immunodeficiency being the prototype (Table 1).

Depending on the disease group to which the patient belongs, preparation for marrow transplantation must have differen considerations. In patients with certain forms of severe combined immunodeficiency where the cells that are precursors for the lymphoid compartments seem to be lacking neither myeloablation nor immunosuppression is necessary. In other patients with SCID, poorly or abnormally developed cells may need to be eliminated if full correction of the disease is to be achieved with marrow from an immunologically normal HLA-matched sibling donor, but immunosuppression is not so crucial. The latter consideration seems to be especially important when marrow from an HLA matched relative or haploidentical parental or sibling donor is to be employed. Thus, preconditioning of patients with SCID may not be required or the cellular ablation need only concern a relatively small residual population of T cells and/or an abnormal population of B lymphocytes. For treatment of patients with other forms of primary immunodeficiency disease, both myeloablation and immunosuppression and, indeed, in some instances profound immunosuppression may be needed.

For patients with aplastic anemia, the prime consideration is effective immunosuppression since the disease process responsible for the aplasia often on its own has ablated much of the hematopoietic system. Immunosuppression is a further paramount consideration because patients with this disease often have been repeatedly transfused and may thus have been sensitized to antigens present on the hematopoietic cells of the HLA matched sibling donor (62).

Further, evidence from our own extensive investigations (63-66) as well as those of others often indicates that the pathogenesis of the aplastic anemia may involve lymphoid cells and immune reactions that damage or inhibit development of hematopoietic elements. Even when syngeneic marrow transplants are used to treat aplastic anemia, the graft fails 50% of the time when immunosuppressive agents are not given but succeeds nearly 100% of the time when immunosupressive agents have been given to the patient in preparation for the marrow transplant (67).

Thus, for successful marrow transplantation with allogeneic and even syngeneic donors, effective immunosuppressive treatment is paramount. The most widely used preparative immunosuppressive regimen for aplastic anemia is cyclophosphamide 50 mg/kg/day for four successive days. However, adjuncts to this immunosuppressive regimen are being tested which include total lymphoid irradiation (68, 69), abdominal irradiation (70, 71), Busulfan and cyclosporine (71) plus high dose cyclophosphamide and even cyclophosphamide plus total body irradiation if the hazard of prior immunization or sensitization seems large (70, 72). (See below).

Patients with leukemia have some normal hematopoietic cells, have a significant but variable degree of immunocompetence, but they bear an abnormal malignant clone of cells. All of these must be eliminated if marrow transplantation is to be curative. Thus, myeloablation and immunosuppression are both of paramount importance in the preparative regimen. Lethal or near lethal doses of total body irradiation plus cyclophosphamide 60 mg/kg/day x 2 are most commonly used (73). The dosage of total body irradiation originally employed was 1000 rad TBI given at 5-7 rad/min in a single treatment (73).

A twin cobalt source aimed at both the front and back of the patient was first used (72, 73). Subsequently, a number of different instruments delivering different forms of irradiation have been used. Since radiation toxicity has been a serious complication of these treatments, numerous schemes have been tested to try to identify an ideal means of preparation of leukemic patients for marrow transplantation. These schemes have ranged from hyperfractionation of the irradiation doses given over 3-6 days to six daily divided doses of irradiation given in doses ranging from 1200-1400 rads TBI (74). In other centers a single daily dose of fractionated irradiation given each day over 5-6 days with a total of 1200-1400 rads is now commonly used (75). Efforts are aimed at maximizing the destruction of leukemic cells while doing minimal damage to the other tissues of the body. Such treatment achieves immunosuppression sufficient to permit the marrow graft to be accepted in almost every instance. But, to make certain, in addition to this near lethal dose of total body irradiation for treatment of leukemia by marrow transplantation, most therapists also employ cyclophosphamide usually given in a dose of 60 mg/kg/day x 2.

For patients with enzymatic defects or congenital hematopoietic disorders who are to be treated by total body irradiation, the object must be both to eliminate the abnormal hematopoietic cells and the stem cells from which these cells could be repopulated and also to achieve effective immunosupression. This goal has also been accomplished by total body irradiation plus cyclophosphamide preparation (49). Alternatively, and now more popularly, a treatment of busulfan which is myeloablative plus cyclophosphamide which is immunosuppressive and which had been developed for marrow transplantation in rats by Santos and his colleagues (76) has been used. This approach was applied first to humans in our laboratories and clinics for treatment of Wiskott-Aldrich syndrome (77) and now is enthusiastically endorsed by others. In this preparative regimen, the busulfan is given in a dose of 2-3 mg/kg/day for four days followed by cyclophosphamide 50-60 mg/kg/day for four days (77, 78).

Marrow Transplantation

Once the marrow recipient has been prepared, marrow is removed from the histocompatible donor within 24 hours of the completion of the radiation therapy or after a minimun interval of 24 hours following completion of cyclophosphamide therapy. Usually the marrow aspiration is performed under general anesthesia. The marrow is aspirated from multiple sites from the posterior iliac crest by using a regular bone marrow aspiration needle. The marrow obtained is collected into a sterile receptacle with saline containing preservative-free heparin to prevent clotting of the marrow. Many small aspirates of marrow from different sites are recommendend to minimize contamination of the marrow with peripheral blood. The latter contains T lymphocytes which, in turn, increase the risk of graft-versus-host disease. 300-800 cc of marrow is harvested from the multiple puncture sites depending upon the size of the recipient and donor. The aim is to obtain a sufficient number of cells to provide a marrow cell dose of 2×10^8 - 5×10^8 nucleated cells/kg. This cell dose appears generally to be adequate to achieve engraftment of hematopoietic cells (79). It is estimated that 1 ml of marrow mixed with a minimun of peripheral blood will yield a cell count of $20\text{-}30 \times 10^8$ nucleated cells. Therefore, the required quantity of marrow suspension is estimated according to the number of cells needed for a particular patient. Even though an ideal cell dose is important to assure achievement of a graft, the donor's safety is considered of paramount importance in the procedure; therefore, no more than 10% of total blood volume should be taken. To minimize the risk to the donor and to optimize harvest of adequate quantities of marrow, an autologous whole blood transfusion is usually given to the donor during the procedure. Blood for this purpose is donated by the prospective bone marrow donor 3-4 weeks prior to the marrow transplantation procedure.

Once harvested, the marrow is filtered through metallic sieves first with the size of 300 nm and then 200 nm to remove fatty particles, bony particles and clots. The filtered marrow is then transferred to a transfusion bag and slowly infused intravenously into the recipient over 3-4 hours.

Hazard to Donor

Since a primary aim of medicine is to avoid inflicting injury, it is of great importance that the procedure of marrow transplantation be safe for the healthy donor who provides the marrow for transplantation. Using the methods currently in practice, marrow transplantation has represented only minimal hazard for the donor.

Graft Versus Host Disease

Even though matched for major histocompatibility antigens, the donor-recipient pair is likely to be mismatched at minor histocompatibility loci and thus to carry a significant risk of graf-versus-host disease. Only with marrow transplants between identical twins can graft-versus-host reaction be completely avoided. Therefore, until recently, intravenous methotrexate prophylaxis developed by Storb et al. (81) has been routinely employed to prevent graft-versus-host disease (82). The standard schedule for giving methotrexate is 15 mg/m^2 on day one after the transplant and then 10 mg/m^2 on day 3, 6, 11 and weekly thereafter for 100 days. Sometimes the schedule is altered depending upon the rate at which hematopoietic reconstitution occurs in the bone marrow of the recipient. The beneficial effect of this treatment for humans has been questioned since despite this treatment, 30-70% of patients treated by marrow transplantation from an HLA MLC-matched sibling donor develop graft-versus-host disease to some degree (83). At present, other agents and techniques are also being investigated to try to provide a regimen that can obviate graft-versus-host disease to some degree (83). At present, other agents and techniques are also being investigated to try to provide a regimen that can obviate graft-versus-host-disease, a most serious complication of marrow transplantation. Donor cells are usually fully engrafted 3-4 weeks post-transplantation and have proliferated in adequate numbers in the marrow to make the recipient independent of red cell transfusion. It then may be considered safe to discharge the patient from a protective environment.

Immunodeficiency and Infection

Although hematological recovery has been well launched at this time, the patient remains immunocompromised for a much longer period (84-86). If the post-transplantation course is uncomplicated, immunological functions recover completely 6 to 8 months after transplantation. During this period of immunodeficiency, the patient is at risk of aquiring viral, bacterial, fungal and protozoal infections. These infectious complications may be lethal (87). Recent studies have established that hyperimmune gammaglobulin given IV or intravenous pooled immune globulin IVIG can provide significant protection from systemic infection, pneumonitis, and pneumonia caused by the life threatening infection with the cytomegalovirus (88, 89). Similarly, prophylactic use of trimethaprim sulfasoxizole given for 100 days beginning 50 days post-transplantation provides significant protection against Pneumocystis carinii pneumonia (90, 91).

Marrow Transplantation for Severe Combined Immunodeficiency Disease (SCID)

The application of bone marrow transplantation to cure primary immunodeficiency disease was launched in 1968 (92) when Gatti et al. (44, 46, 47) were presented a family in which there had been 12 male infant deaths from severe combined immunodeficiency disease (SCID). The propositus of this family was a five-month-old male child who had characteristic findings of SCID with a family history which established a sex-linked recessive mode of inheritance. This male patient was treated using bone marrow from an HLA B, C, D, Dr locus matched female sibling donor which corrected his defective T cell and B cell immunity functions. However, associated with an HLA mismatch at the A locus and perhaps contributed to by and ABO blood group mismatch, the patient developed a GVHR which was complicated by aplastic anemia. A second marrow transplant was given which in turn switched the blood type from the patient's genetic A to the donor's genetic 0 type and all the dividing cells of the marrow became those attributable to the donor (46). This patient, now 17 years of age weighing more than 175 pounds, is perfectly healthy and vigorous with no unusual susceptibility to infection. His immunological functions and even his subpopulations of lymphocytes are able to function quite normally and he is in every way a normal young man who has been fully reconstituted by the bone marrow transplant given to him as an infant (50).

Bone marrow transplantation from a histocompatible sibling donor has proven to be curative in most patients with severe combined immunodeficiency in whom it has been atempted when an HLA-matched sibling donor is available and it is now the treatment of choice for all forms of SCID. More than 75 such patients with SCID have thus been transplanted with marrow from genotypically identical sibling donors throughout the world. Only 10% have developed clinically significant graft versus host disease. The only failures of this treatment reported were patients whose infections could not be controlled. Several patients developed overwhelming pneumonia after having been immunologically reconstructed while having an infection with a microorganism which was not or could not be eliminated from the body and especially from their lungs (50). In these instances, the overwhelming pneumonia that developed appears to have been consequent to the immunologic reaction of the immunocompetent cells from the graft with the entrenched infecting organisms (50). In the early days, this happened with Pneumocystis carinii infection. More recently it has been attributable to virus infections which could not be eliminated. Thus, prior to marrow transplantation for SCID, it is of greatest importance to eliminate if at all possible any existing infections prior to the transplantation-especially if these involve the lungs.

Of importance as well is the absolute necessity to avoid giving patients with SCID, prior to or during the marrow transplantation, transfusions of blood or blood products that have not been irradiated. The hazard of GVHD is great when blood products containing allogeneic T lymphocytes have been given and this tragedy must be avoided (92).

When a histocompatible sibling donor is available, immunosuppressive therapy is not required in most instances. The patients regularly become promptly engrafted and T cell development attributable to the donor develops rapidly. If the patient has the form of SCID in which B lymphocytes are lacking, B cells of donor origin also develop and plasma cells, antibody production and immunoglobulins of all classes are produced which are attributable to the donor cells. However, if the patient has a population of B lymphocytes initially, B cell engraftment of donor types is often not achieve. Regularly in these instances, collaborative interaction between donor T lymphocytes and the host B lymphocytes occurs and effective immunologic functions including antibody production and normal circulating levels of immunoglobulins of all classes develop quite normally (93).

Severe combined immunodeficiency disease is invariably attributable to a genetically inherited disorder. It may be X-linked or autosomal recessive in nature. Therefore, because siblings may be involved with the disease process, the likelihood of having an HLA-matched sibling donor who is perfectly normal is lessened. Carrier sibling donors probably are suitable because thus far no great differences in correction of disease by bone marrow transplantation have been attributable to the carrier state in families with other X-linked or autosomal recessive disease. Since a fully matched sibling donor is available for marrow transplantation of such children only about 25% of the time, alternative approaches to correct this disease have been developed. HLA-matched relative donors have now been used repeatedly in these children as have marrow donors partially but imperfeclty matched at the MHC. Full reconstruction has been achieved in several such cases. With this approach, a suitable donor has been located in approximately 8-10% of the patients who do not have an HLA matched sibling donor (94-96).

During the past few years, we have been struggling further to develop suitable treatment methods for children with SCID who do not have a matched sibling donor. Stem cells from fetal liver (97, 50) or marrow from histoincompatible, haploidentical parental or sibling donors (98, 99, 50) have been used to permit correction of the immunodeficiency in a high proportion of children with SCID who do not have an HLA-matched sibling donor. On a very few occasions, this disease has also been corrected with bone marrow from a donor in the general population who was as well-matched as possible at the MHC (100, 101). Such a donor must be suitably matched with recipient, preferably at all analyzable determinants of the MHC. With efforts such as those made at the Westminister Hospital in London to establish large panels of potential bone marrow donors completely defined at the MHC (101), this possibility may become a reality more frequently.

At present, much effort is being placed on treatment of the more than 60% of children with SCID who have neither an HLA-matched sibling, or HLA-matched near relative donor by using marrow from haploidentical parental or sibling donors after first depleting the marrow of alloreactive cells (98, 99). This approach to marrow transplantation is extensively considered below.

Wiskott-Aldrich Syndrome

Bone marrow transplantation has also been successfully performed to treat other genetically determined immunodeficiencies. One of these is the still highly lethal Wiskott-Aldrich syndrome. This disease is an X-linked recessive disorder featured by the triad of eczema, thrombopenic purpura, and severe immunodeficiency (102). These patients have abnormally small plateletes, rapid destruction of platelets, defective T lymphocyte development, low numbers of T lymphocytes, defective antibody production, especially for polysaccaride antigen, rapid destruction of antibodies low IgM levels and defective function of certain mononuclear cells (102, 103). They often die early in life as a consequence of bleeding, infection, or development of malignant tumors (102-104). The latter are especially tumors of the B lymphocyte lineage. This highly lethal disease was first partially corrected in 1968 about the same time we first corrected SCID by marrow transplantation. In the patient with Wiskott-Aldrich syndrome, bone marrow transplantation was achieved with marrow from a healthy HLA matched sibling following preparation with cyclophosphamide in the super lethal dose of 60 mg/kg/day for four days (45). The child's immunologic functions were corrected but the platelet abnormality remained. Subsequently, Parkman et al. (49) corrected completely all abnormalities using a preparative myeloablation with procarbazine plus total body irradiation and immunosuppression with A.T.G. This treatment corrected both the hematological and immunologic abnormalities of the Wiskott-Aldrich syndrome.

We have employed a regimen of Busulfan 2 mg/kg/day for four days plus cyclophosphamide 50/mg/kg/day for four days (77). This regimen is both adequately myeloablative and immunosuppressive and has now permitted successful marrow transplantation regularly in Wiskott-Aldrich syndrome (104). Such successful marrow transplantation has completely corrected all of the hematological and immunologic abnormalities in Wiskott-Aldrich syndrome in a number of patients. In the patients which we know about who have been treated in this way, eleven of eleven have been cured of both the immunologic and hematologic consequences of Wiskott-Aldrich syndrome (104). Megakaryopoiesis and platelet production is now normal, the patients are free of bleeding and all immunological functions studied including antibody production, T cell function, IgM levels have been returned to normal. Whether such treatment will abbrogate the hazard of malignancy in these patients remains to be seen but it is a consummation eagerly to be anticipated.

Kostman's Severe Neutropenia

Kostman's syndrome is a disease transmitted as an autosomal recessive trait. It is associated with profound and persistent neutropenia and markedly enhanced susceptibility to infection. When the marrow cells of these patients are cultured by the soft agar technique, they may show sufficient numbers of neutrophil-monocytic colonies, but study of the colonies reveals that neutrophils do not mature appropriately in these colonies and true polymorphonuclear leukocytes are not found (105,106). Nonetheless, this immunodeficiency disease has been successfully treated following a preparative regime consisting of antithymocyte globulin, procarbazine and total body irradiation followed by transplantation with marrow from a histocompatible sibling (107).

Chronic Granulomatous Disease of Childhood

This disease, which is characterized by recurrent skin infections, granulomatous and pyogenic pulmonary disease, and lymphadenopathy also with granulomatous and pyogenic inflammation. The infecting organisms are regularly catalase positive bacteria or fungi. The metabolic defect in these children is failure to activate the hexose monophosphate pathway, generate activated states of oxygen and induce H_2O_2 production (108-110). This disease was treated with an apparent transient success using only cyclophosphamide for preparation. However, no clear evidence of sustained corrective graft was presented (111). A patient prepared, however, with ATG procarbazine and large dose total body irradiation got a sustained graft which produced correction of the faulty phagocytic-killing function as well as the metabolic defect which characterized the patients (112).

Osteopetrosis

Osteopetrosis or Marble Bone Disease is an awful disease that is transmitted as an autosomal recessive trait. It is due to a defective function of the osteoclasts which fail to normally remodel the bones. As a consequence, these patients experience progressive loss of vision and hearing as the bony structures encroach on the acoustic and optic nerves. In addition, progressive hematopoietic failure ensues as the medullary cavities of the bone are progressively obliterated. Osteopetrosis in man and laboratory animals are both associated with defective thymus function as well as defects of lymphocyte functions including defective natural killer cell function (113-116). Histocompatible marrow transplants which produce lasting hematopoietic replacement are achieved following myeloablation with Busulfan plus cyclophosphamide immunosuppression. All of the abnormal immunologic functions as well as correction of growth, conversion to negative calcium balance and restoration of normal, properly located, hematopoiesis have been repeatedly corrected by marrow transplantation in these patients (115,116). If the transplanted marrow does not produce a sustained hematopoietic graft but only a transplant of osteoclasts, the graft produces only transient correction of the abnormal bone metabolism without immunologic correction, correction of thymic function, sustained return to normal bone growth and sustained correction of hematopoiesis and natural killer cell function is not achieved (115). Thus, for long-term success in treatment of this disease by bone marrow transplantation, a full hematopoietic replacement must be achieved. This was also the case in the experimental studies (115).

Chediak-Higashi Anomaly

Marrow transplantation has also been extended to correct other immuno-hematological diseases. For example, patients with the Chediak-Higashi anomaly (117) have been corrected following cytoreduction and immunosuppression with cyclophosphamide, total body irradiation and marrow transplantation from a histocompatible sibling donors.

Immunodeficiency and Cartilage-Hair Hypoplasia

A patient with cartilage-hair syndrome with immunodeficiency has also been completely corrected after marrow transplant from histocompatible donor (118). In this defect, deficiencies of neutrophil numbers and functions and deficiencies of lymphocyte numbers and functions were all corrected by a regimen employing Busulfan for myeloablation, cyclophosphamide for immunosupression, followed by bone marrow transplantation. Complete correction of all of these abnormalities was accomplished following marrow transplantation.

Blackfan-Diamond Syndrome

A patient with Blackfan-Diamond syndrome who failed to produce erythroid cells normally was corrected hematologically by marrow transplant from a histocompatible sibling donor following preparation with anti-thymocyte globulin, procarbazine and total body irradiation (119).

Constitutional Anemias

Congenital constitutional anemias including classical Fanconi's anemia may be transmitted as autosomal recessive or autosomal dominant disorders in which heterozygotes sometimes express manifestations of the disease. The classical form is associated with somatic manifestations including skeletal abnormalities, delayed renal development, and hyperpigmentation of the skin. They have progressive pancytopenia of insidous onset. These patients are predisposed to develop malignancies especially myeloid leukemias. They are also known to have impaired DNA synthesis and a striking chromosomal instability especially following the preparative regimens such as those needed for marrow transplantation. With improved understanding of their inordinate susceptibility to irradiation of alkylating agents associated with the chromosomal instability. Preparative regimens using very small doses of alkylating agents and total body irradiation are being employed with success (120, 121).

Leukemias

The largest number of cases for whom marrow transplantation has been used as a therapeutic modality are patients with various forms of leukemia. Between the years of 1969-1976, marrow transplantation was applied to treatment of patients who were also being treated with conventional antileukemic therapy (72). One hundred patients suffering with leukemia were transplanted after being given 1000 rads total body irradiation plus cyclophosphamide (60 mg/kg/day x 2). They were transplanted with marrow from healthy HLA identical siblings. Only 13 patients survived and were disease-free after five years without chemotherapy (72). By contrast, 33% of patients who received marrow from identical twins had disease-free long-term survivals (122, 123, 73). The difference in survival of HLA matched sibling transplants and identical twin transplants was attributed to increased mortality of the allogeneic marrow transplant recipients due to graft-versus-host reaction. Relapse of leukemia occurred frequently in both groups whether the transplantation was done with allogeneic or syngeneic marrow. Since these results with bone marrow transplantation yielded a small improvement over chemotherapy in acute myelogenous leukemia, Thomas and his associates began to treat patients by marrow transplantation during their first remission (123).

Long-term Disease-free Survival in Leukemia

In 1979, Thomas et al. reported for the first time that long-term disease-free survival could be achieved in 63% of patients with acute myeloid leukemia transplanted in first remission (123). Similar results were reported from other centers (124-134). The average disease-free survival varied from 50-70% over follow-up periods which ranged from 2-5 years. In this group, relapse of the disease was observed in only 10-20% of cases. Results differed with the age of the recipient and the stage of the disease at which the marrow transplantation had been carried out. For example, with marrow transplantation in first remission, the projected long-term survival in patients in the age group 2-10 years has been as high as 80%. It has been approximately 70% in patients aged 11-20 years, 55% in those 21-30 years and 40% in patients aged 31-50 years.

Stage of disease at which the marrow transplant is done is also important in determining the final outcome. Results when marrow transplantation was performed in patients with active acute non-lymphoblastic leukemia are not as good as when the marrow transplant is done during a first remission. The projected long-term survival is 45% which is not much different from results obtained when the transplant was done during the first relapse (131-136). The findings suggest that an advantage is obtained by undertaking marrow transplantation during first remission.

Chemotherapy or Bone Marrow Transplantation in Acute Non-Lymphoblastic Leukemias

A few years ago in patients with acute non-lymphoblastic leukemia, chemotherapy yielded remission in only 40-60% of the patients and only 30%-50% sustained a remission which lasted for one year. More recently, however, with more intensive induction regimens coupled with consolidation and maintenance regimens patients with AML sustain remission for more than one year 70% of the time (135-139). More than 50% now survive in continuous remission for a median of 19 months. Results reported from several centers for patients transplanted for non-lymphoblastic leukemia in first remission indicate long-term disease-free survivals in younger patients are achieved in more than 70% of the patients. Although marrow transplantation for leukemia contains some risk of relapse just as with chemotherapy, the duration of intensive therapy which lasts only about 4-6 weeks in the marrow transplant group is short compared to the usual 16 months to two years necessary in those treated by chemotherapy without marrow transplantation. Although present evidence suggests the superiority of marrow transplantation over chemotherapy for treatment of acute non-lymphoblastic leukemia (139), comparative trials must be continuously carried out because the treatments are constantly changing.

Acute Lymphoblastic Leukemia

In acute lymphoblastic leukemia chemotherapy will permit apparent cures in at least 50% of patients. This seems especially true in children (140, 141). However, once relapse has occurred, especially while the patient is on maintenance therapy, the outlook for long-term survival even with marrow transplantation is not good even though a remission can be induced with chemotherapy. Marrow transplantation for treatment of patients with acute lymphoblastic leukemia in second or subsequent remission offers the possibility of a cure in some 25-30 percent of the patients. Indeed, the survival curve appears to plateau at 27% (139-141). A prospective study reported by Johnson et al. (138) showed that marrow transplantation had significant advantage over chemotherapy for those who have relapsed at least once. Similar observations have been reported from other centers. The major problem for these patients is relapse of disease that is attributable to host type leukemia cells (the leukemic clone) and the question of continuing chemotherapy following marrow transplantation has been addressed. Again, as in acute non-lymphoblastic leukemia, when resutls were analyzed according to stage of the disease, survival was better when marrow transplantation was carried out during hematologic remission. Dinsmore et al. (140) reported a projected two year survival of 67.1% and disease-free survival in 62.5% of such patients. Patients who underwent marrow transplantation in second or subsequent remissions had a projected two year disease-free survival of 26.7%. Bone marrow transplantation carried out in patients during relapse of lymphoblastic leukemia can expect a very long disease-free survival in only 10-20% of cases. Early mortality in these patients has the same causes as in acute non lymphoblastic leukemia. Delayed mortality is usually attributable to relapse of the leukemia. It can be concluded that a significant proportion of patients may achieve extended disease-free survival following allogeneic marrow transplantation for ALL when the transplant is done during second remission of the leukemia, but long-term survival is much less likely when the patients must be transplanted during leukemic relapse or when transplanted even in remission after multiple relapses.

Considering the excellent results with marrow transplantation during a second remission of ALL and the remarkable results obtained by marrow transplantation during first remission of AML, it now seems reasonable to recommend that marrow transplantation should be carried out in all younger patients with high risk acute lymphoblastic leukemia during first remissions (140). A recent study reported by Scott et al. (141) showed actuarial survival of patients with high risk ALL with marrow transplantation during remission to be 57% which compares very well to the 34% achieved in the chemotherapy group.

Chronic Myeloid Leukemias

Marrow transplantation has also been used as an effective treatment for patient with chronic mylogeneous leukemia in both chronic and accelerated phases. With conventional chemotherapy, the median survival of patients with CML is approximately three years and less than 20% survive five years. Survival from the onset of the accelerated phase is only 3-6 months in most studies (142).

Relatively early data from several centers indicated favorable results in patients with CML in chronic phase given marrow transplantation from an HLA identical sibling donor (143). Actuarial survival curves show 70% long-term survivals without relapse. Actuarial survival for patients transplanted in accelerated phase is 24%. The latter result, though disappointing, still compares most favorably with results achieved using conventional chemotherapy (143, 145, 151). Clearly, bone marrow transplantation must now be evaluated in controlled trials involving large numbers of patients with extended follow-up before it can be recommendend as routine for treatment of CML. The early results, however, seem most encouraging.

Other Malignancies

Patients with non-Hodgkin's lymphoma have also been treated successfully with high dose chemotherapy, total heavy irradiation followed by identical twin transplant. In one study, 4/7 patients have been in remission for 2.25-12.25 years post-transplant (146). Most recently, marrow transplant has also been applied following high dose chemotherapy and total heavy irradiation to treat the patients with multiple myeloma (147), hairy cell leukemia (148) and myelofibrosis (149, 150).

Thus, marrow transplantation has come of age as a therapeutic modality for a variety of acute and chronic leukemias and is being tested as a potential approached to treatment of other malignant diseases of the hematopoietic system. It seems likely that this approach to hematopoietic malignancies will be further developed in the years ahead. Improved cytoreduction and more complete killing of the malignant cells will probably increase the need for concomitant marrow transplantation. These improved results from marrow transplantation in the treatment of leukemia using matched sibling donor transplants have been responsible for a veritable explosion in the development of marrow transplantation services throughout the world. This is true because the diseases for which allogeneic marrow transplantation can now be employed are much more common than the relatively rare immunodeficiency and congenital hematopoietic disorders for which marrow transplantation was first employed just a few years ago.

Aplastic Anemias

Abundant evidence also indicates that all the forms of aplastic anemia which are listed on Table X can now be successfully treated by bone marrow transplantation. Even when aplastic anemia apparently has its pathogenesis in the immunologically-based destruction or suppression of hematopoietic development, sufficiently intensive myeloablation plus immunosuppression permits successful marrow transplantation.

Severe aplastic anemia characterized by granulocyte count < 500/cu/mm, platelet count < 20,000 corrected reticulocyte count < 1% in the presence of a grossly hypocellular marrow is lethal for more than 80% of affected patients. Indeed, 50% of such patients will die within the first six months of this form of aplastic anemia (151). Supportive care with transfusions, steroids and androgens have not improved prognosis (152). As mentioned above, the first successful use of allogeneic marrow transplantation to treat and cure aplastic anemia was carried out during treatment of a complication of the immunologic reconstruction of the first patient treated for SCID. A second marrow transplant was given to this patient which provided a durable hematopoietic graft, switched the patient's blood type from A to O and established a chimeric state in which all of the marrow blood and lymphoid cells of the recipient can be shown to be attributable to the female sibling donor. This graft has remained fully functional and the source of all the patient's blood cells, hematopoietic cells and lymphoid cells for 16 years.

By the mid 1970's, it had been shown that severe aplastic anemia, not complicating SCID, could also be successfully treated by transplantation of marrow from an HLA identical sibling donor (153). This modality of therapy has now been established as treatment of choice for young unsensitized patients with severe aplastic anemia (154). Unfortunately, marrow rejection occurs in some 30% of the cases. The rejections appear to be primarily attributable to sensitization of the patient to donor antigens by the random blood transfusions that have been used (155) for treatment of the severe anemia. Patients who did not receive transfusion prior to marrow transplantation have sustained engraftment more than 80% of the time and can be expected to be long-term survivors without re-developing the aplastic anemia (156). Other factors which seem to play a role in sustaining engraftment and long-term survival are: age, race, and HLA phenotype. However, it now appears that these obstacles to successful marrow graft in aplastic anemia can all be overcome by giving more intensive immunosuppression in treatment of the disease prior to the transplant (156, 157).

To permit successful marrow engraftment in patients with AA, several intensive imunosuppressive preparative regimes are now being used. Aplastic patients prepared with cyclophosphamide, 60 mg/kg/day x 2, plus 1000 rads rarely reject their marrow graft. However, survival is not ideal with this regimen due to the side effects attributable to preparation. However, total body irradiation using lung shielding, abdominal irradiation (71), and total lymphoid irradiation (69, 70) have all been used in conjunction with cyclophosphamide to reduce the incidence of bone marrow graft rejection and to improve long term survival in patients with aplastic anemia who have an HLA matched sibling donor.

Hemoglobinopathies

With the continuous improvement in support system and improved understanding of means to cope with the pitfalls of marrow transplantation, this modality of treatment can be considered for care of disease that are not so immediately lethal as the diseases for which marrow transplantation has been used to date. For example, treatment of the highly morbid and ultimately lethal Thalassemia major has been successfully begun using marrow from a histocompatible sibling donor (158, 159) who was free of the disease. It seems certain that this approach will be rapidly expandend in the future and soon will encopass many other hemoglobinopathies. Progress in developing the most optimum myeloablative and immunosuppressive regimens must be continued, but the great promise of this approach for treatment of diseases like severe sicklecell anemia we fell certain will soon be addressed.

Mucopolysaccharidoses

The group led by John Hobbs at the Westminister Hospital in England (160) has attempted marrow transplantation as treatment for the mucopolysaccaridoses. They have given marrow transplants to patients with Hurlers syndrome following myeloablative Busulfan plus immunosuppressive cyclophosphamide using siblings, parent or even matched unrelated donors from their large marrow donor panel at Westminister. The levels of iduronidase in these patients has been restored from very low levels characteristic of patients with full-blown Hurler's disease to the near normal range present in heterozygotes. Improvement in appearance and delay in progression of the skeletal abnormalities has been observed without clear evidence that the progression of the central nervous abnormality can be prevented. This result was probably to be expected in light of the "experiment of nature" which had earlier been observed with fraternal twin cattle chimeras which showed correction of the systemic mucopolyssacaride dysmetabolism without evidence of inhibition of the progression of the central nervous system disease (161).

Patients with Type VI mucopolysaccharidosis have also had their disease treated by bone marrow transplantation using a matched sibling donor. The result was to achieve normalization of the enzyme arylsufatase B activity, regression of characteristic corneal clouding and of the characteristic hepatosplenomegaly (162).

Gaucher's Disease

In 1982, Ginns et al. (163) reported successful engraftment of compatible allogeneic bone marrow from an HLA matched sibling donor which was used for treatment of Gaucher's disease after myeloablative treatment with Busulfan and immunosuppression with cyclophosphamide. The Gaucher's cells disappeared and the patient was said to have been improved.

Explorational treatment of other disease using marrow transplantation is now being attempted, and it can be certain that as marrow transplantation with HLA matched donor becomes progressivley safer, further extension of this therapeutic modality to more and more otherwise untreatable highly morbid or ultimately lethal disease will be attempted. As mentioned above, Table 1 lists 50 diseases for which marrow transplantation has been tried and we count nearly 40 of these in which marrow transplantation should be the treatment of choice. Numerous problems, however, remain to be solved before marrow transplantation has been perfected. At the present time, many of these problems are under intensive investigation, and as a consequence, it can be promised that marrow trasnsplantation will continue to develop for application to more and more diseases and to more and more patients who have diseases in which its use has been shown to be of value at the present writing.

Obstacles for Successful Marrow Transplantation and the Progress Made to Overcome These Problems

During the last three decades, much progress has been made to understand the science and art of marrow transplantation. In spite of extensive investigation, many problems remain which still restrict the application of marrow transplantation include: Lack of suitable donor, graft-versus-host disease, infections, interstitial pneumonia, graft rejection, and recurrence of malignant disease. Each of these problems are under scientific and medical attack, and in the sections to follow we will attempt to define some of the advances being made toward their solution.

Lach of Histocompatible Sibling Donor

Until recently, marrow transplantation was almost exclusively used in patients having a histocompatible sibling donor. According to Mendelian inheritance, only 1 of 4 siblings should be histocompatible donor. Thus with American families being approximately 2-3 siblings in size, a donor can be identified in approximately 40% of instances. For and additional 10% of patients, a suitably matched relative may be found. This frequency is a function of family size and a small contribution of genetic disequilibrium with respect to HLA determinants. At best, there remain > 50% of patients who might need marrow transplantation but who lack histocompatible sibling or family donor. Engraftment of HLA disparate marrow leads to severe graft-versus-host disease which would cause significant morbidity and very high mortality. Donor disparate with the recipient at HLA-A, C and/or B on one haplotype who share the HLA-D locus with the recipient have now been successfully used for bone marrow transplantation without lethal graft-versus-host disease (164). In some instances, a donor selectively mismatched one at the D locus has also been engrafted without producing lethal graft-versus-host disease (164).

The existence of certain common HLA-A, B and D haplotypes also permits occasional identification of HLA phenotypically identical unrelated donors (100, 101). To date, only a small number of such cases have been reported do have been successfully transplanted with marrow from an unrelated histocompatible donor. This limited experience, however, indicates the feasibility of such transplants and large panels of donors are being tissue typed to permit this important contribution to the extension of marrow transplantation (101). However, at present, lack of a sufficient number of such large panels and lack of fully computerized HLA banks keep efforts to identify histocompatible unrelated donors laborious, time-consuming and expensive. Therefore, efforts for identifying histocompatible donors for the majority of patients is restricted to investigation of close family members when the patient has a common tissue type.

The 50% of the patients with lethal diseases who otherwise could be treated by giving them a marrow transplant but who lack a histocompatible sibling or relative donor are now being offered histoincompatible marrow transplantation. This has been made possible by depletion of alloreactive T cells and potentially alloreactive T cells from the bone marrow inoculum. This approach derived from the original research of Delta Uphoff (165). She showed that transplantation of hematopoietic precursors derived from the fetal liver could sometimes be used to cure fatal irradiation without producing graft-versus-host disease. Transplantation of these immature hematopoietic cells from fetal liver prior to appearance of immunocompetent cells at this site into a lethally irradiate H-2 incompatible recipient in mice sometimes produced long-term chimeras without graft-versus-host disease. Stutman et al. (166) showed that transplantation of thymus from parental to F_1 mice often induces graft-versus-host disease in neonatally thymectomized F_1 hybrid mice. However, extending Uphoff's findings, Tulunay et al. (167) showed that fetal liver could regularly be used to permit survival of fatally irradiated mice if the H-2 disparate fetal liver was taken from a donor prior to its having developed post-thymic cells (168). If post-thymic cells are present in the fetal liver inoculum, a fatal graft-versus-host reaction can ensue thought the post-thymic cells may not be immunocompetent when inoculated. Yunis et al. (169) extended these findings and showed that even neonatal spleen cells or spleen cells from older neonatally thymectomized mice could be used to protect against lethal irradiation without producing graft-versus-host disease if the spleen cells were completely free of post-thymic immunoincompetent precursors plus immunocompetent cells. Such transplants of hematopoietic cells that crossed major histocompatibility barriers without producing graft-versus-host reactions showed that hematopoietic grafts might be achieved safely if methods could be developed to free the grafts of post-thymic immunoin-competent post-thymic cells (170). Müeller-Ruchholtz and his collaborations (171-183) were the first to achieve this feat in rats using heteroantisera pre-pared in rabbits which could permit elimination from the marrow of both post-thymic and what they called immediate pre-thymic precursor cells. Jo and Good (184) confirmed these findings. The radiation chimeras produced in this way were regularly mixed chimeras and were fully competent im-munologically in every way. Von Boehmer et al. (185) carried out experiments with parent + F_1 hybrids in which they showed that mismatched bone marrow which otherwise would produce lethal graft-versus-host disease, purged of Thy-1 positive T lymphocytes with anti-Thy-H complement could be infused after lethal irradiation without producing graft-versus-host reaction. Onoe et al. (186), Krown et al. (187) and Coico et al. (188) showed that full radiation chimeras could be produced without any graft-versus-host reaction whatever if the marrow cells had been purged of unwanted post-thymic cells bearing the Thy-1 antigen. Striking immunologic reconstruction occurred in these fully allogeneic chimeras. Reisner et al. (189) showed that similar purging of bone marrow and spleen could also be achieved using plant lectin agglutination coupled with differential centrifugation to separate the unwanted mature T cells from the bone marrow stem cell population. Subsequently, Vallera et al. (61) confirmed these findings and added the evidence that total body irradiation is a more effective preparation for such T cell purged marrow grafts than total nodal irradiation and that marrow not possessing T lymphocytes is more readily resisted by incompletely immunosuppressed mice than marrow grafts possessing T lymphocytes (61). Onoe et al. (186, 190-193), Krown et al. (187) and Coico et al. (188) have made extensive studies of the correction of immunocompetence by bone marrow transplantation when donor and recipient host are mismatched at the MHR. These fundamental studies have set the stage for extension of bone marrow transplantation using hematopoie-tic resources other than those of HLA matched sibling, HLA matched close relative or phenotypically matched donors from the general population.

Keightly et al. (194) and now a number of others (194-196) applied fetal live transplants to correct the immunodeficiency of children with SCID. In our efforts we found it necessary also to transplant fetal thymus from the same fetus who donated the liver or an irradiated piece of thymus obtained from young patients undergoing cardiac surgery (197). Several patients with SCID have been successfully and impressively corrected immunologically by this technique without producing any GVHD whatever. It is, however, required that the fetal liver be obtained from a fetus younger than 12 weeks of embyoni-zation. Such liver graft are completely lacking in post-thymic cells.

A total of 23 transplants of liver with or without thymus from fetuses of less than 12 weeks gestation were given to eight patients with SCID.

Engraftment of lymphoid precursor was doumented in 9 of the 23 trans-plants by HLA typing. Sustained engraftment was achieved in six cases. The children with SCID exhibited variable degrees of resistance to engraftment of these allogenic hematopoietic cells and four patients in this group required immunosuppression with anti-thymocyte globulin and cyclophosphamide to achieve transplantation of the liver graft.

With all of these experiences, it became clear that although fetal tissues could be used and could occasionally be life-saving in clinical therapy and provide immuno-hematologic reconstitution, fetal liver cannot be a reliable or legitimate source of stem cells. The difficulties of tissue procurement are too great; problems with the cooperative interaction of donor and host cells yield incomplete immunologic reconstruction too often; problems of achievement of engraftment because of incompletely understood host resistance and inadequate cell numbers are just too difficult. From these clinical experiments and from the basic experiments with animals, it was indicated that histoincompatible hematopoietic cells which did not possess alloreactive T cells could be used for hematopoietic tissue transplantation without producing graft-versus-host disease. They, thus, might not induce graft-versus-host disease or other immunosuppressions following preparative irradiation. Similar methods have recently been applied successfully to humans. To avoid the problems with engraftment that are due to lack of homology and genetic restrictions, a partially matched or haploidentical parental donor's marrow that has been depleted of mature T cells but contains stem cells, which can develop into both hematopoietic cells and all the lymphoid cells, is used.

Depletion of alloreactive T cells from human marrow has been accomplished by using several different techniques. Reisner et al. (59, 198-202) developed a lectin based agglutination technique that employed soybean agglutination plus differential centrifugation following rosetting with sheep red blood cells. With this technique, we and several colleagues we have trained to use the method have transplanted 35 patients with severe combined immunodeficiency from haplo-nonidentical donors. Complete immunological reconstitution without graft-versus-host disease has been achieved on some 20 occasions and another 10 achieved impressive partial immunologic reconstruction. There were five deaths and only one of these could be attributed to graft-versus-host reaction. Indeed, no other instances of significant graft-versus-host reaction occurred in this group. A single additional mild GVHR was recognized among all the other 34 patients, and even that one could be attributed ot the fact that the sheep red blood cells were aged when employed for the second phase of the lectin separation (50). However, general applicability of this approach has been somewhat difficult because the marrow transplant lacking mature lymphocytes and mature T lymphocytes is somewhat more difficult to transplant from a haploidentical donor and requires greater myeloablation and immunosuppression than is required for a matched sibling donor in whom all populations of cells are present in the marrow (206). Other techniques have also now been explored for haploidentical marrow transplantation.

The method we have employed extensively in the mouse, namely use of monoclonal antibodies against surface antigens on T lymphocytes, has also been adapted by the group headed by Schlossman and his young associates at Harvard to purge marrow of the unwanted T lymphocytes. Reinherz et al. (203) reported the successful reconstitution of immunological functions in a patient with severe combined immunodeficiency using haploidentical marrow. This patient, however, developed a severe graft-versus-host reaction that was subsequently treated systemically using monoclonal antibodies against T cell surface antigens. Subsequently, this approach fo purging marrow with a monoclonal antibody against a cell surface T cell antigen has also been applied by several grops to treat patients with leukemia using haploidentical parental or sibling marrow when the patient lacked a histocompatible marrow donor (204, 205). This approach if not used with great care has introduced the drastic complication of B cell lymphoma when T lymphocytes alone are removed from the marrow inoculum leaving B cells infected with EBV unopposed in the marrow inoculum.

Another possible source of hematopoietic precursors cells to be used for histoincompatible transplant is culture of marrow stem cells, which have potential to produce different hematopoietic lineages (207, 208). This approach has already been applied successfully to produce hematological and immunological reconstruction after fatal irradiation in an animal model system and may ultimately be developed for human use (208).

All of these methods and their variation, for example the more simplified version of our lectin-separation method which uses only sheep red blood cell rosetting that has been employed by Kersey and his associates at Minnesota (209) or their adaptation of anti-T immunotoxin (210, 61) have exactly the same underlying principal — namely that bone marrow transplantation can be accomplished without graft-versus-host reaction if the bone marrow or other hematopoietic resource has been purged of the post-thymic immunocompetent as well as committed precursor cells. When this has been achieved, development of T-lymphocytes in the recipient must be carried all the way from their beginning as stem cells to fully competent lymphocytes. Such patients and animals are tolerant of both donor and recipient histocompatibility antiens and fully reactive to third party histocompatibility determinants (186, 191). By using parental or sibling haploidentical donors, virtually everyone who needs a bone marrow transplant can now be given this option if this approach can be perfected. One problem with mismatched haploidentical donors in leukemic patients has been that the grafts sometimes fail to take. We have found, indeed, that such grafting often requires a more intense immunosuppressive or myeloablative regimen than do matched sibling transplants (206).

Management of Graft-Versus-Host Disease

In the preceding section we considered how to make available a suitable donor for everyone needing a marrow transplantation. In large part, this is a matter of how to prevent graft-versus-host reaction. Thus, our discussion above was concerned with avoidance of the GVHR. In this section we will consider graft-versus-host reaction in a different context and will ephasize its treatment and prevention when allogeneic immunocompetent cells have been given.

Except for identical twin transplants, graft-versus-host disease occurs in all forms of marrow transplants. Even in HLA histocompatible matched sibling marrow transplants, graft-versus-host disease occurs with high frequency. It is a greater problem when a phenotypically identical parent or unrelated person is the donor. In spite of attempts to prevent graft-versus-host disease by treatment with Methotrexate (MTX) or cyclophosphamide as prophylaxis, a high proportion of patiens given an HLA matched marrow transplant develop evidence of acute or chronic graft-versus-host disease or they develop acute graft-versus-host disease which progresses to become chronic graft-versus-host disease.

In experimental animals this phenomenon has been studied in a neonatal model (26), in a model in the neonatally thymectomized mouse (211), in parent to F_1 hybrid models (13, 26, 22), in sublethally irradiated mice or rat models (22, 26), and in models where host defenses are greatly compromised by chemoimmunosuppression. In all forms of graft-versus-host disease, the basic mechanism is that the recipient must not have capacity to recognize the donor cells as being foreign or to reject these cells. Thus, the immunocompetent foreign cells of the donor that cannot be rejected recognize cells of the host as foreign, react to these cells, and produce inflammation and cell destruction in the recipient (22, 26, 211). The most prominent lesions are produced in the skin, intestinal mucosa, liver, bone marrow, lymphoid tissues and in the epithelium of the pharynx, esophagus and salivary glands. In parent to F_1 hybrid models, the F_1 recipient cannot recognize foreign cells and thus cannot react to the parental cell antigens as foreign. The transplanted parental cells on the other hand are stimulated by antigens in the F_1 recipient and the GVH reaction ensues. If, on the other hand, spleen cells from the hybrids are transplanted to the parent strain, the parental immune system will recognize the foreign antigens of the hybrid and reject the transplanted tissue. No graft-versus-host reaction occurs. If the recipient is a neonate or has been thymectomized or irradiated, the foreign cells are not rejected and so are free to attack cells of the recipient; because, they do not recognize or attack the cells of the parent strain. F_1 donor cells may be successfully engrafted into parent strain without inducing any graft-versus-host disease (22, 26, 211, 212). Therefore, it has been established that graft-versus-host disease (GVHD) results from an interaction of donor's immunocompetent T cells (which contaminate the marrow inoculum) with recipient's histocompatibility antigens. The T cells scrutinize recipient cell antigens and then react by direct cytotoxicity or through secondary mechanisms to produce the clinical damage of acute graft-versus-host disease (22, 213). T cells are essential for initiation of graft-versus-host disease. After interacting with recipient antigens, they release a variety of lymphokines, e.g. IL-2, interferon chemotactic factors and macrophage activating factors which can in turn recruit and activate both donor and recipient mononuclear cells, i.e. macrophages, monocytes, PMN's and natural killer cells. It is reported, though not documented in human experience, that administration of irradiated third party spleen cells may increase lethality of GVHD as a consequence of either specific stimulation of cytotoxic T cells or by inducing production of IL-2 which may expand the effector T cell pool (22, 213). The onset of acute graft-versus-host disease is a function of the time required for the infused lymphocytes to proliferate and differentiate. Acute GVHD sometimes progresses to chronic graft-versus-host disease which is also a function of the immunoaggression of lymphocytes in the marrow inoculum. Failure to develop chronic GVHD may be attributable to the appearance of suppressor cells which regulate the capacity of donor lymphocytes to respond to the recipients histocompatibility antigens. Alternatively, it may be due to clonal deletion of potentially alloreactive donor lymphocytes. When graft-versus-host disease occurs, the severity of the disease depends upon the number of immunocompetent cells that have been infused and the degree of histoincompatibility between donor and recipient.

Acute Graft-Versus-Host Disease

The clinical presentation in acute GVHD in humans represents a distinc clinicopathological syndrome characterized by inflammatory disease of skin, liver and gut. It develops within 100 days following marrow transplantation and occurs in approximately 35-70% of patients who undergo marrow transplantation from a matched histocompatibile sibling donor.

A frequent initial presentation is as an erythematous maculopapular rash which regularly involves the palms and soles. The rash can be present as distinct maculopapular lesions, or if severe, it may become confluent and in the worst cases is widespread and may develop bullous lesions. The liver often shows functional abnormalities as reflected in hyperbilirubinemia and enzyme abnormalities. In severe cases the GVHR may lead to total functional failure of the liver. Pathologically, GVHR is associated with marked cellular infiltration in the portal triads coupled with cellular cytotoxicity of lymphoid cells for hepatic cells and bile duct cells (212).

Gut involvement often begins with crampy pain, nause, frequent stools and then progresses to watery and bloody diarrhea, which may be of enormous volume and which regularly persists despite cessation of oral alimentation (212).

Cutaneous histopathology comprises lymphocytic invasion of the dermis and epidermis. Basic lesions, besides cell infiltration into the epidermis, include lymphocyte-epithelial satelite necrosis, appearance of mummified cells in the corneal layer and basilar cellular necrosis and vacuolization (212, 215). It has been graded from I to IV by Glucksberg (214) and Lerner et al. (215). Grade I changes are characterized by epidermal and basal cell vacuolar degeneration. Grade II lesions comprise separation and edema of basal cells coupled with eosinophilic body formation or mummified cells. Grade III changes include separation of the cells at the dermal-epidermal junction. Grade IV represents frank epidermal denudation. Infiltration with mononuclear cells may vary in amount in the different stages of the disease.

Histpathology of the gut in Grade I disease shows cryptic cell necrosis. Grade II reveals striking flattening of the villous architecture and infiltration of the lamina propria and smooth muscle layers with inflammatory cells. Grade III is featured in focal denudation of the mucosa and Grade IV is defuse mucosal denudation (215-217).

Histological changes in the liver in acute GVHD involves degenerative changes in hepatic cells, infiltration of peripheral area of the lobules with mononuclear cells, bile duct cell necrosis and atypia plus cholestasis (214, 218).

Clinical staging of acute graft-versus-host disease is based on the histopathological findings observed by Clucksberg et al. (214), Lerner et al. (215), Sale et al. (216) and Epstein et al. (217) and the correlation of histopathologic changes with clinical presentation. The various organ involvement also has been arbitrarily divided in four stages to assess the grade and severity of graft-versus-host disease.

Diagnosis of Graft-Versus-Host Disease

A patient presenting with any of the above mentioned clinical manifestations must have histological study to confirm the diagnosis of GVHD. In the majority, a punck skin biopsy is adequate. However, when hepatic or gut abnormalities of unknown origin persist even in the absence of skin rash within the first four weeks post-transplant, biopsies of these organs may be required to establish the diagnosis. Venocclusive disease of the liver is a common serious disorder which complicates marrow transplantation in patients with graft-versus-host disease. Indeed, it may rival viral hepatitis and severe GVHD in frequency (218).

Treatment of Graft-Versus-Host Disease

Treatment of acute graft-versus-host disease of Grade II to IV involves administration of methylprednisolene (2-3 mg/kg/day). However, if no response occurs with corticosteroid treatment, anti-thymocyte globulin has also proved helpful in controlling graft-versus-host disease (219). it is given in a dosage of 10-15 mg/kg/day for six days.

Both adrenal steroid treatment and ATG, individually, have been effective in controlling acute GVHD to a certain extent (220). No difference in efficacy or in survival between these two therapeutic modalities has been established cyclosporine has also been used as a treatment for acute graft-versus-host disease (221) but also does not show clear evidence of superiority over steroidal or ATG treatment (221). Treatment of acute graft-versus-host disease may also employ use of indomethacin, or azathioprin which appears to improve management of the acute form of the disease. It surely often permits effective use of smaller and safer doses of prednisone (222).

Because treatment of the severe forms of GVHD is often inadequate, prophylactic administration of methotrexate in low doses for the first 100 days post-transplantation has quite regularly been employed in an effort to reduce the incidence and severity of GVHD. This medication has been shown to be effective in marrow transplanted in dogs (223). However, in humans, despite the methotrexate therapy, 35-70% develop GVHS. Further, a recent report by Smith (224) showed that a short course (4 doses) of methotrexate may produce results as good as those observed with the 100 day regimen in preventing acute and chronic graft-versus-host disease.

Attempts to further reduce GVHD by prophylactic administration of antithymocyte globulin have not been successful (225, 226). However, prophylactic administration of a combination of methotrexate, steroids and anti-thymocyte globulin seemed actually to reduce the severity of GVHD and prevent GVHD more than methotrexate alone but it did not improve overall survival (227). A randomized comparative trial of cyclosporine and methotrexate (221) for prophylaxis showed overall survival of 60% in transplant patients. In patients with acute non-lymphoblastic leukemia, the incidence of GVHD was significantly less in the cyclosporinegroup. However, renal toxicity produced by the cyclosporine was a compromising factor. In this study, increased incidence of relapse of the leukemia which could be attributed to the cyclosporine treatment was not seen.

Other factors have also been noted to be significant in reducing graft-versus-host disease. In animal studies the microbial environment may significantly influence expression of GVHD (228). When lethally irradiated germ-free animals are given bone marrow cells from a germ-free donor, no GVHD was observed in one strain combination that produced 100% fatality of GVHD in conventional mice (228). An attempt was made to relate this finding to human (220) patients with aplastic anemia transplanted over a 10-year period on a regular hospital floor without decontamination or after decontamination in a laminar air flow isolation. Thirty-nine percent of the patients transplanted on the regular hospital ward without decontamination developed Grade II-IV graft-versus-host disease whereas only 23% of cases transplanted in laminar air flow (LAF) rooms following decontamination developed significant graft-versus-host disease. Moreover, survival of the patients increased to 86% in the decontaminated LAF group as compared to 68% in the non-decontaminated group cared for on the regular hospital ward (229). These differences were statistically significant.

A more promising approach for prevention of graft-versus-host disease even when HLA matched donors are employed may be to eliminate alloreactive T cells from donor marrow in vitro prior to inoculation. This has been achieved by use of soybean lectin separation coupled with multiple cycles of rosetting and differential centrifugation mentioned above. Alternatively, monoclonal antibodies or monoclonal antibodies plus ricin have been used.

In each of these techniques, as mentioned earlier, lymphocytes are removed from the marrow. With the lectin separation, B cells and pre-B cells are also completely removed as are the T lymphocytes. Thus, reconstitution of the immune system must occur entirely from early precursor cells. Studies are under way at present to evaluate effectiveness of this approach and also to compare the tempo of reconstruction of such grafts as compared to unmanipulated marrow grafts when donor and recipient are matched at MHC (230). Similarly, studies are being carried out to compare marrow transplantation with and without prior treatment with monoclonal anti-T cell antibodies in both matched and mismatched transplants (230). Already, however, the monoclonal antibody technique has run into one serious obstacle in that a threateningly high proportion of marrow transplants where the marrow has been treated in vitro with monoclonal anti-T cell antibodies have developed B cell lyphomas (204, 231). This complication has rarely occurred in patients whose marrow has been treated with soybean agglutination plus E-rosetting to remove T lymphocytes.

Current research places considerable emphasis on development of the most appropriate and best means of avoiding graft-versus-host disease. It is hoped that if marrow transplantation can be performed without complicating graft-versus-host disease, that the mortality of the marrow transplantation can be greatly reduced. Progress toward this goal is being made in both experimental and clinical systems.

Graft-versus-host reaction and graft-versus-host disease have been only a very minimal problem when marrow transplantation has been used to treat patients with severe combined immunodeficiency disease. In leukemia patients, patients with aplastic anemia and patients with inborn errors of metabolism, or congenital hematopoietic disorders, on the other hand, graft-versus-host reaction and graft-versus-host disease have occurred frequently and have been of virtually the same severity and life threatening quality. What is the explanation for this rather striking clinical difference? The explanation is to be found in the experimental evidence which shows that graft-versus-host disease may be very much more severe and may be a much more lethal disease when it occurs in animals that have been subjected to total body irradiation or cytotoxic chemicals. In mice, lethal and severe graft-versus-host disease is produced in animals matched at MHC only when the animals have been prepared with irradiation or alkylating agents in large doses. The best explanation for these findings may be that the sites of assault by the T lymphocytes in graft-versus-host disease are also the very sites where much of the damage is produced by irradiation or cytotoxic chemicals. Although these issues seem clear, the clinical differences between patients with SCID and all the other groups treated by bone marrow transplantation may still require further explanation.

Chronic Graft-Versus-Host Disease

Approximately 30% of the long-term survivors of bone marrow transplantation develop chronic GVHD (232). GVHD is considered chronic when it persists 100 days after the marrow transplant. This is a disorder which has many features of certain autoimmune diseases and which involves multiple organs and systems. Clinical presentations include malar erythema, skin reticulosis, hyperpigmentation, atrophy, ulceration and fibrosis. It is associated with a dermatomyosis-like disease and is thus associated with rather striking limitation of joint movement. Other presenting features include alopecia, photosensitivity, oral ulcerations, polyserositis, scleroderma, xerophthalmia, and xerostomia. There can be extensive liver disease which lead to cholestasis. Lung involvement may occur which leads to restrictive and obstructive pulmonary disease. Gut involvement may be revealed by desquamating esophagitis and strictures. The musculoskeletal system shows inflammation of muscles, tendons and even of synovial membranes (232, 233).

Autoimmune hemolytic anemia and a spectrum of other autoimmune diseases as well as aplastic anemia can be other presentations of chronic GVHD. Immunological abnormalities occurring in chronic GVHD include hypergammaglobulinemia, immunoglobulin M paraproteinemia, presence of multiple autoantibodies, elevated circulating immune complexes, and impaired cell-mediated immunity. Return of immunocompetence following marrow transplantation is severely retarded by active chronic graft-versus-host disease, which is further compromised by the efforts to treat this disease that may render these patients unusually susceptible to gram positive infections (234, 235). Chronic graft-versus-host disease appears to be a syndrome of disordered immune regulation which includes both immunodeficiency and autoimmunity.

Predisposing factors for chronic GVHD

The features which predispose for chronic graft-versus-host disease include increasing age of the patient; severe acute graft-versus-host disease and administration with the marrow transplant of buffy coat leukocyte transfusions which have not been irradiated (236).

Diagnosis

Skin biopsy usually establishes the diagnosis of chronic graft-versus-host disease. Sometimes oral mucosal biopsy and lacrimal histology and measurement of lacrimal gland function may help to establish the diagnosis. However, the diagnosis is usually readily established on clinical grounds. Appearance of the skin and multiple organ involvement as well as involvement of multiple systems occurring more than 100 days after the bone marrow transplantation signals the presence of this disorder.

Dermopathological analyses in the early phase of chronic GVHD shows hyperkeratosis, epidermal hypertrophy along with cellular infiltration of dermis and epidermis by lymphocytes. Further, there may be lichenoid changes in the basal epithelial layers. In later stages of the disease, epidermal fibrosis and atrophy occur. Biopsy of the oral mucosa reveals mucositis and necrosis of the squamous cells. Sometimes a blind biopsy of the skin presents evidence of subclinical chronic GVHD (237).

Treatment

Before 1977, treatment for chronic GVHD was regularly unsatisfactory. Fewer than 20 percent of patients who developed this disease survived without disability. However, at present, persistent rather gentle treatment with prednisone 1 mg/kg/every other day coupled with imuran or cyclophosphamide 1.5 mg/kg/day of each drug permits salvage of 80% of patients and most escape without residual disability (225, 235).

Prevention of chronic graft-versus-host disease has not been often attempted. Forman et al. (236) reported less than 10% chronic graft-versus-host disease when patients were kept on prednisone for 6-18 months, whereas Rindgen et al. (237) reported no beneficial effect of prophylactic steroid therapy.

The possibility that GVHD may contribute to a graft-versus-leukemia effect of bone marrow transplantation is provocative. Experimentally, there can be no question that graft-versus-keukemia is a demonstrable phenoma (238). Weiden et al. (239) reported that relapse of leukemia following allogeneic transplantation is 2.5 times less frequent in patients who develop Grade II-IV graft-versus-host disease, than in patients given allogeneic marrow transplantation without GVHD. Recipients of marrow from an identical twin also have a twofold increase in risk of recurrence as compared to recipients of an allogeneic marrow transplant (240). Whether a decreased incidence of relapse of the disease is attributable to development of cytotoxic T cells destructive of minimal residual leukemia or to the production of lymphokines, which like interferon exert anti-tumor influences is unclear. Alternatively, the graft-versus-leukemia effect might be attributable to the introduction of a newly reconstructed immunological system which has greater genetic disparity from the leukemic cells than was the host immune system. Indeed, other modes of action of potential resistance genes introduced by virtue of the greater genetic distance which also can favor occurrence of graft-versus-host reaction remains to be determined by subsequent investigations. GVHD surely could contribute to graft-versus-leukemia influences but thus far this has not been established nor has a mechanism been defined. It would be most important if a graft-versus-leukemia effect could be shown not to require the adverse consequences of graft-versus-host disease.

Infections and Bone Marrow Transplantation

In bone marrow transplantation, intercurrent or opportunistic infections represent a major problem and they are encountered frequently whether transplantation is undertaken for immunodeficiency, hematological malignancy, marrow failure, or for congenital hematologic abnormality. Depending upon the disease and the status of the disease, time of the marrow transplantation and the time following marrow transplantation the kinds of infection that occur are quite different.

A patient who is being treated by marrow transplantation for severe combined immunodeficiency may present with dissemination mucocutaneous candidiasis or with a disseminated respiratory virus infection, e.g. due to respiratory syntitial virus, adenovirus, influenza or parainfluenza viruses. Alternatively the patient may be admitted with a parasitic pulmonary infestation caused by pneumocystis carinii or may have gastro-intestinal disease attributable to Giardia lamblia or cryptosporidiosis. Often such children are admitted when moribund or semi-moribund and marrow transplantation as curative treatment must be considered in a context of the presence of these life threatening infections. Despite the existence of such infections, these patients may not exhibit the manifestations of such infectious diseases that are expected in an immunologically intact person. In the immediate post-transplantation period reconstitution of immunological functions occurs, and sometimes quite promptly. These patients may then react against the infective agent and full expression of disease may become overwhelming. If the infectious process cannot be effectively treated with antibiotics, chemotherapeutics or antibodies, an unfortunate fatal outcome may occur. In the days prior to recognition of SCID, Pneumocystis carinii infection of course destroyed patients with SCID. Such patients might exhibit cough, mild pulmonary infiltration and minimal cyanosis coupled with rapid respirations for prolonged periods. Ultimately, they would of course die of the infection. Following successful treatment of SCID by bone marrow transplantation, however, several such children were promptly and dramatically reconstructed immunologically only to experience development of a fulminant, overwhelming pneumonia due to the pneumocystes organisms. As the immunological reconstruction took place, the indolent Pneumocystis infection was transformed by reconstruction of the immunological functions into a pneumonia which reflected both the infestation by the parasite and the host's newly developed capacity to express an immunological reaction against the extensive parasitosis. Similarly, with a number of forms of virus infections, the reaction of the immunologically reconstructed host transformed a persistent infection into overwhelming disease. Bacterial infections, virus infections aand parasitic infestations have all exhibited this dramatic change as the immunological system is reconstructed. Thus, it is prudent if at all possible in patients with SCID first to eliminate any persisting infections. Or, if it is not possible, to eliminate the infection prior to marrow transplantation to reduce the magnitude of infection.

Measures which have proved useful to eliminate or reduce such infections in these immunodeficient children have included intensive antibiotic therapy, effective antifugal therapy, antiparasitic treatment, e.g. with Trimethaprim sulfamethoxizole, and more recently inhalation therapy with antiviral compounds such as Ribovirin®. Treatment of persistent virus infection with very large doses of intravenous immunoglobulins, hyperimmune gammagloblins to prevent or treat CMV infection, and even treatment of persistent EB virus infection or Herpes virus infection with one of the newer antiviral agents, e.g. Acyclovir all seem to be helpful.

A patient with leukemia in remission and in stable condition may be at great risk of infections in the post-transplantation period. This vulnerability is attributable to the iatrogenic immunodeficiency or to the neutropenic state created by myeloablation and immunosuppression, essential measures to make marrow transplantation successful. These measures often open the door to the life threatening infection. In aplastic anemia, a patient may have infection prior to marrow transplantation due to severe and persistent neutropenia. Such a patient may experience dissemination of infectious disease following immunosuppression if antimicrobial therapy has been inadequate. Therefore, prior to initiation of the marrow transplantation procedures, it is imperative that attempts be made to recognize and identify active or smoldering infections, infestations and even to record colonization with potential patogens. Therapy for existing disease and prophylaxis for potential disease must if possible be imposted prior to immunosuppression and myeloablation.

Infections which appear soon after the transplantation procedure usually appear during the period of profound myelosuppression characterized by marked neutropenia. Besides neutropenia, myeloablation may produce damage to the mechanical barriers to infection. For example, ulceration of the mucosal lining of the upper or lower gastrointestinal tract may occur as a consequence of irradiation damage or injury by toxic myeloreductive or immunosuppressive medication. Such damage may foster incubation of potential pathogens into the tissues or bloodstream. Even normal flora of the gut can become pathogens under the condition of immunosuppression especially when body surfaces have been compromised.

Therefore, during the early post-transplant period, infections can be caused by almost any organism. These may include gram negative or gram positive, aerobic or anaerobic bacteria, fungi of many varieties or many different viruses with which the patient may be colonized, any one of these organisms and often more than one systemic circulation or undefended tissues and organs of the body (241).

Another source of infection during the early post-transplant period which occurs as a consequence of the neutropenic state (neutrophil $< 500/mm^2$ from 2-4 weeks post-transplant) is an indwelling access line used for long-term intravenous treatments (242, 243), alimentation and in restoration of essential fluids, blood products and/or medications. Particularly threatening infections which commonly infect such plastic tubings these days and produce frequently fatal bacteremias and septicemias are the slime producing normal skin flora, e.g. Staphylococcus epidermis (224). Although most of the time bacteremia resolves on treatment alone, many times removal of the catheter may be necessary especially when sepidermidis is the culprit. Early recognition of such infection and early initiation of aggressive broad spectrum antibiotic therapy, often even before identification of an offending pathogen, have produced the best results in management of such neutropenic patients (245). Use of prophylactic granulocyte transfusions remains controversial (246, 247). Laminar flow isolation, decontamination and maintenance on prophylactic non-absorbable antibiotics has proved to yield both decreased morbidity and decreased mortality from infections (248, 249).

Control of infection, decontamination and provision of protective laminar flow isolation environment, besides decreasing morbidity, has now been shown to yield long-term disease-free survival in 82% of patients receiving marrow transplantation for aplastic anemia (249). This figure is significantly higher than the 65% survival achieved when these prophylactic measures are not employed. Patients so managed also seem to have a lower incidence of graft-versus-host disease compared to a group who received either prophylactic granulocytes or were given no measures to protect against infection (249). However, no improvement in survival was noted in patients undergoing marrow transplantation for leukemia, although morbidity was reduced significantly. Thus, the current state of the art which yelds maximum opportunity for full hematological reconstruction following marrow transplantation with minimal morbidity and mortality necessitates treatment of existing pathogens where possible, decontamination for potential pathogens on skin and in the gut, laminar air flow isolation and early vigorous treatment for established pathogens and even intensive treatment for presumed pathogens wherever possible.

Fungal infections often occur in patients who are colonized with fungus and who have had prolonged neutropenia and have been treated with multiple antibiotics. Most such infections are due to one of several different species of Candida. A smaller number may be due to Aspergillus or an infection with an occasional histoplasmosis, cocidiomycosis, or mucoromycosis occurring. These fungal infections usually occur during the early stages following transplantation before the marrow has recovered. Alternatively, they may be seen in patients with acute or chronic graft-versus-host disease who are being treated with immunosuppressive therapy to inhibit expression of the graft-versus-host disease.

Use of oral nystatin, ketoconazole and Clotrimazole have produced a reduction in colonization (248), but they have not been effective in eliminating the colonizing fungi. Thus, no satisfactory prophylaxis against fungal infections exists. Thus, any patient who is febrile and neutropenic and who is or has been treated with antibacterial chemotherapy nor antibiotics should be suspected of having fungal invasion. This is true even when cultures are negative. The only satisfactory therapy for fungal invasion and fungemia is Amphotericin B.

This drug, unfortunately, is toxic and often produces significant damage to the kidneys. It may be myelosuppressive and can even inhibit platelet function (250).

Viral infections due to DNA viruses, e.g. herpes viruses, adenoviruses, papovaviruses, may also be observed during the early stage following marrow transplantation. Such infections may also be opportunistic in later stages following transplantation. Rarely, these viruses produce localized disease. However, most often the virus infection in these patients becomes disseminated, leading to viral pneumonia which often produces a lethal outcome if effective therapy cannot be instituted promptly.

For the first week or two following marrow transplantation, a common viral infection is that caused by a Herpes simplex virus of types I or II. Adenovirus, Parainfluenza virus or Epstein-Barr Virus (EBV) infections are also frequent at this time. At present, it is difficult to establish the diagnosis of EBV infection since this virus cannot be readily cultured (251). However, fever and hepatic dysfunction can often be attributed to EBV infection (252). Reactivation on EB Virus infection from a latent state is thought to be common in marrow transplantation patients.

Herpes simplex is a virus for which clinical and laboratory diagnosis is easily made. Significant improvement in treatment has recently been possible following introduction of new agents effective against the Herpes simplex virus (253). In a double blind study in which Acyclovir, 10 mg/kg/day, was used for prophylaxis of Herpes simplex infection in seropostive patients, 100% were protected while 50% of placebo controls developed evidence of infection. At the time of entry into this study, five patients were secreting EBV in their saliva, and while being given this treatment, all five stopped secreting the virus. Thus, a seropositive patient for HS or EB herpes virus should be placed on Acyclovir prophylaxis in full therapeutic dosages prior to initiation of immunosuppression for bone marrow transplantation.

Beginning about three weeks post-transplant, the risk of these viruses is dominant. At this time CMV becomes a major life threatening agent. Infection with CMV usually appears about three weeks after transplant and patients may excrete virus as long as a year. The incidence of CMV infection has been as high as 50% in transplanted patients, and infection with this virus is one of the leading causes of death in patients given marrow transplants. Seropositive patients are at higher risk of developing active infections than are seronegative patients. However, a seronegative patient receiving bone marrow from a seropositive donor may be at even greater risk (254). It is presumed that most exogenous infections with CMV are acquired from leukocytes containing blood products, including granulocyte transfusions. Patients may be asymptomatic, or may present with fever, hepatitis, pneumonia, leukopenia, graft suppression or even graft rejection (255) as consequences of CMV infection.

At present, no drug or biological treatment has been shown to be effective for CMV virus infection. In a study (256) of treatment of biopsy-proven CMV positive pneumonia, 21 allogeneic marrow graft recipients were given high dose Acyclovir or Acyclovir in combination with alpha-interferon. No consistent influence on survival, virus titer in lung or shedding of the virus was observed. Thus, this mode of therapy was not adequate for the treatment of CMV pneumonia in allogeneic transplant recipients. However, Acyclovir therapy was reported by another group to be effective for prevention of disease attributable to CMV infection (257).

CMV Prophylaxis

Perhaps the most promising direction for effective management of CMV infections has been the use of intravenous CMV hyperimmune globulin in which donors to the IVIG pool were selected because they had a high titer of antibodies against the cytomegalovirus. In a randomized control trial, not one patient developed interstitial pneumonia and no patient became infected with CMV who had been given the hyperimmune gammaglobulin preparation. Simultaneous randomized controls showed the usual high incidence of CMV infection and interstitial pneumonia (88). These are indeed impressive results which appear to indicate that CMV infection and serious consequences of CMV infection can be prevented by use of hyperimmune gammaglobulin preparations. In another study (89) in which the intravenous gammaglobulin preparation was prepared from a very large pool of unselected donors, gammaglobulin administration produced a significant decrease of interstitial pneumonia attributable to CMV infection Although this prophylaxis reduced the frequency of CMV infection, this effect was not significant. However, evidence of disease (89) attributable to the CMV virus infection was significantly reduced.

Thus, from both of these studies, one must conclude that prophylactic use of intravenous gammaglobulin preparations containing high titers of antibody against the cytomegalovirus can greatly inhibit CMV infection and/or the development of disease attributable to CMV. Since CMV infection and its consequent interstitial pneumonia represent a major cause of death in patients treated by bone marrow transplantation, this is a major step forward in development of marrow transplantation as a safe therapeutic modality.

Another prophylactic measure for CMV is of promise against CMV infection in transplantation patients. This is to select CMV negative blood donors to avoid primary infection with CMV during the pre- and post-transplantation period. This approach is somewhat expensive, and the feasibility of providing blood and blood products certified as being free of CMV has been questioned. This approach, however, is being attempted in several blood centers and its efficacy may depend on the frequency of CMV infection in the donor pool of a particular area (258, 259).

Varicella Zoster

Infection with varicella-zoster virus generally appears six weeks or more following transplantation and this infection may occur as frequently as 50% in patients who have undergone marrow transplantation. In the majority, the infection is restricted to a single dermatome; however, in 30% of the patients subjected to treatment with immunosuppressive regimens for chronic graft-versus-host disease, the disease becomes disseminated and sometimes has devastating consequences. In only 15% is the disease a primary varicella infection. Therefore, use of antiviral agent therapy has not been adequate to arrest the disease. Restoration of immunological function is of course the best preventive measure. Recently, however, impelling evidence indicating that intravenous gammaglobulin containing high titers of antibody against the Varicella-Zoster organism has revealed in controlled trials that IVIG can prevent primary infections with Varicella-Zoster infection, but it seems likely now that even IVIG can achieve this end as well. What effect IVIG may have on reactivation of V-Z infection will have to be determined by control clinical trial. It seems likely that disseminated infection can be prevented when these preparations of gammaglobulin are given to patients undergoing marrow transplantation (260).

Other Viruses

Adenovirus infection is being recognized in increasing numbers of bone marrow transplantation patients. These infections can take place at any stage after the transplantation and large numbers of patients have symptomatic virus excretion (261, 262). In many, the patients present with pneumonia, nephritis, or both. Rotovirus infections and enterovirus are also common causes of diarrhea in marrow transplantation patients (263). Papovavirus (e.g. the BK virus) has been found in association with hepatic dysfunction (264). Coxsackie viruses, Echo viruses, rubella virus, though not common, have also been recognized to cause severe and often fatal infection in patients undergoing bone marrow transplantation (265).

Pneumocystis Pneumonia

Pneumocystic carinii is another common cause of pulmonary infection in marrow transplanted patients. It commonly occurs 6-8 weeks after the transplant has been given. However, with the use of pre-transplant and post-transplant prophylaxis with trimethoprim sulpha (91, 104), this disease can be prevented in a great majority of cases. In the few cases in which pneumocystis pneumonia does emerge in spite of prophylactic therapy, early diagnosis and treatment with larger doses of trimethoprim sulfamethoxizole or pentamadine are indicated and are often effective.

Thus, to prevent the infectious complications of marrow transplantation to the greatest extent possible, a variety of prophylactic regimens can be given.

Further, to permit effective treatment of infections that do occur, it is vital that diagnosis be extablished early and therapeutic measures be instituted promptly. Prompt institution of theraphy should never compromise specific microbial diagnosis. When cultures and pathology specimens have been taken, empiric treatment based on surveillance cultures, the state of the transplant, the knowledge of the likely pathogen from experience with the time particular infections are likely to occur post-transplantation and the clinical and laboratory features of each infection are all helpful in directing the therapies which are most likely to be effective.

Interstitial Pneumonia

Interstitial pneumonia is the most common cause of fatal outcome in patients undergoing allogeneic marrow transplants. Historically, 60-70% of the patients undergoing allogeneic transplant for leukemia developed interstitial pneumonia. This complication had a high fatality rate. In 40% of the cases of I.P., the cause may be attributable to bacterial or fungal infections. These are often treatable. The commonest cause of I.P. has been cytomegalovirus pneumonia and this disease still produces the highest mortality of all forms of interstitial pneumonia. This is because no effective treatment exists once the virus has been introduced or reactivated and disease established. However, as indicated above, prevention is now promising and use of CMV negative blood donor may avoid the complication in many patients.

Interstitial pneumonia may also be due to Herpes simplex, adenovirus, Echo virus, or Respiratory syncytial virus and these have all been discussed above. Interstitial pneumonia due to Pneumocystis carinii has decreased significantly since trimethoprim sulpha has become available, and even once recognized, this disease can be treated successfully.

Some patients develop interstitial pneumonia late in the course of the transplantation and no infectious agent can be identified. The latter form of idiopathic interstitial pneumonia has been shown often to be attributable to irradiation. In a comparative study of syngeneic and allogeneic marrow transplant, the incidence of the idiopathic form of pneumonia proved to be the same (265). In one study of twin transplants where the incidence of idiopathic interstitial pneumonia was compared in one group given Cyclophosphamide plus a single large dose of total body irradiation and a group given Ciclophosphamide with fractionated total body irradiation, the incidence of interstitial pneumonia was reported to be 50% less in those given the fractionated total body irradiation (265).

In another study (266), comparison of the incidence of interstitial pneumonia in a group who were given hyperfractionated total body irradiation plus partial lung shielding showed only 20% developed interstitial pneumonia, compared to 60% in those given a single large dose of total body irradiation. According to this report, hyperfractionated total body irradiation with partial lung shielding reduced the incidence of interstitial pneumonia presumably by reducing irradiation injury to the lung. This report also suggested that the two year survival rate had been increased and the leukemia relapse rate decreased due to increased anti-leukemic effect of the pre-transplant cytoreduction that was attributable to the hyperfractionated total body irradiation.

Graft Rejection

Graft rejection has not been a major problem in allogeneic marrow transplantation for leukemia. By contrast graft rejection has been the cause of marrow transplantation failure in 20% or more cases of aplastic anemia. Rejection of a bone marrow graft is signaled by persistence or recurrence of aplastic anemia in the post-transplant period. Rejection is documented by the relatively abrupt replacement of donor derived hematopoietic and lymphoid elements with lymphoid cells of host origin. It has been shown in experimental animals, as well as in a clinical setting, that most instances of marrow graft rejections are associated with Cyclophosphamide-resistant host lymphocytes which have derived from previous sensitization to minor donor alloantigenic determinant through blood transfusion (267, 268). The incidence of graft rejection in untransfused patients is less than 10% whereas in patients who have been given many transfusions experience graft rejection in 30-59% of the cases if the preparation for transplantation involves only Cyclophosphamide (269, 270). However, since 10-15% of unsensitized and 30-50% of sensitized patients with AA reject their grafts, various options have more recently been explored to overcome the problem of graft rejection. Multiagent-immunosuppression using anti-thymocyte globulin, procarbazine and Cyclophosphamide has been employed successfully to transplant sensitized patients (270). Whereas in other centers, a combination of chemotherapy with radiation therapy has been utilized to overcome the problem of graft rejection (69, 70), the Seattle group has used Cyclophosphamide alone to condition the patients with severe aplastic anemia. In their analysis, graft rejection was rarely observed in patients who were given a high dose of marrow cells (270). The role of donor buffy coat cell was studied in transplanting transfused aplastic anemia patients (155). In this study, a high incidence of engraftment occurred (155, 272). However, there was also a high incidence of morbidity due to graft-versus-host disease. These results suggest that to ensure the engraftment in sensitized or unsensitized aplastic anemia patients, a combination of Cyclophosphamide plus total lymphoid irradiation or thoraco-abdominal irradiation or another combination immunosuppressive preparative regimen should be and can be used without compromising the survival due to other complications (271).

As mentioned earlier, in leukemic patients treated by marrow transplantation engraftment of allogeneic marrow cells following Cyclophosphamide (120 mg/kg) and total body irradiation of 1000 rads or 1200 to 1500 rads of fractionated total body irradiation is sufficiently immunosuppressive to permit engraftment of a histoincompatible donor's hematopoietic and lymphoid cells. Graft rejection is rarely observed.

The new capability of removing alloreactive T cells and potential alloreactive T cells from the bone marrow inoculum and of grafting histoincompatble marrow in a recipient following multi-agent chemotherapy plus fractionated total body irradiation without graft-versus-host disease is exiciting. But unexplained graft failure has become a significant problem (206). This problem can be overcome by further immunosuppression and a second marrow transplant from the same or from another donor. To achieve regular grafting of histoincompatible hematopoietic precursor cells that have been depleted of immunocompetent T cells requires more intensive immunosuppressive therapy than is required to achieve grafting with an HLA matched sibling donor.

CONCLUSIONS

In conclusion, bone marrow transplantation has opened new avenues for treatment of many human disease. Particularly, treatment of certain genetically determined immunodeficiency diseases and lethal congenital hematologic disorders, leukemias and all forms of aplastic anemias has become possible. Management of each of these groups of diseases has been revolutionized by this rapidly developing therapeutic modality. Progress over the past fifteen years to perfect marrow transplantation has made this treatment increasingly a safer and more effective therapy. Consequently, this addition to the therapeutic armamentation is being rapidly extended and delivered to an ever increasing population of patients throughout the world. Improving chemotherapy and antibiotic prophylaxis and immunological prophylaxis to prevent bacterial, fungal, viral, and protozoal infection, improved preparative irradiation for cytoreduction and immunosuppression, earlier use of marrow transplantation to avoid immunization to the transplanted marrow, more general application of laminar flow isolation and use of mismatched and matched marrow purged of post-thymic T lymphocytes and their immediate precursor to avoid graft-versus-host reactions-all are making significant contributions to improving the outlook for patients treated by marrow transplantation. The development in experimental systems and application to humans of the methods of marrow purging makes the possibility of being able to provide a bone marrow donor for every patient who needs marrow transplantation now seem most proximal. Thus, marrow transplantation can now be undertaken using any of the following donors: identical twins, HLA matched sibling donors, HLA matched family members donors, HLA matched donors that can be found in large panels in the general population, haploidentical parent or haploidentical sibling donors where the marrow has been purged of post-thymic and other hazardous cells by: 1. lectin-based fractionation; 2. monoclonal anti-T cell antibodies; 3. monoclonal antibody cocktails. This new possibility opens additional horizons for marrow transplantation. However, in spite of these advances bone marrow transplantation remains a demanding field-almost a discourse of its own in which clinical skills, medical resiliency and dogged determination are crucial to success. Thus, for the most part, marrow transplantation is still used primarily to treat otherwise lethal diseases. It is, however, now possible to begin to consider explorations that will establish marrow transplantation as a valid approach to cellular engineering that can correct many additional diseases which carry a high morbidity and high mortality in the long run. Such diseases encompass the several hemoglobinopathies, autoimmune disorders, most of the genetically determined immunodeficiencies, and many other inborn errors of metabolism. Perhaps with a little additional analysis, the possibility of being able to introduce resistance genes will be a reality and such acquired immunodeficiencies as AIDS may be treated by marrow transplantation. Only time will tell how far the development of marrow transplantation can be taken. Already this approach is taking a rightful place in the medical armamentarium and it appears to have much to contribute to medical care of many diseases and disorders in the years ahead.

REFERENCES

1. Medawar, P.B., The behaviour and fate of skin autografts and skin homografts in rabbits. *J. Anat.* 78: 176, 1944.
2. Medawar, P.B., Experimental study of skin grafts. *Br. Med. Bull.* 3: 79, 1945.
3. Billingham, R.E., Brent, L. and Medawar, P.B., Actively acquired tolerance of foreign cells. *Nature* 172: 603, 1953.
4. Gorer, P.A., The detection of antigenic differences in mouse erythrocytes by the employment of immune sera. *Br. J. Exp. Biol.* 17: 42, 1936.
5. Gorer, P.A., The genetic and antigenic basis of tumour transplantation, *J. Pathol. Bacteriol.* 44: 691, 1937.
6. Gorer, P.A., The antigenic basis of tumour transplantation. *J. Pathol. Bacteriol.* 47: 231, 1938.
7. Jacobson, L.O., Marks, E.K., Robson, M.J., Gaston, E.O., and Zirkle, R.E., The effect of spleen protection on mortality following irradiation *J. Lab. Clin. Med.* 34: 1638, 1949.
8. Jacobson, L.O., Simmons, E.L., Marks, E.K. and Eldredge, J.H., Recovery from irradiation injury. *Science* 113: 510, 1951.
9. Lorenz, E., Congoon, C.C., and Uphoff, D.E., Modification of acute irradiation injury in mice and guinea pigs by bone marrow injections. *Radiology* 58: 863, 1952.
10. Jacobson, L.O., Evidence for a humoral factor (or factors) concerned in recovery from radiation injury: A review. *Cancer Res.* 12: 315, 1952.
11. Barnes, D.W.H., and Lautit, J.F., What is the recovery factor of the spleen? *Nuclear* 12: 68, 1954.
12. Heim, L.R., Yunis, E.J. and Good, R.A., Pathogenesis of graft-versus-host reaction, I. Influence of thymectomy and adrenalectomy on development of lymphopenia. *Proc. Soc. Exp. Biol. Med.* 139: 793, 1972.
13. Simonsen, M., Graft versus host reactions. Their natural history and applicability as tools of research. *Prog. Allergy* 6, 349, 1962.
14. Thomas, E.D., Ashely, C.A., and Loehte, H.L., Homografts of bone marrow in dogs after lethal total body irradiation. *Blood* 14: 720, 1959.
15. Mathé, G., Transfusion et grefte de cellules myeloides chez l'homme. In *Biological Problems of Grafting,* P. 314. Liège, Univ. Liège, 1959.
16. Mathé, G., Jammet, H., Pendic, B., Schwarzenberg, L., Duplan, J.F., Maupin, B., Latarjet, R., Larrieu, M.J., Kalic, D., and Djukie, L., Transfusions et grettes de moelle osseuse homologue chez des homains a haute dose accidentellment, *Rev. Franc. Stud. Clin. Biol.* 4: 226, 1959.

17. Mathé, G., Jammet, H., Playfair, J., and Amiel, J.L., Irradiation Totale et grette de moelle osseuse chez l'homme. *In C.R. 8th Congr. Soc. Europ. Hemat. Bale.,* p. 67, Karger, 1962.
18. Barnes, D.W.H., Ilbery, P.L.T., and Lontit, J.F., Incidence of secondary disease in radiation chimera. *Nature (London)* 177: 452, 1956.
19. Bekkum, D.W. van, and Vos, O., Immunological aspects of homo and heterologous bone marrow transplantation in irradiated animals. *J. Cell. Comp. Physiol.* 50: 139, 1957.
20. Bekkum, D.W. van, Vos. O., and Weyzen, W.W.H., The pathogenesis of the secondary disease after foreign bone marrow transplantation in γ-irradiated mice. *J. Nat. Cancer Inst.* 23: 75, 1959.
21. Cole, L.J., and Graver, R.M., Studies on the mechanism of the secondary disease. *Radiat. Res.* 12: 398, 1960.
22. Elkins, W.L., Cellular immunology and pathogenesis of graft-versus-host reactions. *Prog. Allergy* 15: 78, 1971.
23. Simonsen, M., Graft-versus-host studies in experimental animals. In *Immunobiology of Bone Marrow Transplantation* (B. Dupont and R.A. Good, Eds.), pp. 3-7. Grune and Stratton, New York, 1976.
24. Cohen, J.A., Vos, O., and van Bekkum, D.W., The present status of radiation protection by chemical and biological agents in mammals. In *Advances in Radiobiology* (G.C. de Heresy, A.G. Forssberg and J.D. Abbot, Eds.), p. 134. Edinburg, Oliver and Boyd, 1957.
25. Santos, G.W., and Cole, L.J., Effects of donor and host lymphoid and myeloid tissue injections in lethally γ-irradiated mice with rat bone marrow. *J. Nat. Cancer Inst.* 21: 279, 1958.
26. Heim, L.R., Martinez, C., and Good, R.A., Cause of homologous disease. *Nature* 214: 26, 1967.
27. Yunis, E.J., Good, R.A., Smith, J., and Stutman, O., Protection of lethally irradiated mice by spleen cells from neonatally thymectomized mice. *PNAS (OSA)* 71.6, 2544, 1974.
28. Yunis, E.J., Martinez, C., and Good, R.A., Increased graft versus host susceptibility of thymectomized recipients. *Proc. Soc. Exp. Biol. Med.* 124(2): 418, 1967.
29. Snell, G.D., Histocompatibility genes of the mouse. II. Production and analysis of isogenic resistant lines. *J. Nat. Cancer Inst.* 21: 843, 1958.
30. Dausset, J., Leuco-agglutinin. IV. Leuco-agglutinins and blood transfusion. *Vox. Sang.* 4: 190, 1954.
31. Dausset, J., Iso Leuco Anticorps. *Acta Haematologice Basel 20:156, 1958.*
32. *Van Rood, J.J., Leucocyte grouping, a method and its application. Thesis.* Drukkerij Pasmas, Den Haag, 1962.
33. Ceppellini, R., and van Rood, J.J., The HL-A system. I. Genetics and molecular biology. *Seminars in hematology* 11:233, 1974.
34. Amos, D.B., Genetic and antigenetic aspects of human histocompatibility systems. *Adv. Immunol.* 10:251, 1969.
35. Terasaki, P.I., Auk, M.S., Bernoco, D., Opelz, G., Mialey M.R., Overview of the 1980 International Histocompatibility Workshop. In *Histocompatibility Testing* (P.I. Tesaraki, ed.), p. 1. Los Angeles, CA, UCLA Tissue Typing Laboratory, 1980.
36. Festenstein, H., and Demant, P., HLA and H_2 basic immunogenetics, biology and clinical relevance. In *Current Topics in Immunology (J. Tuore, Ed.),* p. 212. Edward Arnold, London, 1978.
37. Shapiro, F., Martinez, C., and Good, R.A., Homologous skin transplantation from F_1 hybrid mice to parent strains. *Proc. Soc. Exp. Biol. Med.* 101:94, 1959.
38. Mariani, T., Martinez, C., Smith, J.M., and Good, R.A., Induction of immunologic tolerance to male skin isografts in female mice subsequent to neonatal period. *Proc. Soc. Exp. Biol. Med.* 101:596, 1959.
39. Mariani, T., Martinez, C., and Good, R.A., Studies of sex-linked histo-incompatibility in inbred mice, Role of age and production of immunological tolerance. *Int. Arch. Allergy Appl. Immunol.* 16, 216, 1960.
40. Martinez, C., Shapiro, G., and Good, R.A., Essential duration of parabiosis and development of tolerance to skin homografts in mice. *Proc. Soc. Exp. Biol. Med.* 104, 256, 1960.
41. Shapiro, F., Martinez, C., Smith, M., and Good, R.A., Tolerance of skin homograft induced in adult mice by multiple injections of homologous spleen cells. *Proc. Soc. Exp. Biol. Med.* 106:472, 1961.
42. Good, R.A., Martinez, C., and Gabrielsen, A.E., Progress toward transplantation of tissues in man. *Adv. Pediatr.* 13:93, 1964.
43. Good, R.A., and Bach, F.H., Bone marrow and thymus transplant: Cellular engineering

to correct primary immunodeficiency. In *Clinical Immunobiology,* Vol. 2, (F.H. Bach and R.A. Good, Eds.). *Academic Press,* New York, 1974.

44. Gatti, R.A., Meuwissen, H.D., Allen, H.D., Hong, R., and Good, R.A., Immunological recognition of sex-linked lymphophenic immunological deficiency. *Lancet* 2:1366, 1968.
45. Bach, F.J., Albertine, R.J., Joo, P., Anderson, J.L.Y., and Bortin, M.M., Bone marrow transplantation in a patient with the Wiskoh-Aldrich syndrome. *Lancet,* 1:1364, 1968.
46. Gatti, R.A., Meuwissen, J.H., Terasaki, P.I., and Good, R.A., Recombination within the HL-A locus. *Tissue Antigens* 1:239, 1971.
47. Meuwissen, H.J., Rodey, G., McArthur, J., Pabst, H., Gatti, R., Chilgren, R., Hong, R., Frommel, D., Coifman, R., and Good, R.A., Bone marrow transplantation. Therapeutic usefulness and complications. *Am. J. Med.* 51:513, 1971.
48. Thomas, E.D., Bone marrow transplantation. In *Clinical Immunobiology* (F.H. Bach and R.A. Good, Eds.), pp. 1-32. *Academic Press, New York,* 1974.
49. Parkman, R., Rappaport, D., Geha, R., Cassady, R., Levey, R., Nathan, D.G., Belli, J., and Rosen, F., Complete correction of the Wiskott-Aldrich syndrome by allogeneic marrow transplantation. *N. Engl. J. Med.* 298:921, 1978.
50. Good, R.A., Kapoor, N., and Reisner, Y., Bone marrow transplantation. An expanding approach to treatment of many diseases. *Cell. Immunol.* 82:36, 1983.
51. Bortin, M.M, and Bortin, M.M., Personal Communication, 1984.
52. Graze, P.R., and Gale, R.P., Autotransplantation for leukemia and solid tumors. *Transplant Process.* 10:177, 1978.
53. Deisseroh, A., and Abrams, R.A., Role of autologous stem cell reconstitution in the intensive therapy of resistant neoplasm. *Cancer Treatment Reports* 63:461, 1979.
54. Dicke, K.A., Zander, A., Spitzer, G., et al., Autologous bone marrow transplantation in relapsed adult acute leukemia. *Lancet* i (8115): 514-7, 1979.
55. Kaizer, H., Stuart, R.K., Colvin, M., Korbling, M.D., Wharam, M.D., and Santos, G.W., Autologous bone marrow transplantation in acute leukemia: A pilot study utilizing in vitro incubation of autologous marrow with 4-hydroperoxy cyclophosphamide (4HC) prior to cryopreservation. *Proc. Am. Asso. Cancer Res. and Am. Soc. of Clin. Oncology* 22:483, 1981.
56. Santos, A.W., and Kaizer, H., Current status of autologous marow transplantation. In *Cancer Achievements, Challenges and Prospects for the 1980s* (J.H. Buchenal and H.F. Oettgen, Eds.), p. 673. Grune and Stratton, New York, 1981.
57. Trigg, M.E., and Poplack, D.G., Successful transplantation in mice of leukemic bone marrow incubated with cytotoxic anti-leukemic antibodies. *Exp., Hematol.* 25. 9(9):96, 1981.
58. Trigg, M., Billing, R., Sondel, P., Erickson, C., and Hong, R., In vitro treatment of donor bone marrow with anti-E rosette antibody and complement prior to transplantation. *Abstract #0136, J. Cell. Biochem., Suppl.* 7A, 1983, p. 57.
59. Reisner, Y., Differential agglutination by soybean agglutinin of human leukemia and neuroblastoma cell lines, Potential application to autologous bone marrow transplantation. *Proc. Natl. Sci. USA* 80(21):6657-61, 1983.
60. Vitteta, E.S., Krolick, K.A., and Uhr, J.W., Neoplastic B cells as target for antibody ricin A chain immunotoxin. *Immunol. Rev.* 62:159, 1982.
61. Vallera, D.A., Youle, R.J., Neville, D.M., and Kersy, J.H., Bone marrow transplantation across major histocompatibility barriers. V. Protection of mice from lethal graft-versus-host disease by pre-treatment of donor cells with monoclonal anti-Thy 1,2 coupled to the toxin ricin. *J. Exp. Med.* 155:949, 1982.
62. Storb, R., Prentice, R.L. and Thomas, E.D., Treatment of aplastic anemia by marrow transplantation from HLA identical sibling, prognostic factors associated with graft-versus-host disease and survival. *J. Clin. Invest.* 59:625, 1977.
63. Kagan, W.A., Ascensao, J.A., Pahwa, R., Hansen, J.A., Goldstein, G., Valera, E.B., Incefy, G.S., Moore, M.S., and Good, R.A., Aplastic anemia: presence in human bone marrow of cells that suppress myelopoyesis. *Proc. Natl. Acad. Sci USA* 73:2890, 1976.
64. Kagan, W.A., Ascensao, J.L., Fialk, M.A., Coleman, M., Valera, E.B., and Good, R.A., Studies on the pathogenesis of aplastic anemia. *Am. J. Med.,* 66:444, 1979.
65. Ascensao, J., Pahwa, R., Kagan, W., Hansen, J., Moore, M., and Good, R.A., Aplastic anemia: evidence for an immunological mechanism. *Lancet* 1:699, 1976.
66. Kagan, D.A., Fialk, M.A., Coleman, M., Ascensao, J.L., Valera, E., and Good, R.A., Studies on the patogenesis of refractory anemia. *Am. J. Med.* 68:381, 1980.

67. Gale, R.P., Marrow transplantation in twins with aplastic anemia. Submitted. *(N. Eng. J. Med.*, 1981).
68. Appelbaum, F.R., Fefer, A., Cheever, M.A., Sanders, J.E., Singer, J.W., Adamson, J.W., Mickelson, E.M., Hansen, J.A., Greenberg, P.D., and Thomas, E.D., Treatment of aplastic anemia by bone marrow transplantation in identical twins. *Blood.* 55:1033, 1980.
69. Ramsay, N.K.C., Kim, T.C., Nesbit, M.E., Krivit, W., Coccia, P.F., Levitt, S.H., Woods, W.G., and Kersey, J.H., Total lymphoid irradiation and cyclophosphamide for bone marrow transplantation for severe aplastic anemia. *Blood.* 55:344, 1980.
70. Gluckman, E., Devergie, A., Dutreix, A., Dutreix, J., Boiron, M. and Bernard, J., Bone marrow grafting in aplastic anemia after conditioning with cyclophosphamide and total body irradiation with lung shielding. *Hamatol. Bluttransfus.* 25:339, 1980.
71. Gluckman, E., Barrett, J., Arcese, W., Devergie, A., and Degoulet, P., Bone marrow transplantation in severe aplastic anemia. A survey of European Group for Bone Marrow Transplantation. *Br. J. Hématol.* 49:165, 1981.
72. Thomas, E.D., Bone Marrow transplantation. In *Cancer: Achievements, Challenges and Prospects for the 1980's* (J.H. Burchenal, and H.F. Oettgen, eds.), Vol. 2, p. 625. Grune and Stratton, New York, 1981.
73. Fefer, A., Cheever, M.A., Thomas, E.D., Appelbaum, F.R., Buckner, C.D., Clift, R.A., Glucksberg, H., Greenberg, P.D., Johnson, F.L., Kaplan, H.G., Sanders, J.E., Storb, R., and Weiden, P.L., Bone marrow transplantation for refractory acute leukemia in 34 patients with identical twin donors. *Blood,* 57:421, 1981.
74. Shank, B., Chu, F.C.H., Dinsmore, R., Kapoor, N., Kirkpatrick, D., Teitelbaum, H., Reid, A., Bonfiglio, P., Simpson, L., and O'Reilly, R.J., Hyperfractionated total body irradiation for bone marrow transplantation. III. Results in seventy leukemia patients with allogeneic transplants. *Int. J. Radiat. Oncol. Biol. Phys.* 7(8):1109, 19081.
75. Buckner, C.D., Clift, R.A., Tomhas, E.D., Sanders, J.E., Stewart, P.S., Storb, R., Sullivan, K.M., and Hackman, R, Allogeneic marrow transplantation for acute non-lymphoblastic leukemia in relapse using fractionated total body irradiation. *Leukemia Res.* 6:389, 1982.
76. Tutschka, P.J. and Santos, G.W., Bone marrow transplantation in the Busulfan-treated rat. III. Relationship between myelosuppression and immunosuppression for conditioning bone marrow recipients. Transplantation 24(1):52-62, 1977.
77. Kapoor, N., Kirkpatrick, D., Blaese, R.M., et. al. Reconstitution of normal megakaryocytopoiesis and immunologic function in Wiscott-Aldrich syndrome by marrow transplantation following myeloablation and immunosuppression with Busulfan and cyclophosphamide. *Blood* 57:692, 1981.
78. Santos, G.W., Tutschka, P.J., Beschorner, W.E., Burns, W.H., Bias, W.B., Elfenbei, G.J., Kaizer, H., Saral, R., Sensenbrenner, L.L., Stuart, R.K., Marrow transplantation in acute nonlymphocytic leukemia (ANL) following Busulfan (BU) and cyclophosphamide (CY). *Blood* 58(1):176a (Abst.), 1981.
79. Lowenburg, B., Dicke, K.A., van Bekkum, D.W., and Dooren, L.J., Quantitative aspects of fetal liver cell transplantation in animals and man. In *Immunobiology of Bone Marrow Transplantation* (B., Dupont and R.A. Good). *Grune and Stratton,* New York, 1976, p. 179.
80. Bortin, M.M., and Buckner, C.D., Major complications of marrow harvesting for transplantation. *Exp. Hematol.* 2(10):916, 1983.
81. Storb, R., Epstein, R.B., Graham, T.C., and Thomas, E.D., Methotrexate regimens for control of graft-versus-host disease in dogs with allogeneic marrow grafts. *Transplantation* 9:240, 1970.
82. Thomas, E.D., Bryant, J.I., and Buckner, C.D., Clift, R.A., Fefer, A., Johnson, F.L., Neiman, P., Kamberg, R.E., and Storb, R., *Lancet* 1:1310, 1972.
83. Glucksberg, H., Storb, R., Fefer, A., Buckner, C.D., Neiman, P.E., Clift, R.A., Lerner, K.G., and Thomas, E.D., Clinical manifestations of graft-versus-host disease in human recipients of marrow form HLA matched sibling donors. *Transplantation* 18:295, 1974.
84. Pahwa, S.C., Pahwa, R.N., Friedrich, W., O'Reilly, R.J., and Good, R.A., Abnormal humoral immune responses in peripheral blood lymphocyte culture of bone marrow transplant recipients. *Proc. Natl. Acad. Sci. USA* 79:2663, 1982.
85. Friedrich, W., O'Reilly, R.J., Koziner, B., Gebhard, Jr., D.F., Good, R.A., and Evans, R.L., T-lymphocyte reconstitution in recipients of bone marrow transplants with and without GVHD: Imbalances of T-cell subpopulations having unique regulatory and cognitive functions. *Blood* 59:696, 1982.
86. Witherspoon, R.P., Matthews, D., Storb, R., Atkinson, K., Cheever, M., Deeg, H.J.,

Doney, K., Kalefleisch, J., Noel, D., and Prentice, R., Recovery of in vivo cellular immunity after human marrow grafting: Influence of post-grafting and acute graft-versus-host disease. *Transplantation* 37:145, 1984.

87. Winston, D.J., Gale, R.P., Meyer, D.V., and Young, L.S., Infectious complications of human bone marrow transplantation. *Medicine* 58:1, 1979.

88. O'Reilly, R.J., Reich, L., Gold, J., Kirkpatrick, D., Dinsmore, R., Kapoor, N., and Condie, R., A randomized trial of intravenous hyperimmune globulin for prevention of cytomegalovirus (CMV) infections following marrow transplantation: preliminary results. *Transplant. Proc.* 15(1):1405, 1983.

89. Winston, D.J., Ho, W.G., Lin, C.-H., Budinger, M.D., Champlin, R.E., and Gale, R.P., Intravenous immunoglobulin for modification of cytomegalovirus infections associated with bone marrow transplantation. Preliminary results of a controlled trial. *Am. J. Med.* 76(3A):128-133, 1984.

90. Springmeyer, S.C., Sylvestri, R.C., Sale, G.E., Peterson, D.L., Weems, C.E., Huseby, J.S., Hudson, L.D., and Thomas, E.D., The role of transbronchial biopsy for diagnosis of diffuse pneumonia in immunocompromised marrow transplant recipients. *Am. Rev. Resp. Dis.* 126:763, 1982.

91. Good, R.A., Unpublished observations.

92. Hong, R., Gatti, R.A., and Good, R.A., Hazards and potential benefits of blood transfusion in immunological deficiency. *Lancet* 2:388, 1968.

93. O'Reilly, R.J., Kapoor, N., Pollack, M.S., Chaganti, R.S., Dupont, B., Kirkpatrick, D., Pahwa, S., and Reisner, Y., Immunologic function in patients transplanted for severe combined immunodeficiency selectively engrafted with donor T lymphocytes. *Behring Inst. Mitt.* 70:187, 1982.

94. Koch, C., Henriksen, K., Juhl, F., Wiik, A., Faber, V., Andersen, V., Dupont, B., Hansen, G.S., Svejgaard, A., Thomsen, M., Ernst, P., Killmann, S.A., Good, R.A., Jensen, K., and Muller-Berat, N.: Bone marrow transplantation from an HL-A non-identical but mixed-lymphocyte-culture identical donor. *Lancet* 1:1146, 1973.

95. Hansen, J.A., Good, R.A., and Dupont, B., HLA-D compatibility between parent and child: Increased occurrence in severe combined immunodeficiency and other hematopoietic disease *Transplantation* 23:366, 1977.

96. Dupont, B., O'Reilly, R.J., Pollack, M.S., and Good, R.A., use of HLA genotypically different donors in bone marrow transplantation. *Transplant. proc.* 11:219-224, 1979.

97. O'Reilly, R.J., Pahwa, R., Sorell, M., Kapoor, N., Kapadia, A., Kirkpatrick, D., Pollack, M., Dupont, B., Incefy, G.S., Iwatas, T., and Good, R.A., Transplantation of foetal liver and thymus in patients with severe combined immunodeficiencies. In *The Immune System: Functions and Therapy of Dysfunction;* Proceedings of the Serono Symposia, Vol. 27 (G. Doria and A. Eshkol, Eds.), pp. 241-253, *Academic Press,* New York, 1980.

98. Reisner, Y., Kapoor, N., Kirkpatrick, D., Pollack, M.S., Cunningham-Rundles, S., Dupont, B., Hodes, M.Z., Good, R.A., and O'Reilly, R.J., Transplantation for severe combined immunodeficiency with HLA-A, B, D, Dr incompatible parental marrow cells fractionated by soybean agglutinin and sheep red blood cells. *Blood* 61:341, 1983.

99. Reisner, Y., Kapoor, N., Pollack, S., Friedrich, W., Kirkpatrick, D., Shank, B., Csurny, R., Pollack, M.S., Dupont, B., Good, R.A., and O'Reilly, R.J., Use of lectins in bone marrow transplantation. Advances in Bone Marrow Transplantation, *UCLA Symposia,* 1983.

100. O'Reilly, R.J., Dupont, B., Pahwa, S., Grimes, E., Smithwick, E.M., Pahwa, R., Schwartz, S., Hansen, J.A., Siegal, F.P., Sorell, M., Svejgaard, A., Jersild, C., Thomsen, M., Platz, P., L'Esperance, P., and Good, R.A., Reconstitution in severe combined immunodeficiency by transplantation of marrow from an unrelated donor. *N. Engl. J. Med.* 297:1311, 1977.

101. Hobbs, J.R., Bone marrow transplantation for inborn errors. *Lancet,* 2:709, 1981.

102. Cooper, M.D., Chase, H.P., Lowman, J.T., Krivit, W., and Good, R.A., Wiskott-Aldrich syndrome: An immunologic deficiency disease involving the afferent limb of immunity. *Am. J. Med.* 44:499, 1968.

103. Blaese, R.M., Strober, W., Levy, A.L., and Waldmann, T.A., Hypercatabolism of IgG, IgA, IgM and albumin in the Wiskott-Aldrich syndrome. *J. Clin. Invest.* 50:2331, 1971.

104. Kapoor, N., et al., Unpublished observations.

105. L'Esperance, P., Brunning, R., and Good, R.A., Congenital neutropenia, In vitro growth of colonies mimicking the disease. *Proc. Natl. Acad. Sci. USA* 70:669, 1973.

106. Falk, P.M., Rick, K., Feig, S., Stiehm, E.R., Golde, D.W., and Cline, M.J., Evaluation

of congenital neutropenic disorders by in vitro marrow culture. *Pediatrics* 59:739, 1977.

107. Rappeport, J.M., Parman, R., Newburger, P., Camitta, B.M., Chusid, M.J., Correction of infantile agranulocytosis (Kostmann's syndrome) by allogeneic bone marrow transplantation. *Am. J. Med.* 68:605, 1980.

108. Holmes, B., Page, A.R., and Good, R.A., Studies of the metabolic activity of leukocytes from patients with a genetic abnormality of phagocytic function. *J. Clin. Invest.* 46:1422, 1967.

109. Johnston, R.B., Jr., Keele, B.B., Jr., and Misra, H.P., Role of superoxide anion generation in phagocytic bactericidal activity. Studies with normal and chronic granulomatous disease leukocytes. *J. Clin. Invest.* 55:1257, 1975.

110. Curnette, J.T., Whitte, D.M., and Babior, B.M., Defective superoxide production by granulocytes from patients with chronic granulomatous disease. *N. Engl. J. Med.* 290:593, 1977.

111. Westminister Hospital Bone Marrow Transplant Team. Bone marrow transplant from an unrelated donor for chronic granulomatous disease. *Lancet* 1:210, 1977.

112. Rappeport, J.M., Newburger, P.E., Goldblum, R.M., Goldman, A.S., Nathan, D.G., and Parkman, R., Allogeneic bone marrow transplantation for chronic granulomatous disease. *J. Pediatr.* 101(6):952, 1982.

113. Seaman, W.E., Gindhart, T.D., Greenspan, J.S., Blackman, M.A., and Talal, N., Natural killer cells, bone and the bone marrow: Studies in estrogen-treated mice and in congenitally osteopetrotic (mi/mi) mice. *J. Immunol.* 122:2541, 1979.

114. Milhand, G., Labat, M., Parant, M., Damais, C., and Chedid, L., Immunological defect and its correction in the osteopetrotic mutant rat. *Proc. Natl. Acad. Sci USA* 74:339, 1977.

115. Sorrell, M., Kapoor, N., Kirkpatrick, D., Rosen, J.F., Chaganti, R.S.K., Lopez, C., Dupont, B., Pollack, M.S., Terrin, B.N., Harris, M.B., Vine, D., Rose, J.S, Goossen, C., Lane, J., Good, R.A., and O'Reilly, R.J.: Marrow transplantation for juvenile osteopetrosis. *Am. J. Med.* 70:1280, 1981.

116. Coccia, P.F., Krivit, W., Cervenka, J., Clawson, C., Kiersey, J.H., Kim, T.H., Nesbit, M.E., Ramsay, N.K., Warkentin, P.I., Teitelbaum, S.L., Kahn, A.J., and Brown, D.M., Successful bone marrow transplantation for infantile malignant osteopetrosis. *N. Engl. J. Med.* 302:701, 1980.

117. Virelizier, J.L., Lagrue, A., Durandy, A., Arenzana, F., Oury, C., Griscelli, C., and Reinert, P., Reversal of natural killer defect in a patient with Chediak Higashi syndrome after bone marrow transplantation. *N. Engl. J. Med.* 306:1055, 1982.

118. Sorrell, M., Kapoor, N., Pahwa, R., et al., Correction of combined immunodeficiency and agranulocytosis in a patient with cartilage hair hypoplasia by marrow transplantation. *Clin. Immunol. Immunopathol.* (in press), 1984.

119. August, C.S., King, E., Aithens, J.H., et al., Establishment of erythropoiesis following bone marrow transplantation in a patient with congenital hypoplastic anemia (Diamond-Blackfan). *Blood* 48:491, 1976.

120. Gluckman, E., Devergie, A., Schaison, A., Bussel, A., Berger, R., Sohier, J., and Bernard, J., Bone marrow transplantation in Franconi's anemia. *Br. J. Haematol.* 45:557, 1980.

121. Deeg, H.J., Storb, R., Thomas, E.D., Appelbaum, F., Buckner, D., Clift, R., Doney, K., Johnson, L., Sanders, J.F., Stewart, P., Sullivan, K.M., Witherspoon, R.P., Fanconi's anemia treated by allogeneic marrow transplantation. *Blood* 61(5):954-9, 1983.

122. Fefer, A., Buckner, C.D., Thomas, E.D., Cheever, M.A., Clift, R.A., Glucksberg, H., Neiman, P.E., and Storb, R., Care of hematologic neoplasia with transplantation of marrow from identical twins. *N. Eng. J. Med.* 297:146, 1977.

123. Thomas, E.D., Buckner, C.D., Clift, R.A., Fefer, A., Johnson, F.L., Neiman, P.E., Sale, G.E., Sanders, J.E., Singer, J.W., Shulman, H., Storb, R., and Weiden, P.L., Marrow transplantation for acute nonlyphoblastic leukemia in first remission. *N. Engl. J. Med.* 301:597, 1979.

124. Poweles, R.L., Morgenstern, G., Clink, H.M., Hedley, D., Bandini, G., Lumley, H., Watson, J.G., Lawson, D., Spence, D., Barrett, A., Jameson, B., Lawler, S., Kay, H.E., and McElwain, T.J., The place of bone marrow transplantation in acute myelogenous leukemia. *Lancet* 1:1047, 1980.

125. Blume, K.G., Beutler, E., Bross, K.J., Chillar, R.K., Ellington, O.B., Fahey, J.L., Farbstein, M.J., Forman, S.J., Schmidt, G.M., Scott, E.P., Spruce, W.E., Turner, M.A. and Wolf, J.L., Bone marrow ablation and allogeneic marrow transplantation in acute leukemia. *N. Engl. J. Med.* 302:1041, 1980.

126. Mannoni, P., Vernanti, J.P., Rodet, M., Rochant, H., Bracgeh, T., Tournesac, A.,

Feuilhade, F., Bierling, P., Dreufus, B., Marrow transplantation for acute non-lymphoblastic leukemia in first remission. *Blood* 41:220, 1980.

127. Santos, G.W., Tutschka, P.J., Beschorner, W.E., et al., Marrow transplantation in acute non-lymphocytic leukemia (ANL) following Busulfan (BV) and cyclophosphamide (CY). Blood 58(1):176A, 1981 (Abst.).

128. Gale, R.P., For the transplantation biology unit. A prospective controlled trial of bone marrow transplantation versus chemotherapy in acute myelogenous leukemia. *Blood* 58(1):173A, 1981 (Abst.).

129. Dinsmore, R., Kirkpatrick, D., Flomenberg, et al., Allogeneic marrow transplantation (BMT) for acute non-lymphoblastic leukemia (ANLL). *Blood* 60(1):595A, 1982 (Abst.).

130. Buckner, C.D., Clift, R.A., Thomas, E.D., Sanders, J.E., Stewart, P.S., Storb, R., Sullivan, K.M., Hackman, R., Allogeneic marrow transplantation for patients with acute non-lymphoblastic leukemia in second remission. *Leukemia Res.* 6:359, 1982.

131. Applebaum, F.R., Clift, R.A., Buckner, C.D., Stewart, P., Storb, R., Sullivan, K.M., and Thomas, E.D., Allogeneic marrow transplantation for acute non-lymphoblastic leukemia after first relapse *Blood* 61:949, 1983.

132. Bortin, M.M., Gale, R.P., and Ram, A.A., For the Advisory Committee of the Registry. Factors associated with early mortality following allogeneic bone marrow transplantation for acute myelogeneous leukemia. A report from the International Bone Marrow Registry. *Transplant. Proc.* 15(1):1389, 1983.

133. Deeg, H.J., Storb, R., Thomas, E.D., et al., Marrow transplantation for acute non-lymphoblastic leukemia in first remission: Preliminary results of a randomized trial comparing cyclosporin and methotrexate for the prophylaxis of graft-versus-host disease. *Transplant. Proc.* 15(1):1385, 1983.

134. Weinstein, H.J., Mayer, R.J., Rosenthal, D.S., Camitta, B.M., Coral, F.S., Nathan, D.G., and Frei, E., Treatment of acute myelogeneous leukemia in children and adults. *N. Engl. J. Med.* 303:473-8, 1980.

135. Preisler, H., Browman, G., Henderson, E., Hruniuk, W., Freeman, A., Treatment of acute myelogeneous leukemia. Effect of early intensive consolidation. *Proc. Am. Asso. Cancer. Res.* 21:443, 1980.

136. Gale, R.P., Foon, K.A., Cline, M.J., Zighelboim, J., Acute leukemia study group. Intensive chemotherapy for acute myelogenous leukemia. *Ann. Intern. Med.* 94:753, 1981.

137. Mauer, A.M., Therapy of acute lymphoblastic leukemia in childhood. *Blood* 56:1, 1980.

138. Johnson, F.L., Thomas, E.D., Clark, B.S., Chard, R.L., Hartmann, J.R., and Storb, R., A comparison of marrow transplantation to chemotherapy for children with acute lymphoblastic leukemia in second or subsequent remission. *N. Engl. J. Med.* 305(15):846-51, 1981.

139. Woods, W.G., Nesbit, M.E., Ramsay, N.K., Krivit, W., Kimt, T.H., Goldman, A., McGlare, P.B., and Kersey, J.H., Intesive therapy followed by bone marrow transplantation for patients with acute lymphocytic leukemia in second or subsequent remission: Determination of prognostic factors (A report from the University of Minnesota Bone Marrow Transplantation Team). *Blood* 61(6):1182, 1983.

140. Dinsmore, R., Kirkpatrick, D., Flomenberg, N., Gulati, S., Kapoor, N., Shank, B., Reid, A., Groshen, S., and O'Reilly, R.J., Allogeneic bone marrow transplantation for patients with acute lymphoblastic leukemia. *Blood* 62(2):381, 1983.

141. Scott, E.P., Forman, S.J., Spruce, W.E., et al., Bone marrow ablation followed by allogeneic bone marrow transplantation for patients with high risk acute lymphoblastic leukemia during complete remission. *Transplant. Proc.* 15(1):1395, 1983.

142. Strychmans, P.A., Current concepts in chronic myelogenous leukemia. *Seminars Hematology* 11:101, 1974.

143. Champlin, R., Ho, W., Arenson, E., and Gale, R.P., Allogeneic bone marrow transplantation for chronic myelogeneous leukemia in chronic or accelerated phase. *Blood* 60:1038, 1982.

144. Champlin, R., Ho, W., Winston, D.J., et al., Allogeneic bone marrow transplant for chronic myelogeneous leukemia in chronic and accelerated phase. *Transplant. Proc.* 15(1):1401, 1983.

145. McGlave, P.B., Arthur, D.C., Weisdorf, D., Kim, T., Goldman, A., Hurd, D.D., Ramsay, N.K., and Kersey, J.H., Allogeneic bone marrow transplantation for accelerated chronic myelogeneous leukemia. *Blood* 63(1):219-22, 1984.

146. Applebaum, F.R., Fefer, A., Cheever, M.A., Buckner, C.D., Greenberg, P.D., Kaplan, H.G., Storb, R., and Thomas, E.D., Treatment for non-Hodgkin's lymphoma with marrow transplantation in identical twins. *Blood* 58:509, 1981.

147. Osserman, E.F., Dire, L.B., Dire, J., Sherman, W.H., Hersman, J.A., and Storb, R., Identical twin marrow transplantation in multiple myeloma. *Acta Haematologica* 68:215, 1982.
148. Cheever, M.A., Fefer, A., Greenberg, P.D., Appelbaum, F., Armitage, J.O., Buckner, C.D., Sale, G.E., Storb, R., Witherspoon, R.P., and Thomas, E.D., Treatment of hairy cell leukemia with chemoradio therapy and identical twin bone marrow transplantation. N. Engl. J. Med. 307:479, 1982.
149. Smith, J.W., Shulman, H.M., Thomas, E.D., and Fefer, A., Bone marrow transplantation for acute myelosclerosis. *Cancer* 48:2198-203, 1981.
150. Wolf, J.L., Spruce, W.E., Bearman, R.M., Forman, S.J., Scott, E.P., Fahey, J.L., Farbstein, M.J., Rappaport, H., and Blume, K.G., Reversal of acute (malignant) myelosclerosis by allogeneic bone marrow transplantation. *Blood.* 59:191, 1982.
151. Lynch, R.E., Williams, D.M., Reading, J.C., and Cartwright, G.E., The prognosis in aplastic anemia. *Blood* 45:517, 1975.
152. Camitta, B.M., Thomas, E.D., Nathan, D.G., Gale, R.P., Kopecky, K.J., Rappeport, J.M., Santos, G., Gordon-Smith, E.C., and Storb, R., A prospective study of Androgen and bone marrow for treatment of severe aplastic anemia. *Blood* 53:504, 1979.
153. Camitta, B.M., Storb, B., and Thomas, E.D., Aplastic anemia: Pathogenesis, diagnosis, treatment and prognosis II. *N. Engl. J. Med.* 306:712, 1982.
154. Storb, R., Thomas, E.D., Buckner, C.D., Clift, R.A., Deeg, H.J., Fefer, A., Goodell, B.W., Sale, G.E., Anders, J.E., Singer, J., Stewart, P., Marrow transplantation in thirty untransfused patients with severe aplastic anemia. *Ann. Intern. Med.* 92:30, 1980.
155. Storb, R., Doney, K.W., Thomas, E.D., et al., Marrow transplantation with or without donor buffy coat for 65 transfused aplastic anemia patients. *Blood* 59(2):236, 1982.
156. Storb, R., Thomas, E.D., Buckner, C.D., et al., Marrow transplantation in thirty untransfused patients with severe aplastic anemia. *Ann. Int. Med.* 92:30, 1980.
157. Elfenbein, G.J., Mellits, E.D., and Santos, G.W., Engraftment and survival after allogeneic bone marrow transplantation for severe aplastic anemia. *Transplant Proc.,* Vol. XV(1):1412, 1983.
158. Thomas, E.D., Buckner, C.D., Sanders, J.E., et al., Marrow transplantation for Thalassaemia. *Lancet* ii:227, 1982.
159. Lucarelli, G., Izzi, T., Polichi, P., et al., Bone marrow transplantation in Thalassemia. *Exp. Hematol.* 11 (Suppl.): 101, 1983.
160. Hobbs, J.R., Hugh-Jones, K. Barrette, A.J., et al., Reversal of clinical features of Hurler's disease and biochemical impairment after treatment by bone marrow transplant. *Lancet* ii:709, 1981.
161. Jolly, R.D., Thompson, K.G., Murphy, C.E., Manktelow, B.W., Bruere, A.M., and Winchester, B.G., Enzyme replacement therapy an experiment in nature in a chimeric mannosidosis calf. *Pediatr. Res.* 10:219, 1976.
162. Krivit, W., Kersey, J., Pierpoint, M.E., Tsai, M., Filipovich, L., Nesbit, M.E., Ramsay, N.K.C., Desnick, R.J., Bone marrow transplantation as treatment for Maroteaux Lamy syndrome (type VI) mucopolysaccharidosis. *Blood* 60 (Suppl.): 170a, 1982.
163. Ginns, E.J., Rappeport, J.M., Brady, R.O., Rosen, F.S., Nathan, D.G., Parkman, R., Barranger, J.A., Correction of glucocerebrosidase deficiency in Gaucher's Disease by bone marrow transplantation. *Blood* 60(Suppl.): 168a, 1982.
164. Hansen, J., Clift, R.A., Beatty, P.G., Michelson, E.M., Nisperos, B., Martin, P.J., Thomas, E.D., Marrow transplantation from donor othr than HLA genotypically-identical sibling. In UCLA Symposia on Molecular and Cellular Biology. New Series: Recent Advances in Bone Marrow Transplantation 53:0127, 1983.
165. Uphoff, D., Preclusion of secondary phase of irradiation syndrome by inoculation of fetal hematopoietic tissue following lethal total body x-irradiation. *J. Nat. Cancer Inst.* 20:625, 1958.
166. Stutman, O., Yunis, E.J., Teague, P.O., and Good, R.A., Graft-versus-host reactions induced by transplantation of parental strain thymus in neonatally thymectomized F_1 hybrid mice. *Transplantation* 6(4):514, 1968.
167. Tulunay, O., Good, R.A., and Yunis, E.J., Protection of lethally irradiated mice with allogeneic fetal liver cells: Influence of irradiation dose on immunologic reconstitution. *Proc. Natl. Acad. Sci. USA* 72:4100, 1975.
168. Stutman, O., Yunis, E.J., and Good, R.A., Studies on thymus function. I. Cooperative effect of thymic function and lymphohemopoietic cells in restoration of neonatally thymectomized mice. *J. Exp. Med.* 132:583, 1970.

169. Yunis, E.J., Fernandes, G., Smith, J., and Good, R.A., Long survival and immunologic reconstitution following transplantation with syngeneic or allogeneic fetal liver and neonatal spleen cells. *Transplant. Proc.* 8:521, 1976.
170. Good, R.A., Clin. Bull, 1967.
171. Muller-Rucholtz, W., Wotge, W.U., Muller-Hermelink, H.K., Bone marrow transplantation in rats across strong histocompatibility barrier by selective elimination of lymphoid cells in donor marrow. *Transplant Proc.* 8:537, 1976.
172. Joh, K., Tsuei, L., Good, R.A., and Oettgen, H.F., Adherent suppressor cells in the blood of cancer patients. *Proc. Am. Soc. Cancer Res.,* 20:115, 1979 (Abst.).
173. Von Boehmer, H., Sprent, J., and Nabholz, M., Tolerance to histocompatibility determinats in tetraparental bone marrow chimeras. *J. Exp. Med.* 141:322, 1975.
174. Onoe, K., Fernandez, G., and Good, R.A., Humoral and cell-mediated immune response in fully allogeneic bone marrow chimera in mice. *J. Exp. Med.* 151:115, 1980.
175. Krown, S.E., Coico, R., Scheid, M.P., Fernandes, G., and Good, R.A., Immune function in fully allogeneic mouse bone marrow chimeras. *Clin. Immunol. Immunopathol.* 19:268, 1981.
176. Coico, R., Krown, S.E., Good, R.A., and Hoffmann, M.K., Helper cell factors restore antibody responses of allogeneic bone marrow chimeras: Evidence for ineffective cellular interactions. *J. Immunol.* 128(4):1590, 1982.
177. Reisner, Y., Itzicovitch, L., Meshorer, A., and Sharon, N., Hematopoietic stem cell transplantation using mouse bone marrow and spleen cells fractionated by lectin. *Proc. Natl. Acad. Sci USA* 75:2933, 1978.
178. Muller-Ruchholtz, W., Muller-Hermelink, H.K. & Wottage, H.U., Induction of lasting hemopoietic chimerism in a zenogeneic (rat-mouse) model. *Transplant. Proc.* 9, 517 1979.
179. Muller-Ruchholtz, W., Wottage, H.U., Muller-Hermelink, H.K., Bone marrow transplantation in rats across strong histocompatibility barriers by selective elimination of lymphoid cells in donor marrow. *Transplant. Proc.* 8, 537, 1976.
180. Muller-Ruchholtz, W., Wottage, H.U., Muller-Hermelink, H.K., «Restitution potential of allogenetically or zenogenetically grafted lymphocyte-free hemopoietic stem cells» in Immunobiology of Bone Marrow Transplantation, ed. by S. Thierfelder, H. Rodt, H.J. Kobl (Springer Verlag, Berlin, Heidelberg, 1980), pp. 153-177.
181. Muller-Ruchholtz, Blanck, M., Wottage, H.U., Muller-Hermelind, H.K., Specific immune suppression in adult mice across K-I-D fully allogeneic histo-incompatibility barriers induced by lymphocyte-free bone marrow cells. *Transplant. proc.* 8, 603, 1981.
182. Muller-Ruchholtz, W., Blanck, M., Wottage, H.U., Ulrichs, K., Muller-Hermelink, H.K., Relevance of prethymic precursor cells for GVHR prevention in rat and mouse fully allogeneic combinations. *Transplant. Proc.* 15, 1463, 1963.
183. Wottage, H.U., Hensen, J.M., Muller-Ruchholtz, W., Bone marrow chimerism-determined restriction of genetic restriction: Acquired cooperation of MHC different cells. *Transplant. Proc.,* 15, 203, 1983.
184. Joh, K., Tsuei, L., Good, R.A., Oettgen, H.F., Adherent suppressor cells in the blood of cancer patients. *Proc. Amer. Soc. Cancer Res.,* 20, 115, 1979.
185. Von Boehmer, H., Sprent, J. and Nabholz, M., Tolerance to histo-compatibility determinants in tetraparental bone marrow chimeras. *J. Exp. Med.* 141:322, 1975.
186. Ono, K., Fernandez, G., and Good, R.A., Humoral and cell-mediated immune response in fully allogeneic bone marrow chimera in mice. *J. Exp. Med.* 151:115, 1980.
187. Krown, S.E., Coico, R., Scheid, M.P., Fernandes, G., and Good, R.A., Immune function in fully allogeneic mouse bone marrow chimeras. *Clin. Immunol. Immunopathol.* 19, 268, 1981.
188. Coico, R., Krown, S.E., Good, R.A., and Hoffmann, M.K., Helper cell factors restore antibody responses of allogeneic bone marrow chimeras. Evidence for ineffective cellular interactions. *J. Immunol.* 128(4):1590, 1982.
189. Reisner, Y., Itzicovitch, L., Meshorer, A., and Sharon, N., Hematopoietic stem cell transplantation using mouse bone marrow and spleen cells fractionated by lectin. *Proc. Natl. Acad. Sci USA* 75:2933, 1978.
190. Onoe, K., and Good, R.A., Immune responses in fully allogeneic chimera. *Proc. Japan Soc. Immunol.* 9:45, 1979.
191. Onoe, K., Yasumizu, R., Oh-ishi, T., Kakinuma, M., Good, R.A., and Morikawa, K., Restricted antibody formation to sheep erythrocytes of allogeneic bone marrow chimeras histoincompatible at the K end of the H-2 complex. *J. Exp. Med.* 153, 1009, 1981.
192. Onoe, K., Fernandes, G., Shen, F.-W., and Good, R.A., Sequential changes of thymocyte

surface antigens with presence or absence of graft-versus-host reaction following allogeneic bone marrow transplantation. *Cell. Immunol.* 68:207, 1982.

193. Onoe, K., Yasumizu, R., Oh-ishi, T., Kakinuma, M., Good, R.A., Fernandes, G., and Morikawa, K., Specific elimination of the T lineage cells: Effect of in vitro treatment with anty-Thy 1 serum without complement on the adoptive cell transfer system. *J. Immunol. Methods* 49:315, 1982.

194. Keightley, R.G., Lawton, A.R., Cooper, M.D., and Yunis, E.J., Successful fetal livery transplantation in a child with severe combined immuno-deficiency. *Lancet* 2:850, 1975.

195. Buckley, R.H., Reconstitution: grafting of bone marrow and thymus. In *Progress in Immunology* (B. Amos, ed.), p. 1061. *Academic Press, New York, 1971.*

196. O'Reilly, R.J., Kapoor, N., and Kirkpatrick, D., Fetal tissue transplants. for severe combined immunodeficiency. Their limitation and functional potential. In *Primary Immunodeficiencies* (M. Seligmann and W.H. Hilzig, Eds.), p. 419. Amsterdam, Elsevier-North Holland, 1980.

197. Iwata, T., Incefy, G.S., Cunningham-Rundles, C., Smithwick, E., Geller, N., O. Reilly, R.J., and Good, R.A., Circulating thymic horman activity in patients with primary and secondary immuno-deficiency diseases. *Am. J. Med.* 71:385, 1981.

198. Reisner, Y., and Sharon, N., Cell fractionation by lectins. *Trends Biochem. Sci.* 5:29, 1980.

199. Reisner, Y., O'Reilly, R.J., Kapoor, N., and Good, R.A., Allogeneic bone marrow transplantation usign stem cells fractionated by lectins: VI, in vitro analysis of human and monkey bone marrow cells fractionated by sheep red blood cells and soybean agglutinin. *Lancet* 2:1320, 1980.

200. Reisner, Y., Kapoor, N., Kirkpatrick, D., Pollack, M.S., Dupont, B., Good, R.A., and O'Reilly, R.J., Transplantation for acute leukemia with HLA-A and B non-identical parental marrow cells fractionated with soybean agglutinin and sheep red blood cells. *Lancet* 2:327, 1981.

201. Reisner, Y., Kapoor, N., Hodes, M.Z., O'Reilly, R.J., and Good, R.A., Enrichment for cFU-C from murine and human bone marrow using soybean agglutinin. *Blood* 59:360, 1982.

202. Reisner, Y., Kapoor, N., Kirkpatrick, D., Pollack, M.S., Cunningham-Rundles, S., Dupont, B., Hodes, M.S., Good, R.A., and O'Reilly, R.J., Transplantation for severe combined immunodeficiency with HLA A, B, D, Dr incompatible parental marrow cells fractionated by soybean agglutinin and sheep red blood cells. *Blood* 61-341, 1983.

203. Reinherz, E.Z., Geha, R., Rappeport, J.M., Wilson, M., Penta, A.C., Hussy, R.E., Fitzgerald, K.A., Daley, J.F., Levine, H., Rosen, F.S., and Schlosman, S.F.: Reconsistitution after transplantation with T lymphocyte depleted HLA haplotype mismatched bone marrow for severe combined immuno-deficiency. *Proc. Natl. Acad. Sci USA* 79:6047-51, 1982.

204. Trigg, M., Billing, R., Sondel, P., et al., In vitro treatment of bone marrow with Anti-E rosette antibody and complement prior to transplantations. In UCLA Symposia on Molecular and Cellular Biology, New Series: Recent Advances in Bone Marrow Transplantation 57: 0136, 1983.

205. Ashe and Thompson. Personal communication.

206. Kapoor, N., Jung, L., Bogardis, C., DeBault, L., Muneer, R., Nitschke, R., and Good, R.A., An immunosuppressive, myeloablative preparative regimen adequate for matched sibling transplant, inadequate in histo-incompatible, T cell depleted marrow transplant in leukemia. The Fourth International Symposium on Immunological Monitoring of the Transplant Recipient, p. 6, 1983.

207. Dexter, T.M., Moore, M.A.S., and Sheridan, A.P.C., Maintenance of hematopoietic stem cells and production of differentiated progeny in allogeneic and serum allogeneic bone marrow chimeras in vitro. *J. Exp. Med.* 145:1612, 1977.

208. Dexter, T.M., and Spooncer, E., Loss of immunoreactivity in long-term bone marrow culture. *Nature* 275:135, 1978.

209. Filipovich, N.K.C., Ramsay, P., McGlave, R., Quinones, C., Winslow, C., Heinitz, R.J., and Kersey, J.H., Mismatched bone marrow transplantation (BMT): The Minnesota Experience (UMH). *J. Cell. Biochem.* (Suppl. 7A): 60, 1983 (Abst.).

210. Filipovich, A.H., Vallera, D., Quinonis, R., Youle, R., Neville, D., Kersey, J.H., Bone marrow pretreatment with anti-T cell immunotoxins (IT) for prevention of graft-versus-host disease (GVHD) in human bone marrow transplantation (BM). *Blood* 62(1):221a, 1983.

211. Dalmasso, A.P., Martinez, C., Sjodin, K., Good, R.A., Studies on the role of the Thymectomy in immunobiology. *J. Exp. Med.* 118:1089, 1963.

212. Woodruff, J., Hanson, J., Good, R.A., Santos, G.W., and Slavin, R.E., The pathology of

the graft-versus-host reactions (GVHR) in adults receiving bone marrow transplants. *Transplant. Proc.* 8:675, 1976.

213. Bennett, M. and Hand, A.S., Effect of irradiated spleen cells on severity of graft-versus-host disease. *Transplantation* 26:199, 1978.

214. Glucksberg, H., Storb, R., Fefer, A., Buckner, C.D., Neiman, P.E., Clift, R.A., Lerner, K.G., and Thomas, E.D., Clinical manifestations of graft-versus-host disease in human recipients of marrow from HLA matched siblind donors. *Transplantation* 18:295-304, 1974.

215. Lerner, K.G., Kao, G.F., Storb, R., Buckner, C.D., Clift, R.A., and Thomas, E.D., Histopathology of graft-versus-host reaction (GVHR) in human recipient of marrow from HLA matched sibling donors. *Transplant. Proc.* 6:367-71, 1974.

216. Sale, A.E., Shulman, H.M., McDonald, G.B., and Thomas, E.D., Gastrointestinal graft-versus-host disease in man. A clinicopathological study of the rectal biopsy. *Am. J. Surg. Pathol.* 3:291, 1979.

217. Epatein, R.J., McDonald, G.B., Sale, G.E., Shulman, H.M., and Thomas, E.D., The diagnostic accuracy of the rectal biopsy in acute graft-versus-host disease. A prospective study of thirteen patients. *Gastroenterology* 78:764-71, 1980.

218. Shulman, H.M., McDonald, G.B., Matthews, D., Doney, K.C., Kopecky, K.J., Gauvreau, J.M., and Thomas, E.D., Analysis of hepatic veno occlusive disease and centrolobular hepatic degeneration following marrow transplantation. *Gastroenterology* 79; 1178, 1980.

219. Storb, R., Gluckman, E., Thomas, E.D., Buckner, C.D., Clift, R.A., Fefer, A., Glucksberg, H., Graham, T.C., Johnson, F.L., Lerner, K.G., Neiman, P.E., and Ochs, H., Treatment of established human graft-versus-host disease by anti-thymocyte globulin. *Blood* 44:57, 1974.

220. Doney, K.C., Weiden, P.L., Storb, R., and Thomas, E.D., Treatment of graft-versus-host disease in human allogeneic marrow recipient, a randomized trial comparing anti-thymocyte globulin and corticosteroids. *Am. J. Hematol.* 11:1, 1981.

221. Deeg, H.J., Storb, R., Thomas, E.D., et al., Marrow transplantation for acute lymphoblastic leukemia in first remission: Preliminary results of a randomized trial comparing cyclosporin and methotrexate for the prophylaxis of graft-versus-host disease. *Transplant. Proc.* 15:1385, 1983.

222. Sullivan, K.M., Shulman, H.M., Storb, R., Weiden, P.L., Witherspoon, R.P., McDonald, G.B., Schubert. M.M., Atkinson, K., and Thomas, E.D., Chronic graft-versus-host disease in 52 patients: Adverse natural course and successful treatment with combination immunosuppression. *Blood* 57:267, 1981.

223. Storb, R., Epstein, R.B., Graham, T.C., and Thomas, E.D., Methotoxate regimen for control of graft-versus-host disease in dogs with allogeneic marrow grafts. *Transplantation* 9:240, 1970.

224. Smith, B.R., Parkman, R.P., Lipton, J.M., Nathan, D.G., Rappeport, J.M., Efficacy of short course (four dose) methotoxate following bone marrow transplantation for prevention of graft-versus-host disease. *Blood* 62(1):230a, 1983.

225. Weiden, P.L., Doney, K., Storb, R., and Thomas, E.D., Anti-human lymphocyte globulin for prophylaxis of graft-versus-host disease: A randomized trial in patient with leukemia treated with HLA identical sibling marrow graft.

226. Doney, K.C., Weiden, P.L., Storb, R., and Thomas, E.D., Failure of early administration of anti-thymocyte globulin to lessen graft-versus-host disease in human allogeneic marrow transplant recipients. *Transplantation* 31:141, 1981.

227. Ramsay, N.K.C., Kersey, J.H., Robinson, L.L., Mcglave, P.B., Woods, W.G., Krivit, W., Kim, T.H., Goldman, A.I. and Nesbitt, M.E., Jr., A randomized study of the prevention of acute graft-versus-host disease. *N. Engl. J. Med.* 306:392, 1982.

228. Jones, J.M., Wilson, R., and Bealmear, P.M., Mortality and gross pathology of secondary disease in germ free mouse radiation chimeras. *Radiation Res.* 45:577, 1971.

229. Storb, R., Prentice, R.L., Buckner, C.D., Clift, R.A., Appelbaum, F., Deeb, J., Doney, K., Hansen, J.A., Mason, M., Sanders, J.E., Singer, J., Sullivan, K.M., Witherspoon, R.P. and Thomas, E.D., Graft-versus-host disease and survival in patients with aplastic anemia treated by marrow graft from HLA-identical sibling. Beneficial effect of a protective environment. *N. Engl. J. Med.* 308:302-7, 1983.

230. Reisner, Y., Maparstek, E., Or, R., Polliack, A., Samuels, S., Morecki, S., Weiss, L., Rachmilewitz, E.A., Slavin, S., Bone marrow transplantation for acute leukemia in remission using T-cell depleted HLA identical bone marrow. *Blood* 62(1):228a, 1983.

231. Prentice, H.G., Blacklock, H.A., Janossy, G., Bradstock, K.F., Skeggs, D., Goldstein, G., and Hoffbrand, A.V., Use of anti-T cell monoclonal antibody OKT3 to prevent acute

graft-versus-host disease in allogeneic bone marrow transplantation for acute leukemia. *Lancet* 1:700, 1982.

232. Sullivan, K.M., Dahlberg, S., Storb, R., Shulman, H., Thomas, E.D., Chronic graft-versus-host disese (GVHD): Risk factor analysis in patients surviving > 70 days after marrow transplantation. *Exp. Hematol.* 10:7, 1982 (Abst.).

233. Storb, R., Prentice, R.L., Sullivan, K.M., Shulman, H.M., Deeg, H.J., Doney, K.C., Buckner, C.D., Clift, R.A., Witherspoon, R.P., Appelbaum, F.A., Sanders, J.E., Stewart, P.S., and Thomas, E.D., Predictive factors in chronic graft-versus-host disease in patients with aplastic anemia treated by marrow transplantation from HLA identical siblings. *Ann. Int. Med.* 98:461, 1983.

234. Atkinson, K., Storb, R., Prentice, R.L., Weiden, P.L., Witherspoon, R.P., Sullivan, K., Noel, D., and Thomas, E.D., Analysis of late infections in 89 long-term survivors of bone marrow transplantation. *Blood* 53:270, 1979.

235. Sullivan, K.M., Storb, R., Flournoy, M., Weidin, P., Shulman, H., Deeg, H.J., Witherspoon, R., Thomas, E.D., Preliminary analysis of a randomized trial of immunosuppressive therapy of chronic graft-versus-host disease. *Blood* 60:173, 1982 (Abst.).

236. Forman, S.J., Farbstein, M.J., Scott, E.P., Wolf, J.L., Spruce, W.E., Fahey, J.L., Nademanee, A., and Blume, K.G., Prevention and therapy of graft-versus-host disease. *N. Engl. J. Med.* 307:376, 1982.

237. Ringden, O., Lonnavist, B., Lundgren, A., Gahrton, G., Groth, C.G., Moller, E., Baryd, I., Johansson, B., Pihlstedt, P., and Gullbring, B., Experience with a co-operative bone marrow transplantation program in Stockholm. *Transplantation* 33:500, 1982.

238. Bortin, M.M., Graft versus leukemia. In *Clinical Immunobiology*, Vol. 2, (F.H. Bach and R.A. Good, eds.), p. 287. *Academic Press, New York, 1974.*

239. Weiden, P.L., Sullivan, K.M., Flournoy, M., Storb, R., and Thomas, E.D., Anti-leukemic effect of chronic graft-versus-host disease. Contribution to improved survival after allogeneic marrow transplantation. *N. Engl. J. Med.* 304:1529-33, 1981.

240. Gale, R.P., Bone marrow transplantation in acute myelogenous leukemia in first remission: Evidence for an anti-leukemic effect of graft-versus-host disease. *Exp. Hematol.* 10:20, 1982 (Abst.).

241. Winston, D.J., Gale, R.P., Meyer, D.V., and Young, L.A., Infectious complications of human marrow transplantation. *Medicine*, 58:1, 1979.

242. Hideman, R.O., Buckner, C.D., and Clift, R.A., A modified right atrial catheter for access to the venous system in marrow transplant recipients. *Surg. Gyncol. Obstet.* 148:871, 1979.

243. Sanders, J.E., Hickman, R.O., Aker, S., Hersman, J., Buckner, C.D., and Thomas, E.D., Experience with double lumen right atrial catheter. J. Parent. Nutri. 6:95-9, 1982.

244. Meyer, D., Winston, D., Chapin, M., Gale, R.P., Young, L., and Martin, W.J., Staphylococcus epidermis bacteremia: An emerging problem in immunosuppressed patients in laminar air flow units. 20th Interscience Conference on Antimicrobial Agents and Chemotherapy (Abst # 682), New Orleans, September 1980.

245. Love, L.J., Schimpff, S.C., Schiffer, C.A., and Wiernik, P.H., Improved prognosis for granulocytopenic patients with gram negative bacteremia. *Am. J. Med.* 68:643, 1980.

246. Strauss, R.G., Therapeutic neutrophil transfusions. Are controlled studies no longer appropriate? *Am. J. Med.* 65:1001, 1978.

247. Winston, D.J., Ho, W.G., Young, L.S., and Gale, R.P., Prophylactic granulocytes transfusions during human bone marrow transplantation. *Am. J. Med.* 68:893, 1980.

248. Buckner, C.D., Clift, R.A., Thomas, E.D., et al., infection prophylaxis in marrow transplant recipients. In *Recent Advances of Germ Free Research* (S. Sasaki, A. Ozawa and K. Hashimoto, Eds.), p. 557. Tokyo, Tokai, University Press, 1981.

249. Storb, R., Prentice, R.L., Buckner, C.D., Clift, R.A., Appelbaum, F., Deeg, J., Doney, K., Hansen, J.A., Mason, M., Sanders, J.E., Singer, J., Sullivan K.M., Witherspoon, R.P., and Thomas, E.D., Graft-versus-host disease and survival in patients with aplastic anemia treated by marrow graft from HLA identical siblings. Beneficial effect of a protective environment. *N. Engl. J. Med.* 308:302, 1983.

250. Kutti, J., Zaroulis, C.G., Dinsmore, R.E., Clarkson, B.D., and Good, R.A., A prospective study of platelet-transfusion therapy administered to patients with acute leukemia. *Transfusion* 22:44, 1982.

251. Lange, B., Henle, W., Meyers, J.D., Yang, L.C., August, C., Koch, P., Arbeter, A., and Henle, G., Epstein-Barr virus related to serology in marrow transplant recipients. Int. J. Cancer 26:151, 1980.

252. Sullivan, J.L., Wallen, W.C., and Johnson, F.L., Epstein-Barr virus infection following

bone marrow transplantation. *Int. J. Cancer* 22:132, 1978.
253. Prentice, H.G., Use of acyclovir for prophylaxis of herpes infections in severely immunocompromised patients. *J. Antimicrob. Chemother.* 12:153-9, 1983, Suppl. B.
254. Meyers, J.D., Flournoy, M., and Thomas, E.D., Cytomegalovirus injections and specific cell mediated immunity after marrow transplant. *J. Infect. Dis.* 142:338, 1980.
255. Lopez, C., Simmons, R.L., Mauer, S.M., Najarian, J.S., and Good, R.A., Association of renal allograft rejection with virus infections. *Am. J. Med.* 56:280, 1974.
256. Meyers, J.D., Wade, J.C., McGuffin, R.W., Springmeyer, S.D., and Thomas, E.D., The use of acyclovir for citomegalovirus infections in the immunocompromised host. *J. Antimicrob. Chemother.* 12 (Supp. B):181-93, 1983.
257. Gluckman, E., Lotsberg, J., Devergie, A., Zhad, X.M., Melo, R., Gomez-Morales, M., Nebout, T., Mazeron, M.C., and Perol, Y., Prophylaxis of herpes infections after bone marrow transplantation by oral acyclovir. *Lancet* ii: 706-8, 1983.
258. Bayer, W.L., and Tegtmeier, C.E., The blood donor: Detection and magnitude of cytomegalovirus carrier state and the prevalence of cytomegalovirus antibody. *Yale J. Biol. Med.* 49:5, 1976.
259. Armstrong, D., Ely, M., and Steger. L., Post-transfusion cytomegalo-viremia and persistence of cytomegalovirus in blood. *Infect. Immunol.* 3:159, 1971.
260. Parjani, S.G. et al., Use of passive antibody for varicella prophylaxis in immune suppressed patients. *Am. J. Med.*, in press.
261. Winston, D.J., Gale, R.P., Meyer, D.V., and Young, L.S., Infections complications of human bone marrow transplantation. *Medicine* 58:1, 1979a.
262. Meyers, J.D., and Thomas, E.D., Infection complicating bone marrow transplantation. In *Clinical Approach to Infection in the Immunocompromised Host* (R.H. Rubin and L.S. Young, eds.), p. 507. Plenum Press, New York, 1982.
263. Yolken, R.H., Bishop, C.A., Townsend, T.R., Bolyard, E.A., Bartlett, J., Santos, G.W., and Saral, R., Infectious gastroenteritis in bone transplant recipient. *N. Engl. J. Med.* 306:1009, 1982.
264. O'Reilly, R.J., Lee, F.K., Grossbard, E., Kapoor, N., Kirkpatrick, D., Dinsmore, R., Strutzer, C., Shah, K.V., and Nahmias, A.J., Papovavirus excretion following marrow transplantation. Incidence and association with hepatic dysfunction. *Transplant. Proc.* 13:262, 1981.
265. Appelbaum, F.R., Meyers, J.D., Fefer, A., Fluornoy, N., Cheever, M.A., Greenberg, P.D., Hackman, R., and Thomas, E.D., Non-bacterial non-fungal pneumonia following marrow transplantation in 100 identical twins. *Transplantation* 33:265, 1982.
266. Shank, B., Hopfan, S., Kim, J.M., Chu, F.C., Grossbard, E., Kapoor, N., Kirkpatrick, D., Dinsmore, R. Simpson, L., Reid, A., Chui, C., Mohan, R., Finegan, D., and O'Reilly, R.J., Hyperfactionated total body irradiation for bone marrow transplantation. Early results in leukemia patients. *Int. J. Radiat. Oncol. Biol. Phys.* 7:1109, 1981.
267. Storb, R., Epstein, R.B., Rudolph, R.H., and Thomas, E.D., The effect of donor transfusion on marrow grafts between histocompatible canine siblings. *J. Immunol.* 105:627, 1970.
268. Storb, R., Weiden, P.L., Deeg, H.J., Graham, T.C., Atkinson, K., Slichter, S.J., and Thomas, E.D., Rejection of marrow from DLA identical canine litter mates given transfusions before grafting: Antigens involved are expressed on leukocytes and skin epithelial cells but not on platelets and red blood cells. *Blood* 54:477, 1979.
269. Storb, R., Prentice, R.L., and Thomas E.D., Marrow transplantation for treatment of aplastic anemia. An Analysis of factors associated with graft rejection. *N. Engl. J. Med.* 296:61, 1977.
270. Storb, R., Thomas, E.D., Weiden, P.L., Buckner, C.D., Clift, R.A., Fefer, A., Fernando, L.P., Giblett, E.R., Goddell, E.W., Johnson, F.L., Lerner, K.G., Neiman, P.E., and Sanders, J.E., Aplastic anemia treated by allogeneic bone marrow transplantation. A report on 49 new cases from Seattle. *Blood.* 48:817, 1976.
271. Parkman, R., Rappeport, J., Camitta, B., Levey, R.H., and Nathan, D.G., Successful use of multiagent immunosuppression for bone marrow transplantation of sensitized patients. *Blood* 52:1163-9, 1978.
272. Storb, R., For Seattle Marrow Transplant Team. Decrease in the graft rejection rate and improvement in survival after marrow transplantation for severe aplastic anemia. *Transplant. Proc.* 11(1), 1979.

Adverse Reactions to I.V. Immunoglobulins. A Critical Review

M. Eibl

Institute of Immunology University of Vienna
Borschkegasse 8A - A-1090 Vienna, Austria

INTRODUCTION

Anaphylactoid reactions

The utilization of human immunoglobulin (Ig) preparations in the treatment of patients with humoral immunodeficiencies was soon recognized as efficacious, but severe reactions with convulsions, loss of consciousness, hypotension and high fever were not uncommon (6). In the late seventies, several intravenous (i.v.) Ig preparations became available and apprecciated by physicians and patients. Adverse reactions, less severe, but still occurring at a frequency of 10-15% per patient, were considered a "nuisance" by some investigators (41): steroids were used to prevent those reactions (22) and patients had to be excluded from treatment series (11).

The nature of the different factors responsible for the adverse reactions are not fully known at present. The conclusion made by Barandun that "the presence of complement binding aggregates is thus a prerequisite for an anaphylactoid reaction" (6) based on the evidence that complement activating Ig aggregates do cause reactions - like antigen-antibody complexes - has been expressed even recently in spite of the notion that preparation without any detectable anticomplementary activity have been associated with severe adverse reactions (7).

The assumption that high concentrations of activators of the kinin system could correlate with the rate of adverse reactions in a given preparation has been expressed (2, 3), but data extrapolated from studies using PPF contaminated with different concentrations of prekallikrein activator in patients with cardiac bypass surgery will not necessarily apply for gammaglobulins infused to patients with humoral immunodeficiency syndromes.

The presence of antigen-antibody complexes resulting from an antigenic overload in antibody deficient patients with severe chronic infections and the antibodies infused has been clearly documented. The relevance of these antigen-antibody complexes, which has been emphasized especially for the moderate or mild late reactions which have also been called phlogistic is difficult to assess as long as the quantity and quality of contaminants causing anaphylactoid reactions in a given i.v. Ig preparation cannot be extimated. It will be the subject of this report to give a critical view on these points and to describe experimental models which are thought to be suitable if used properly to detect major contaminants causing anaphylactoid reactions. These animal models are truly empirical, but as long as all the contaminants having the potential of causing reactions have not been systematically studied and identified, it is felt that such animal models can greatly contribute to determine the safety of different i.v. Ig preparations and even individual lots (since clinical experience suggests lot-to-lot variation in certain products).

The adverse reactions caused by immunoglobulin preparations have a rather stereotype symptomatology. The categorization between immediate severe or moderate and later developing moderate or minor reactions indicates the two major features of possible symptomatology (6, 18), but does not help to clarify the etiology of the reaction. Reactions could occur as true anaphylactic reactions. Patients receiving blood products were shown to develop IgE antibodies (44), but such antibodies could never be correlated with adverse reactions. Most of the i.v. Ig preparations contain IgE as well (51), but there is not indication that this has ever caused any side effects. The same is true for antibodies against allotypic determinants on the Ig molecule (43).

Autoantibodies against IgA have been associated with severe transfusion reactions especially in IgA deficient patients with gastrointestinal diseases (8, 46). Patients have been reported to show severe adverse reactions who had antibodies against IgA or β-lipoprotein (12), but several other patients were also identified who had antibodies against IgA in their serum, but did not show adverse reactions when treated with i.v. Ig (28, 42, 25).

The notion that the most severe reactions are seen in patients with the most pronounced impairment of antibody production (6) indicates that the true anaphylactic reactions cannot be a common cause of reactions to occur after i.v. Ig infusions. It appears more likely that most of the adverse effects are anaphylactoid in nature caused by contaminants generating and/or releasing the responsible mediators. Aggregates interacting with Fc receptors and triggering the secretion of prostaglandins (38), platelet activating factor (10, 40), and other mediators are likely to be relevant. Fc receptors could be more reactive in patients with low IgG levels since "uncovered", and this could help to explain these patients' sensitivity. Barandun was first to report in his early study (6) that patients with antibody deficiency syndromes are much more likely to react if given an intravenous infusion of a "standard" immunoglobulin prepared by cold ethanol fractionation for intramuscular (i.m.) use than healthy persons and patients with other diseases including those with chronic infections (with an antigenic load comparable to that seen in the immunodeficient). The clinical picture of the anphylactoid reaction includes tachycardia, tachypnoe, shortage of breath, flushing of the face, feeling of oppression in the chest, lumbar pain, slightly elevated blood pressure, and a rise of temperature about 2 hours after completion of the infusion or later.

Severe reactions are more common in the antibdy deficient group with sudden onset of dyspnoe, nausea, vomiting, circulatory collapse with loss of consciousness, and fever. The same types of reactions have been delineated by several other investigators treating antibody deficient patients with different i.v. Ig preparations (11, 36, 41).

Barandun's conclusion (supported by indirect evidence) that the factor in the Ig preparation leading to untoward reactions was related to its anticomplementary activity has been questioned by other investigators who considered anticomplementary activity as only one of several possible reasons for adverse reactions (41, 45). Their view has been supported by additional observations.

Oligomeric and polymeric IgG do possess anticomplementary activity, but patients can exhibit adverse reactions to i.m. or i.v. administration of gammaglobulin in the absence of demonstrable changes in serum complement levels. On the other hand, serum complement levels can fall without systemic reactions. Pepsin treated Ig preparations known to have very low anticomplementary activity have been associated with severe adverse reactions as well. Further evidence on these lines has been provided by the experience that while the testing for anticomplementary activity has become a standard practice, and most preparations have no demonstrable anticomplementary activity, adverse reactions both mild and severe are still occurring especially in certain groups of patients like the immuno-deficient, those with septicemia, etc.

The possibility that Hageman factor fragments could be responsible for hypotensive reactions has been suggested by Alving et al. (2, 3, 4, 5). Several lots of plasma protein fractions causing hypotensive reactions in patients before, during and after cardiac bypass surgery had higher PKA activity than other non-implicated lots. These data indicated that Hageman factor fragments are potent hypotensive agents, presumably because they trigger the generation of kinins in the recipients. PKA was shown to increase vascular permeability in the guinea pig skin. In the circulation, however, PKA is rapidly inactivated (by C1 inhibitor), and a significant systemic reaction in dogs could not be demonstrated even in animals conditioned with kininase inhibitors (data not shown).

More than 5 years ago, we used several lots of an i.v. Ig preparation with high PKA activity in clinical trials in patients with antibody deficiency syndromes and recurrent infections (13). In these studies, each application has been documented and reported including the information whether a patient had or did not have adverse reactions. Table 1 shows the number and severity of adverse reactions reported with the administration of 6 lots, some with low and some with very high PKA activity applied in the same period. The rate of adverse reactions was fairly low even in the lots having 6.8 and 7.2 times the 100% OOB standard levels.

Thus, no correlation between PKA activity of a given i.v. Ig preparation

TABLE 1. *PKA content and rate of adverse reactions as documented in clinical trials for different lots of i.v. Ig*

Lot	PKA*	Amount applied in clinical trials	N. of doses documented in clinical trials	Adverse reaction reported
1	20	181 500 mg	37	0
2	40	323 885 mg	124	3 (1 severe, 2 moderate)
3	50	127 500 mg	51	0
4	100	23 000 mg	21	0
5	680	503 600 mg	270	1 (slight)
6	720	142 700 mg	47	0

* % activity as estimated in comparison to an OOB reference preparation (100%).

and frequency or severity of adverse reactions following administration could be found. While the application of certain preparations with very high PKA activity in these trials was not followed by adverse reactions, other preparations described as being free of PKA as well as anticomplementary activity have been associated with severe, life-threatening anaphylactoid reactions (11, and A. Ugazio personal communication).

As long as all the substances responsible for adverse reactions are not well characterized, the practical question arises which system could be suitable for the detection of contaminants causing the most severe symptoms, e.g. significant drops in blood pressure and life-threatening bronchospasm.

A sensitive and reliable animal model has long been looked for, but was certainly difficult to establish, the main reason being that the variation in the sensitivity towards substances causing anaphylactoid reactions is as wide in experimental animals as it is in humans. The dog has proven to be the species most sensitive to blood pressure lowering activity, while the guinea pig was the most sensitive to regularly demonstrable bronchospasm.

EXPERIMENTAL SYSTEM

Immunoglobulin preparations used

Immune Serum Globulin (ISG) human for i.m. use (Immuno) was administered as a bolus of 50 mg/kg, injected within 90 seconds. A preparation of an i.v. gammaglobulin (Immuno) was administered as a bolus of 500 mg/kg injected within 90 seconds.

Estimation of changes in blood pressure and airway pressure and drop of peripheral blood leukocytes and thrombocytes in the guinea pig

Male guinea pigs weighing approximately 500 grams were used. After anesthesia with a single dose of 60 mg/kg Nembutal^R i.p., the trachea was cannulated and the catheter connected with a Harvard respirator, type 681. The respiratory volume was adjusted at a respiratory frequence of 80/min. according to the body weight of the animal.

Subsequently, the carotid artery was cannulated and connected through a pressure transducer (Beckman) to a dynograph R 611 (Beckman). A venous catheter was also introduced, and the animals were then allowed to stabilize for 10 minutes. The material to be tested was injected in a 90 second period, and blood pressure, respiratory pressure and leukocyte and thrombocyte counts were monitored for 30 minutes.

Evaluation: Maximal blood pressure within 10 minutes after the injection of the sample, and maximal respiratory pressure within 20 minutes following the injection of the sample were determined. A 30% rise in the systolic, a 40% rise in the diastolic blood pressure, and a 30% rise in respiratory pressure were considered positive. An animal giving a positive reaction in one or more of the systems was considered a reactant.

Test system for hypotonic effects in the dog

The tests were carried out on mongrel dogs of both sexes. Dogs were tranquillized. One hour later anesthesia with 40 mg/kg Nembutal^R was initiated. Catheters were introduced into the carotid artery (for the measurement of blood pressure) and into the jugular vein. The arterial catheter was connected by a pressure transducer (Beckman) to a dynograph (R 611, Beckman), and the instrumentend animal allowed to stabilize for 30 minutes. Blood pressure (systolic and diastolic) was recorded and average (pre-injection) values estimated. The animals were then injected the respective immunoglobulin sample, and a drop of blood pressure of 30% or more was considered positive. Each preparation was tested in 4 dogs.

RESULTS

Guinea pigs responded to a bolus of 50 mg/kg ISG injected within 90 seconds regularly and reproducibly with an elevation of airway pressure 30% or more above the pre-injection level (Fig. 1). In the guinea pig, contrary to the effect observed in dogs, an elevation of blood pressure was observed (Table 2). Such discrepancy between the two species has previously been described with vasoactive substances like histamine.

A purified i.v. Ig preparation (characteristics given in 15) injected as a bolus of 500 mg/kg within 90 seconds did not produce any significant changes. Preliminary experiments indicate that several lots of i.v. Ig which have been

Changes in airway pressure in the guinea pig after injection of an ISG for i.m. use (dose response)

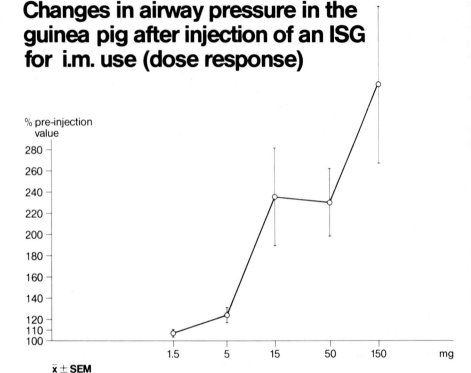

FIG. 1. 4 guinea pigs were injected with a bolus of the respective dose of ISG for each point. Airway pressure was measured with a Harvard respirator and results are expressed as percent pre-injection values. 15 mg/kg and more produced a regular increase in airway pressure in 4 out of 4 responsive guinea pigs.

tolerated by patients without adverse reactions did not produce any changes in these experimental systems. while other preparations implicated in adverse reactions did (Table 2).

30 minutes after the injection of the test preparation, animals were injected a positive reference preparation (Cohn fraction II), which has been shown in preliminary experiments to produce anaphylactoid reactions in the guinea pig with elevation of blood pressure, elevation of airway pressure, drop in leukocyte and thrombocyte count at a dose of 50 mg/kg regularly. Guinea pigs who did not react to a given test preparation and to the subsequent challenge with the positive reference preparation were considered as non-sensitive and therefore unsuitable.

As little as 5 mg/kg of the reference preparation produced a significant lowering of blood pressure in 4 out of 4 responsive dogs (while 15 mg/kg are required to produce an elevation of airways pressure in 4 out of 4 responsive guinea pigs), and a dose-response curve could be established (Figs. 2 and 3).

TABLE 2. *Maximal airway pressure and blood pressure, minimal leukocyte and thrombocyte counts in guinea pigs given different ISG and i.v. Ig preparations.*

Number of animals	Number of reactants	Product & amount	% Maximal blood pressure s/d	% Maximal airway pressure	% Minimal leukocytes	% Minimal thrombocytes
4	4	ISG 1 50 mg/kg	256/ 232 ± 82 ± 73.2	497 ± 199.5	13 ± 5.7	5 ±3.6
4	0	i.v. Ig 2 500 mg/kg	108/ 111 ± 5.2 ± 12.4	100 ± 0	52 ± 0.6	73 ± 6.2
4	1	i.v. Ig 3 500 mg/kg	124/ 128 ± 8.1 ± 17.8	100 ± 0	n.d.	n.d.
4	4	i.v. Ig 4 150 mg/kg	149/ 183 ± 28 ± 40.6	378 ±346.8	40 ±14.9	13 ± 4.9
4	4	i.v. Ig 5 150 mg/kg	178/ 204 ±81.1 ± 86.5	217 ± 89.3	37 ± 9.6	10 ± 1.9

Changes in blood pressure (systolic) in the dog after injection of an ISG for i.m. use (dose response)

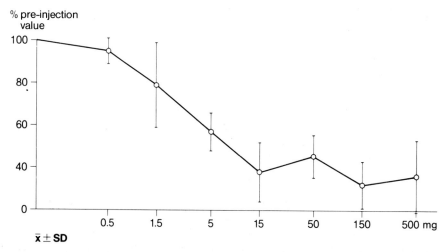

FIG. 2. 4 dogs received a bolus injection of the respective dose of ISG. Blood pressure (systolic) was monitored and results are expressed as percent of the pre-infusion values. 5 mg/kg and more produced a regular increase in airway pressure in 4 out of 4 responsive dogs.

Changes in blood pressure (diastolic) in the dog after injection of an ISG for i.m. use (dose response)

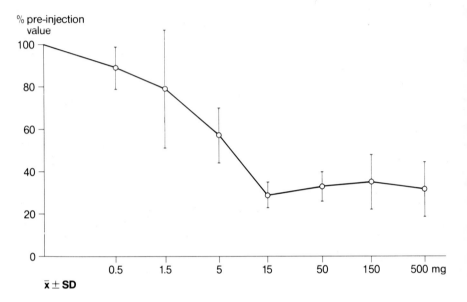

FIG. 3 4 dogs received a bolus injection of the respective dose of ISG. Blood pressure (diastolic) was monitored and results are expressed as percent of the pre-infusion values. 5 mg/kg and more produced a regular increase in airway pressure in 4 out of 4 responsive dogs.

The injection of 500 mg/kg of the i.v. Ig did not induce significant changes in blood pressure. Extensive preliminary experiments as well as the results presented here suggest that these animal models are suitable for the identification of the anaphylactoid potential of any given i.v. Ig preparation (or lot).

Gammaglobulin preparations have been considered to be safe with respect to the transmission of the agent causative of hepatitis B, if single donations of plasma were free of detectable HB_s antigen in a sensitive third generation test, and if appropriate fractionation methodology was used (26). The transmission of viral hepatitis (hepatitis B) has been reported on several occasions before the starting material has regularly been tested (39) and/or in preparations produced under unfavourable circumstances (26).

Gerety et al. demonstrated that, when tested, 0.8% of the lots of ISG prepared between 1962 and 1974 contained HB_s antigen, while none of the lots produced after screening of the starting material had been introduced could be shown to contain this contaminant.

The question of transmission of the agent of non-A, non-B hepatitis by i.v. Ig preparations has recently been addressed by several groups of investigators (30, 33, 37). Lever et al. (32) describe an outbreak of acute non-A, non-B hepatitis among 12 recipients of an i.v. Ig preparation. One patient who had previously been receiving plasma came down with jaundice and greatly raised transaminase serum levels. One other patient reported that he had been mildly jaundiced for a week between infusions. Three biopsies were performed. All of them showed severe lobular hepatities with widespread mononuclear cell infiltration. In general, the inflammatory infiltrate was disproportionate to the amount of liver cell necrosis.

Increased transaminase levels with one case of overt liver disease have been reported in another trial by Ochs et al. (37) in 16 of their patients receiving 400 mg/kg i.v. Ig. 7 of the 16 showed elevated transaminase GPT/GOT levels one to three months after infusion of a new preparation. Only one of those had had high GOT levels before. One of the 7 patients who developed liver disease died of coronary artery disease and had a grossly cirrhotic liver at autopsy. None of the other 6 patients had any symptoms.

Several questions were raised. Was the i.v. Ig contaminated with low dose non-A, non-B virus? Could the manufacturing procedures used in the preparation give rise to infectivity by uncovering masked virus? Furthermore, in this and other situations, the question was asked whether in addition to the problem of transmission of a viral agent, could i.v. Ig trigger pathopysiological mechanism either by reactivation of a silent virus, or could the product by itself cause changes in transaminase levels.

To analyse the effect of repeated infusions of i.v. gamma-globulin (in a dose as used in the therapy of hypogammaglobulinemics), three chimpanzees have been given repeated infusions of i.v. Ig: 600 mg/kg body weight within a 2 week period, and 100 mg/kg weekly thereafter. The animals are being monitored weekly for blood count and differential, T cells and T_4 T_8 subsets, stimulation with mitogens, liver enzymes and liver biopsies. Monitored in parallel were three untreated animals and 3 animals with non-A, non-B hepatitis. Two of the animals treated with i.v. Ig did not have any history of hepatitis, while one animal was known to have had hepatitis B in 1977. From the three untreated animals two had a positive history for hepatitis B. The results of these investigations will be subject of a following report.

Preliminary data regarding GPT levels in the first six months' period show that none of the control chimpanzees and none of the animals treated with i.v. Ig had GPT levels above 2.5 times the upper normal range (GOT levels in 3 animals with non-A, non-B hepatitis exceed the 2.5 times normal range for different lengths of time). The results, event though preliminary, indicate that repeated infusions of the i.v. Ig preparation used do not cause an elevation in GPT levels within a six month period.

We do hope that these studies will provide further valuable information and will allow us to answer at least some of the questions that have been raised concerning the effect of repeated gammaglobulin infusions in the patients.

Acknowledgements

The investigations on anaphylactoid contaminants have been performed in close co-operation with J. Eibl, F. Löblich, T. Mookkenthottathil, and G. Raberger, and the studies on the chimpanzees with G. Eder and H. Wolf. Fruitful discussions with these colleagues is gratefully acknowledged.

REFERENCES

1. Abe, T, and Matsuda, J. (1981): A study of new enzyme immunoassay for quantification of platelet bound IgG and its clinical significance. In: *Immunohemotherapy. A Guide to Immunoglobulin Prophylaxis and Therapy*, edited by U.E. Nydegger, pp. 409-417. Academic Press, London, New York, Sydney, San Francisco.
2. Alving, B.M., Hojima, Y., Pisano, J.J., Mason, B.L., Buckingham, R.E., Jr., Mozen, M.M., and Finlayson, J.S. (1978): Hypotension associated with prekallikrein activator (Hageman-factor fragments) in plasma protein fraction. *N. Engl. J. Med.*, 229:66-70.
3. Alving, B.M., Tankersley, D.L., Mason, B.L., Rossi, F., Aronson, D.L., and Finlayson, J.S., (1980): Contactivated factors: contaminants of immunoglobulin preparations with coagulant and vasoactive properties. *J. Lab. Clin. Med.*, 96:334-346.
4. Alving, B.M., Tankersley, D.L., Mason, B.L., Condie, R.M., and Finlayson, J.S. (1981): Biologic activities of enzymic contaminants in immunoglobulin preparations. In: *Immunohemotherapy. A Guide to Immunoglobulin Prophylaxis and Therapy*, edited by U.E. Nydegger, pp. 161-170. Academic Press, London, New York, Toronto, Sydney, San Francisco.
5. Aronson, D.L., and Finlayson, J.S., (1980): Historical and future therapeutic plasma derivatives (Epilogue). *Seminars in Thrombosis and Hemostasis*, VI:121-139.
6. Barandun, S., Kistler, P., Jeunet, F., and Isliker, H., (1962): Intravenous administration of human γ-globulin. *Vox Sang.*, 7:157-174.
7. Barandun, S., and Morell, A. (1981): Adverse reactions to immunoglobulin preparations. In: *Immunohemotherapy. A Guide to Immunoglobulin Prophylaxis and Therapy*, edited by U.E. Nydegger, pp. 223-227. Academic Press, London, New York, Toronto, Sydney, San Francisco.
8. Bjerrum, O.J., and Jersild, C. (1971): Class-specific anti-IgA associated with severe anaphylactic transfusion reactions in a patient with pernicious anaemia. *Vox Sang.*, 21:411-424.
9. Branigan, E.F., Stevenson, M.M., and Charles, D. (1983): Blood transfusion reaction in a patient with immunoglobulin A deficiency. *Obstetrics & Gynecology*, 61 (Suppl): 47S-49S.
10. Camussi, G., Aglietta, M., Coda, R., Bussolino, F., Piacibello, W., and Tetta, C. (1981): Release of platelet-activating factor (PAF) and histamine. II. The cellular origin of human PAF: monocytes, polymorhonuclear neutrophils and basophils. *Immunology*, 42:191-199.
11. Cunningham-Rundles, C., Day, N.K., Wahn, V., Smithwick, E.M., Siegal, F.P., Gupta, S., and Good, R.A. (1981): Reactions to intravenous gammaglobulin infusions and immune complex formation. In: *Immunotherapy. A Guide to Immunoglobulin Prophylaxis and Therapy*, edited by U.E. Nydegger, pp. 447-450. Academic Press, London, New York, Toronto, Sydney, San Francisco.
12. Day, N.K., Good, R.A., and Wahn, V. (1984): Adverse reactions in selected patients following intravenous infusions of gamma globulin. *Am. J. Med.*, 76:25-32.
13. Delire, M., and Masson, P.L. (1977): The detection of circulating immune complexes in children with recurrent infections and their treatment with human immunoglobulins. *Clin. Exp. Immunol.*, 29:385-392.
14. Eibl, M. (1983): Treatment of defects of humoral immunity. *Birth Defects: Original Article Series*, 19:193-200.
15. Eibl, M.M., Cairns, L., and Rosen, F.S. (1984): Safety and efficacy of a monomeric, functionally intact intravenous IgG preparation in patients with primary immunodeficiency syndromes. *Clin. Immunol. Immunopathol.*, 31:151-160.
16. Ellis, E.F., and Henney, C.S. (1969): Adverse reactions following administration of human gamma globulin. *J. Allergy*, 43:45-54.
17. Gerritz, G., Pirofsky, B., and Nolte, M. (1976): The vasomotor syndrome induced by entravenous (IV) serum immune globulin (SIG). *J. Allergy Clin. Immunol.*, 57:253.

18. Geursen, R.G., Kroh, U., Krump, W., and Scharfe, B. (1982): Ursachen von Nebenwirkungen bei der Anwendung von intravenös applizierbaren Immunoglobulinen. *Beitr. Infusionstherapie klin. Ernähr.*, 9:95-114.
19. Goodwin, J.S., And Webb, D.R. (1980): Review: Regulation of the immune response by prostaglandins. *Clin. Immunol. Immunopathol.*, 15:106-122.
20. Gottlieb, M.S., Schroff, R., Schanker, H.M., Weisman, J.D., Fan, P.T., Wolf, R.A., and Saxon, A. (1981): Pneumocystis carinii pneumonia and mucosal candidiasis in previously healthy homosexual men: evidence of a new acquired cellular immunodeficiency. *N. Engl. J. Med.*, 305:1425-1431.
21. Hammarström, L., Persson, M.A.A., and Smith, C.I.E. (1983): Anti-IgA in selective IgA deficiency. In vitro effects and Ig subclass pattern of human anti-IgA. *Scand. J. Immunol.*, 18:509-513.
22. Hanson, L.A., Björkander, J., Ljunggren, C., Oxelius, V.-A., and Wadsworth, C. (1979): Problems with use of immunoglobulins in treatment of immunodeficient patients. In: *Immunoglobulins: Characteristics and Uses of Intravenous Preparations*, edited by B.M. Alving and J.S. Finlayson, pp. 151-159. US Dept. of Health and Human Services, Public Health Service.
23. Henney, C.S., and Ellis, E.F. (1968): Antibody production to aggregated human γ-G-globulin in acquired hypogammaglobulinemia. *N. Engl. J. Med.*, 278:1144-1146.
24. Homburger, H.A., Smith, J.R., Jacob, G.L., Laschinger, C., Naylor, D.H., and Pineda, A.A. (1981): Measurement of anti-IgA antibodies by a two-site immunoradiometric assay. *Transfusion*, 21:38-44.
25. Invernizzi, F., Balestrieri, G., Consogno, G., Riboldi, P.S., and Tincani, A. (1975): Anti-IgA antibodies in two brothers with selective serum IgA deficiency. *Acta haemat.*, 54:312-320.
26. John, T.J., Ninan, G.T., Rajagopalan, M.S., John, F., Flewett, T.H., Francis, D.P., and Zuckerman, A.J. (1979): Epidemic hepatitis B caused by commercal human immuno-globulin. *Lancet*, i: 1074.
27. Keusch, G.T., Olsson, R.A., and Troncale, F.J. (1969): Asymptomatic hepatitis in adults given γ-globulin for prophylaxis. *Arch. Intern. Med.*, 124:326-329.
28. Koistinen, J., Heikkilä, M., and Leikola, J. (1978): Gammaglobulin treatment and anti-IgA antibodies in IgA-deficient patients. *Brit. Med. J.*, 2:923-924.
29. Lane, R.S., Vallet, L., and Kavanagh, M.L. (1983): Human immunoglobulin for clinical use. *Lancet*, i:357-358.
30. Lane, R.S. (1983): Non-A, Non-B hepatitis from intravenous immunoglobulin. *Lancet*, ii:974-975.
31. Leikola, J., Koistinen, J., Lehtinen, M., and Virolainen, M. (1973): IgA-induced anaphylactic transfusion reactions: a report of four cases. *Blood*, 42:111-119.
32. Lever, A.M.L., Webster, A.D.B., Brown, D., and Thomas, H.C. (1984): Non-A, non-B hepatitis occurring in agammaglobulinaemic patients after intravenous immunoglobulin. *Lancet*, ii:1062-1064.
33. Lever, A.M.L., Webster, A.D.B., Brown, D., and Thomas, H.C. (1985): Non-A, non-B hepatitis after intravenous gammaglobulin. *Lancet*, i:587.
34. Liu, D.T.H., Grzenczyk, B.S., and Pai, R.C. (1979): Removal of anticomplementary activity from human immune serum globulins by treatment with purified human plasmin. *Transfusion*, 19:261-267.
35. Malgras, J., Hauptmann, G., Zorn, J.-J., and Waitz, R. (1970): Mesure de l'activité anti-complémentaire des préparations de gamma-globulines injectables par voie intraveineuse. *Revue Française de Transfusion*, XIII: 173-180.
36. Ochs, H.D., Buckley, R.H., Pirofsky, B., Fischer, S.H., Rousell, R.H., Anderson, C.J., and Wedgwood, R.J. (1980): Safety and patient acceptability of intravenous immune globulin in 10% maltose. *Lancet*, ii:1158-1159.
37. Ochs, H.D., Fischer, S.H., Virant, F.S., Lee, M.L., Kingdon, H.S., and Wedgwood, R.J. (1985): Non-A, non-B hepatitis and intravenous immunoglobulin. *Lancet*, i:404-405.
38. Passwell, J.H., Dayer, J.-M, and Merler, E. (1979): Increased prostaglandin production by human monocytes after membrane receptor activation. *J. Immunol.*, 123: 115-120.
39. Petrilli, F.L., Crovari, P., and De Flora, S. (1977): Hepatitis B in subjects treated with a drug containing immunoglobulins. *J. Infect. Dis.*, 135:252-258.
40. Philp, R.B. (1981): *Methods of testing proposed anti-thrombic drugs.* V. Platelet activating factor (PAF), pp. 114-128. CRC Press, Florida.
41. Pirofsky, B. (1984): Intravenous immune globulin therapy in hypogammaglobulinemia. A review. *Am. J. Med.*, 76:53-60.

42. Rivat, L., Rivat, C., Daveau, M., and Ropartz, C. (1977): Comparative frequencies of anti-IgA antibodies among patients with anaphylactic transfusion reactions and among normal blood donors. *Clin. Immunol. Immunopathol.*, 7:340-348.

43. Ropars, C., Caldera, L.H., Griscelli, C., Homberg, J.C., and Salmon, C. (1974): Anti-immunoglobulin antibodies in immunodeficiencies: their influence on intolerance reactions to gamma-globulin administration. *Vox Sang.*, 27: 294-301.

44. Ropars, C., Geay-Chicot, D., Cartron, J.P., Doinel, C., and Salmon, C. (1979): Human IgE response to the administration of blood components. II. Repeated gammaglobulin injections. *Vox Sang.*, 37:149-157.

45. Rosen, F. (1981): In panel discussion on indications and limitations of immunoglobulin prophylaxis and therapy. In: *Immunohemotherapy. A Guide to Immunoglobulin Prophylaxis and Therapy*, edited by U.E. Nydegger, pp. 451-460. Academic Press, London, New York, Toronto, Sydney, San Francisco.

46. Schmidt, A.P., Taswell, H.F., and Gleich, G.J. (1969): Anaphylactic transfusion reactions associated with anti-IgA antibody. *N. Engl. J. Med.*, 280:188-193.

47. Schwartz, R.S. (1980): Epstein-Barr virus - oncogen or mitogen? *N. Engl. J. Med.*, 302:1307-1308.

48. Skvaril, F., and Gozze, I., (1978): Anticomplementary properties of plasmin-treated human G immunoglobulin and its components. *Int. Archs. Allergy appl. Immun.*, 57: 375:378.

49. Stiehm, E.R., and Fudenberg, H.H. (1965): Antibodies to gammaglobulin in infants and children exposed to isologous gamma-globulin. *Pediatrics* 35:229-235.

50. Thompson, R.A., and Rees-Jones, A. (1979): The antibody deficiency syndrome: a report on current management. *Journal of Infection*, 1:49-60.

51. Tovo, P.-A., Gabiano, C., Roncarolo, M., and Altare, F. (1984): IgE content of commercial intravenous IgG preparations. *Lancet,* i:458.

52. Vyas, G.N., and Fudenberg, H.H. (1969): Isoimmune anti-IgA causing anaphylactoid transfusion reactions. *N. Engl. J. Med.*, 280:1073-1074.

53. Welch, A.G., Cuthbertson, B., McIntosh, R.V., and Foster, P.R. (1983): Non-A, non-B hepatitis from intravenous immunoglobulin. *Lancet,* ii:1198-1199.

Subtle, Antigen-Selective T-Cell Defects as a Cause of Relapsing Purulent Infections of the Upper Respiratory Tract

H.A. Drexhage, E.M. vand de Plassche, M. Kokié and H.A. Leezenberg

*Laboratory for Clinical Immunology, Department of Pathology
and the Department of Oto-rhino-laryngology
Free University Hospital, Amsterdam, NL*

Commensal bacteria, such as unencapsulated Haemophilus influenzae, streptococci and pneumococci, are considered to act as pathogen in relapsing, purulent infections of the respiratory tract (23). Such disorders are not only frequently observed in ENT and pediatric practice but also by the family doctor.

Acute infective respiratory tract diseases are still classified in developed countries as the third commonest cause of death in children aged 1 to 14 months despite a rapid decline in mortality when antibiotics became widely available. It has been estimated that each child acquired about 6 respiratory infections a year (2). There is however a small group of children in whom respiratory infections are even more common and no obvious cause can be found for their relapsing disease. These children in particular seem prone to airways disease at later age. Burrows et al. (6, amongst others) gathered epidemiologic evidence that frequent childhood respiratory illnesses not only led to some permanent impairment of lung function, but that such illnesses also predisposed to a more rapid deterioration of function during adult life and most importantly to a higher susceptibility for bronchial infections. Whether this is a direct result of the childhood illnesses leading to parenchymal destruction, or simply indicates and reflects a lifelong weaknesss of immune mechanisms of the airways remains unclear.

Regarding the adult, relapsing purulent infections of the respiratory tract, often complicated by atopy, consitute approximately 5% of ENT and pul-monologic outpatient consultations (at least in our hospital). Depending on the stage of the disease, the location of the infective focus, sampling methods, and culture conditions the frequency of isolation of the earlier mentioned commensal micro-organisms ranges from 25 to 100% (23). The special characteristics making these organisms important pathogens now are largely unknown, though a few cases have been reported based on well defined deficiencies in humoral immunity (17). In general, however, antibody production is intact and high titers of precipitating antibodies are found (5).

A further proposed mechanism facilitating for instance H. influenzae respiratory tract colonization is the production by the bacteria of a factor hampering ciliary movement of the bronchial epithelium (9). Antigen-antibody complex-mediated reactions (26) as well as atopic reactivity (18) have also been suggested as contributing to the pathogenetic mechanisms.

The role of T-cell mediated immunity (CMI) is not clear. Bacteria such as H. influenzae and streptococci are potent stimulators of the T-cell system (10) and it is therefore likely that CMI plays a part in these infective disorders. Moreover overt disturbances in CMI - as in Di George syndrome - are accompanied by bacterial infections of the respiratory tract. These notions have led us to study both antibody and cell mediated immune mechanisms to three different microbial antigens in 75 adult patients visiting the ENT department of our hospital for unexplained relapsing purulent rhinosinusitis. The inclusion criterium for the study was the lack of permanent response to surgical intervention to improve the drainage of the maxillary and ethmoidal sinuses, and the lack of response to repeated courses of antibiotics.

PATIENTS AND METHODS

Patients with chronically relapsing purulent rhinitis/sinusitis. The group included 75 patients (48 females, 27 males, aged 13 to 73 years, median 38 years) with unexplained chronic suppuration of the upper respiratory tract. All of them showed or had shown positive bacterial cultures on one or more occasions; H. influenzae was present in about 32% of the cases, Streptococcus pneumoniae in about 24%, other streptococci in 14% and staphylococci in 22%. In a few cases Escherichia coli and Branhamella were isolated. Duration of disease varied from 18 months up to approximately 40 years. All of the patients had been treated with several courses of antibiotics, which had given only temporary relief. All had been operated upon to improve drainage of the maxillary and ethmoidal sinuses; in all instances the operation had failed to cure them permanently.

Healthy individuals. This group included 37 healthy laboratory staff (20 females, 17 males, aged 24 to 44 years, median 33 years) with a negative personal and family history for atopy and autoimmunity.

Serum immunoglobulins and H. influenzae antibody titres

The concentration of serum IgG, IgM and IgA was measured by means of commercial available kits. Antibody titres to H. influenzae were estimated by means of a modification of the ELISA-technique, as described for anti-penicillin antibodies by De Haan et al. (8); using 100 μl volumes in U-shaped microtiterplates (Linbro, Flow Lab. Inc. USA). Rabbit anti-human IgG and IgM were purchased from DAKO (Kopenhagen). Horseradish peroxidase conjugated sheep-anti-rabbit IgG was a gift from Dr. D.M. Boorsma, Dept. of Dermatology. 5-amino 2-hydroxybenzoic acid in distilled water (pH 6.0) + 0.005% H_2O_2 was used as colour substrate. All dilutions were made in PBS (pH 7.4) containing 0.05% Tween 20 and 1% bovine serum albumin (BSA). Optimal conditions and dilutions for all the steps involved in the procedure were etablished by checkerboard titrations. After each incubation except the last, the plates were washed 5 times with deionized water containing 0.05% Tween 20.

Optimal coating conditions were found to be 10 μg/ml H. influenzae antigen in 0.1 M sodiumcarbonate buffer (pH 9.6, containing 0.02% NaN3), during 2 hours at 37°C. All subsequent incubations were 30 min. at 37°C. The end point of the reaction was read after the final incubation with substrate for 1 hour at room temperature, followed by 16 hours at 4°C, and expressed as the titre = −2 log dilution of the serum tested.

In absorption experiments, two volumes of serum were mixed with one volume of washed packed H. influenzae and incubated overnight at 4°C. The bacteria were removed by centrifugation (15 min. 3600 g) and the titre of the supernatant was estimate.

Skin tests

Somatic H. influenzae antigen was isolated using a combination of the techniques of Platt and Tunevall as described in detail before (10). This antigen has proven to be suitable for stimulating T-cells and particularly the aggregated form is an excellent dh skin test antigen, both in rats (10) and humans (19).

For use as skin test antigen a suspension of 250 μg aggregated material per milliliter 0.5% phenol in saline was prepared. The antigen was tested for potency in a rat skin test model (10) and only two batches with equal potencies were used throughout the reported studies.

A commercially available preparation of 1% candidal antigen (HAL allergens, Haarlem, The Netherlands) and a commercially available preparation of 100 U of Streptokinase/Streptodornase (SK/SD)/milliliter solvent (Varidase, Lederle, Wayne, Mich.) were also used as skin test antigens, as was PHA, which was obtained from Wellcome Laboratories (Kent, UK). This material was used as a control at a strength of 5 μg/ml saline.

Delayed responsiveness to these antigens was tested by intradermal injection of 0.1 ml of each of these antigen preparations into the forearm. In each patient all four skin tests were carried out at one single occasion. Skin reactions were read at 30 min., 6, 24, 48 and 72 hours and the diameter of induration was recorded.

The criterium for a delayed response was a maximal swelling at 24-48 hours.

We regard such responsiveness as T-cell mediated, firstly because such reactions occur in experimental animals passively sensitized by T-cell transfer (10), and secondly because the histology of such reactions in normal healthy individuals show perivascular lymphocytic infiltrations of mainly T-helper cell phenotype, a feature of delayed skin test hypersensitivity (19).

Lymphocyte proliferative responsiveness to bacteria antigens

Heparinized blood was collected by venopuncture just prior to skin testing. Density-gradient centrifugation was used to isolate mononuclear cells. Cells were washed twice with Hank's balanced salt solution.

Lymphocyte cultures in the presence of 20% pooled human serum were carried out. The lymphoid cells were cultured on Linbro/Titertek microplates (Flow, Irvine, Scotland) using 0.15 ML Hepes-buffered RPMI 1640 (Gibco, Glasgow, Scotland) supplemented with antibiotics. In time-and dose-response curves with cells of five healthy controls the optimal antigen concentration for DNA synthesis to occur was found to be 15 µg/ml culture fluid for both somatic H. influenzae antigen and candidin and 10 U/ml for SK/SD. The optimal time of culture was 6 days. The optimal cell concentration was $10 \times 10^{*}5$ cells per well. The results are expressed in terms of the stimulation indices (SI), i.e. the ratio of the uptake of [3H] thymidine in antigen stimulated/control cultures. The SI of lymphoid cells isolated from neonatal cord blood were measured to determine the nonspecific mitogenic capacity of the bacterial antigens. On three occasions the responder lymphoid cells were depleted of B cells by incubating them on plastic petri dishes coated with Ig (panning technique). This procedure almost completely depleted our suspensions of B cells (13 to 2%). The SI of these depleted suspensions reached the same or even higher levels, indicating the T-cell nature of the test. Proliferative responsiveness to PHA was also measured using a 3-day culture of $4 \times 10^{*}4$ cells with a 5-hr [3H] thymidine pulse.

Two-step MIF-assay with bacterial antigens

The MIF-assay was carried out as described by von Blomberg-v.d. Flier et al. (4) with slight adaptations (14). Lymphoid cells, isolated as described above, were cultured in conical 15 ml tubes ($2.5 \times 10^{*}6$ in 1 ml) in RPMI 1640, supplemented with HEPES, antibiotics and 10% fetal calf serum (FCS). Antigens were added to the cultures to give final concentrations of 0, 5, 10 and 25µg/ml for H. influenzae; 5, 10 and 25 µg/ml for candidin and 1, 5 and 25 I.U./ml for SK/SD. Supernatants (10 min, 2000 x g) were harvested after 3 days of culture (37°C, 5% CO_2 in air), diluted 1:1 with fresh culture medium containing 10% fetal calf serum and tested for MIF activity in a second step.

For this purpose the agarose microdroplet assays was used, the U937 monocytes being indicator cells: a U937 cell pellet (37°C) was suspended ($2 \times 10^{*}7$ cells/ml) in 0.2% agarose (20 mg sea plaque agarose, Marine Colloids, Rockland) dissolved in 1 ml PBS at 120°C and diluted 10x with RPMI 1640 10% FCS and antibiotics. From this suspension 1 µg droplets were placed in flat bottomed microplates using a Hamilton Repeating Dispenser with 0.05 ml gas-tight syringe. After solidifying (19-20 min, 40°C) droplets were overlaid with 100µl of the original culture fluid possibly containing MIF (all tests were carried out in five fold). After incubation of the covered plates during 21 hours at 37°C with 5% CO_2 in air, the migration area was measured using a projection microscope. MIF production was expressed as % migration inhibition: MI = (100 - 100 x (mean area in cultures with bacterial antigen)/(mean area in cultures without bacterial antigen))%.

The U937 cell-line was kindly provided by Dr. G. Garotta (Hoffmann La Roche, Basel). The cell-line was maintained by propagation in RPMI 1640, supplemented with HEPES, glutamine, antibiotics and 10% FCS. U937 cells were harvested in logarithmic growth phase, washed and then utilized as indicator cells in the MIF-assays as indicated above.

Enumeration of peripheral lymphocyte subsets

After isolation lymphoid cells were resuspended in RPMI 1640 containing 5% fetal calf serum. T-cell subsets were estimated by indirect immunofluorescence with mouse anti human monoclonal antibodies (Ortho, New York; Becton, Lakeside) and fluorescein-labelled goat-anti-mouse antiserum (Dako, California). After two washes, wetslide preparations were examined. 200 cells were observed and positively stained cells counted.

B cells were estimated by means of their surface Ig positivity using a commercial available kit based on the binding of B lymphocytes with anti-Ig labelled particles (Immunobeads, Biorad, Richmond, California).

RESULTS

Serum Ig's, H. influenzae specific antibodies, and percentages of circulating B-cells

The levels of serum immunoglobulins were found perfectly normal (fig. 1a) in practically all patients except for a slightly raised IgG, IgM and IgA in a few. Only one case (a female, aged 22 years) out of 36 tested showed a lowered serum IgA. This prevalence for partial IgA deficiency of around 2-3% is comparable to that found in a normal healthy population (15). With regard to specific antibodies of IgG and IgM class to H. influenzae, again near normal levels were found (fig. 1b), indicating that antibody production to one of the important microbes colonizing the respiratory tract of the patient was completely intact. Such observation of a well functioning B-cell system in patients with relapsing rhinosinusitis have been reported by others before (5). The intact B-cell responsiveness was further illustrated by the normal percentages of B-cells (fig. 1c) found in the circulation of practically all patients; only one

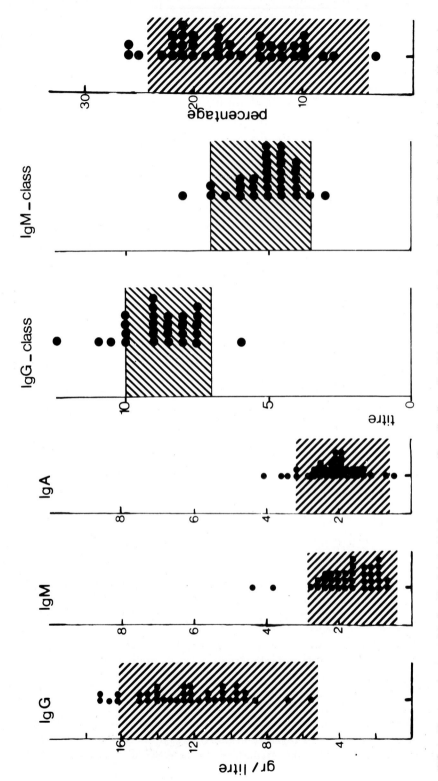

FIG. 1. The serum immunoglobulins (fig. 1a), the H. influenzae specific antibodies (fig. 1b) and the ciruclanting s-Ig+cells (B-cells, fig. 1c) of patients with relapsing purulent rhinosinusitis (●). The hatched area represents the range found in healthy controls. In essence normal levels and percentages were found.

out of 37 (a female, aged 24) showed a lower percentages (3%). She had normal serum IgG, IgM and IgA, but a raised IgE (105 U/ml).

D.H. Skin tests

The microbial skin test antigens (Candidin, SK/SD and the somatic H. influenzae antigen) roughly produced two patterns of reactivity which are shown in fig. 2: a pattern with a maximal swelling at 24-48 hours (normal dh responsiveness) and a pattern which lacked this delayed reactivity (a defective dh responsiveness). 95% of our healthy controls showed normal dh responsiveness) to all three antigens with maximal swellings at 24-48 hours; only one had a defective response to one of the antigens (H. influenzae). In contrast, 44 of our patients (59%) showed a defective dh response; not only to one, but even to more of the antigens tested (25% to two antigens and 2% to all three antigens). Defective dh reactivity to candidin and SK/SD was noted in 71%; to H. influenzae in 32%. In all patients the induration of the skin test to PHA was normal, indicating that the defective T-cell responsiveness was selective for the microbial antigens used and did not reflect a state of general impairment of delayed inflammatory responsiveness.

Lymphocyte proliferative responsiveness

The DNA synthesis of peripheral lymphoid cells in response to the three microbial antigens and PHA was also tested. The data for H. influenzae somatic antigen are shown in fig. 3, the antigen appeared to have slight mitogenic capacity as it stimulated cord blood cells with stimulation indices up to 4.5. 68% of 38 healthy controls showed SI higher than those obtained with cord blood cells (range 4.5-21), which probably indicates the ongoing stimulation with ubiquitous H. influenzae antigen in a normal population. Some of the healthy controls were followed throught time, and strong fluctuations of SI were found ranging from positive to even negative indicating a rapid disappearance from and appearance in the circulation of these antigen-specific lymphoid cells.

Sixty-six percent of the chronic purulent sinusitis/rhinitis patients showed stimulation indices equal to or even higher than those of the healthy controls (range 6-45). This indicates that T-cell proliferative responsiveness is in general intact and that the very high SI probably reflect the very high exposure rates to H. influenzae in some of the patients. There were, however, three patients with persistent negative responses, tests being performed over a period of 6 months, though all were heavily infected with H. influenzae. This persistent negativity might therefore be and indication of a defective microbe-specific T-cell proliferative responsiveness in these few patients.

In essence, proliferative responses obtained with SK/SD and candidin were similar to those for H. influenzae and are hence not shown. PHA responsiveness was found normal in all controls and patients tested.

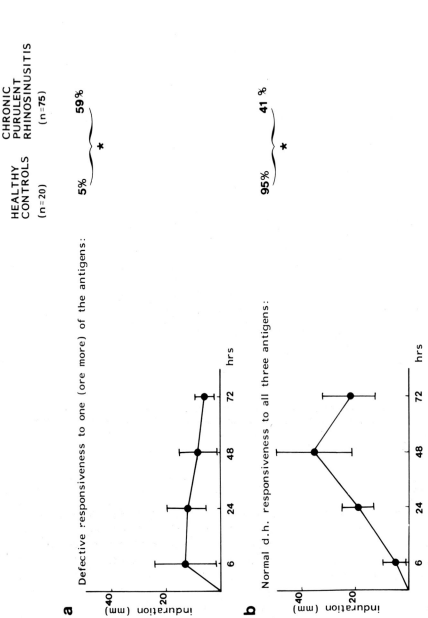

FIG. 2. The skin test reactivity to H influenzae somatic antigen (as an example) in healthy controls and patients with relapsing purulent upper respiratory tract infections. Means (●) +/− s.d. of swelling (induration) in time course are given. * = statistiscally significant difference (p < 0.05, x² test).

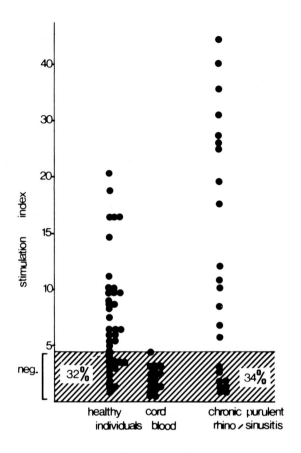

FIG. 3. The stimulation indices of lymphocyte proliferation assays with H. influenzae - one of the important microbes - as stimulatory antigen. Normal to even enhanced proliferation was found.

MIF-assay

Fig. 4 shows the data of the MIF-assay carried out in 39 patients. Patients with a defective dh skin test to either one of the antigens mostly showed an impairment of the in vitro MIF-production to that antigen as well, and in general a good correlation was found between the dh skin test and the MIF-assay (data not shown).

On the whole 76% (16 out of 21) of the skin test defective patients were defective MIF-producers, whereas only 28% (5 out of 18) in the normal skin test group showed this in vitro defect. The in vitro MIF-data further substantiate the microbe-selective defective T-cellular responsiveness of the patients as found in the in vivo skin test assay.

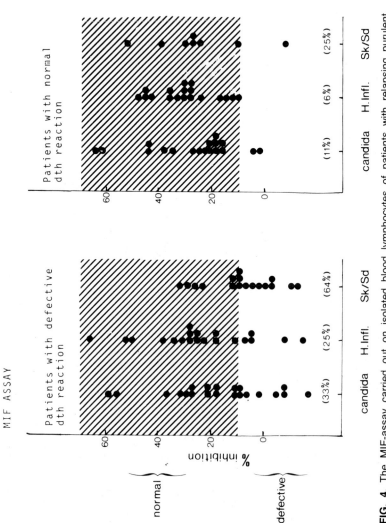

FIG. 4. The MIF-assay carried out on isolated blood lymphocytes of patients with relapsing purulent rhinosinusitis. The data are given for the three separate antigens. The hatched area represents the normal range of inhibition found in healthy controls. Figures in parentheses are the percentages of defective MIF-producers. In the skin test defective group 16 out of 21 (76%) showed defective MIF-production to one or more of the antigens. In the normal skin test group only 5 out of 18 (28%) showed such defective MIF-production.

Marker expression of circulating T lymphocytes

The percentages of circulating lymphoid cells, showing the T-11 marker (E-receptor) was found diminished in our patients, particularly in the group of patients with defective dh skin tests (fig. 5, 35% of defective skin test responders showed percentages lower than 60). In contrast the expression of the T-3 marker was practically normal (only 3 out of 35 showed a marginally lower expression). This discrepancy again indicates a subtle defect in the T-cell system of the patients.

The Leu3a/OKT8 ratio was calculated to get an impression of the balance between T helper and T suppressor function (fig. 5). Elevated ratios (over 2.1) were noted both in the skin test normals (22%) as in the skin test defective group (42%). In the latter it appeared by further exploration that those with a raised Leu3a/OKT8 ratio were mostly the ones who additionally had atopic complaints and an elevated serum IgE (see below).

Other immune disturbances in patients with defective T-cell function

Just over half of the patients with T-cell defects and relapsing suppuration of the upper respiratory tract showed other immunological disorders, such as atopic complaints and atopic skin test reactivity to common allergens as grass pollen and house dust mite. A raised serum IgE (higher than 100 IU/ml) was present in 39% (it must be brought forward that a raised serum IgE was even more prevalent in those with a normal dh skin test - namely in 60% - and atopy might therefore be the prime disturbance for the upper respiratory tract complaints in this group of patients). In 17% of the dh skin test defective patients upper respiratory tract complaints were accompanied by thyroid autoimmune disease including thyroid atrophy treated with thyroxin, recurrent simple sporadic goiter, transient attacks of Graves' disease, and cases of positive thyroid autoantibodies without overt thyroid disease.

27% showed or had shown episodes of recurrent infections of the skin with staphylococci (furunculosis or pyogenic dermatitis), whereas only 10% had or had had episodes of dematophytosis. Most of the patients had first degree relatives with histories of chronic respiratory illnesses (40%) or thyroid autoimmune disease (33%, one of the patients had a mother with polyendocrine autoimmunity).

Antibiotic treatment

A group of ten patients were tested as described before and six were classified as "defective T-cell responders". They were treated with a six-weeks course of doxacyclin (first day 200 mgs, thereafter 100 mgs daily). Bacteria cultured from their nose and throat were invariably sensitive for this antibiotic. In the week after completing the course patients were retested; data are shown in table 1. In none of them T-cell responsiveness, as measured by dh skin test

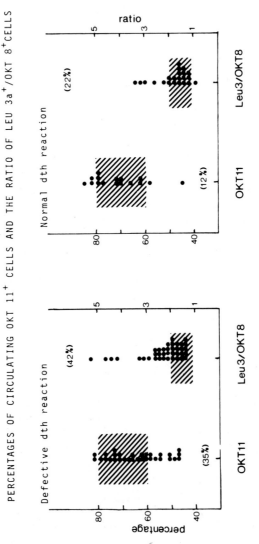

FIG. 5. The percentages of circulating OKT11⁺ positive cells together with the Leu3a to OKT8⁺ cell ratio in patients with relapsing purulent rhinosinusitis. The hatched areas represents the ranges found in healthy controls. In the skin test defective group 35% of patients showed a defective expression of the T11-marker, whereas 42% had raised T-helper to T-suppressor/cytotoxic cell ratios.

TABLE 1. *The skin test and MIF-assay before and after a six-week course of doxacycline in 6 patients with relapsing purulent infections of the upper respiratory tract*

	Pretreatment	Posttreatment
Skin test defect to candidin in:	3/6 (50%)	4/5 (80%)
to Sk/Sd in:	4/6 (66%)	4/6 (66%)
MIF test defect to candidin in:	3/6 (50%)	2/5 (40%)
to Sk/Sd in:	3/6 (50%)	2/5 (40%)
to H. infl. in:	2/6 (33%)	1/5 (20%)

or MIF-assay improved, though suppuration of the respiratory tract stopped and bacterial cultures became negative.

Levamisole treatment

Thirteen patients classified as T-cell defective were put on levamisole (150 mgs, once weekly). Eleven completed a half years course; two stopped due to severe side effects such as skin rashes, fever and nausea. In total 7 complained of such side effects, ranging from mild headache and nausea to fever and severe skin rashes. The beneficial effects of levamisole were however striking, and became evident some 3-4 months after taking the drug. In 7 of the 11 who completed the course purulent secretion stopped and bacterial cultures became negative. Six of these seven were available for T-cell testing: two had become completely normal in dh skin test and MIF-assay, another two showed clear improvements. These results encourage us to undertake a double blind cross over trial with levamisole.

DISCUSSION

All patients in this study had relapsing purulent infections of the upper respiratory tract colonized by predominantly H. influenzae and streptococci, and yet in a considerable proportion T-cell responsiveness to somatic antigen of H. influenzae and to streptokinase/streptodornase as measured by dh skin test and MIF production was found absent. These findings are in agreement with those of Palmer, who studied a group of patients with chronic sinopulmonary disease, which also lacked delayed hypersensitivity to candidin, trichophyton, streptokinase/streptodornase, PPD, or histoplasmin but reacted weakly to DNCB sensitization and challenge.

Though the subject is still controversial (21), delayed skin test reactivity and MIF-production are generally regarded as reflecting the state of protective immunity to chronic bacterial infections (3). Absent T-cell reactivity to bacterial antigen as found in our patients may therefore be a strong indication of a high susceptibility to these bacteria and they might thus be causative for the relapsing purulent infection. Nevertheless, our data in fact only show a relationship between suppuration of the upper respiratory tract and T-cellular defects and they may therefore also be explained in the way that the found T-cellular defects are not a cause but a consequence of the purulent infection. The data, however, obtained in the patients treated with doxacyclin do not support this latter view: the T-cell defects were still present right after treatment when the suppuration had stopped.

The restricted T-cellular defects to bacterial antigens as described here in our patients are reminiscent of the immune defects found in chronic mucocutaneous candidiasis and other dermatophytoses. The underlying abnormalities of the immune system in chronic candidiasis have been described as heterogeneous, though the majority of patients show a defective T-cell system, involving disturbed T-cell cytotoxicity and impaired production of lymphokines (16). The candidiasis sometimes occurs in whole families and is then often accompanied by other immune disturbances such as IgA deficiencies and autoimmune endocrinopathies (1). It is assumed that under these latter circumstances a concomitant defect in the T-cell regulatory system explains the exaggerated endocrine autoantibody production.

A further well-defined disease entity based on T-cellular defects is the relapsing pyogenic dermatitis caused by S. aureus. Apart from defects in dh skin test reactivity to this micro-organism patients often show high levels of serum IgE and atopic dermatitis (14).

It is most remarkable that our patients also showed a high incidence of thyroid autoimmunity and atopy. Such a high prevalence of these disorders in patients with chronic purulent sputum production has been reported before (22). In this respect it is worthy to note the other abnormality in T-cell function in our patients: namely the elvated ratio of T helper to T suppressor/ cytotoxic cells. It is tempting to speculate that such an imbalance in T-cell regulatory function must lead to uncontrolled exaggerated IgE immunoglobulin synthesis (7) which underlies most forms of atopy. It might also bring about the escape of autoimmune B-cell clones (11) giving rise to the thyroid autoimmunity.

Relapsing purulent infections of the upper respiratory tract seem closely related to chronic candidiasis and relapsing chronic dermatitis; first, because both latter disorders are often complicated by purulent infections of the respiratory tract (14, 24); and secondly, a considerable number of our patients (27%) had had periods of pyogenic dermatitis and furunculosis.

The cause of the defects in T-cell function in our patients is speculative. Viruses, notably measles and influenza virus, are able to suppress immune T-cell function and thus pave the way for commensal micro-organisms (12). Well known are the episodes of acute H. influenzae pneumonia accompanying epidemics of influenza. Whether relapsing respiratory infections might evolve due to more sustained T-cell defects after virus infection is unknown. In our group 25% of the patients had a clear history of influenza preceding the onset of their purulent infections of the upper respiratory tract. However, it must be borne in mind that all these patients also had a positive family history for chronic respiratory diseases. Hence, genetic influences probably play a very important role; this is further indicated by the high incidence of chronic respiratory diseases and other immunologic disorders in the first-degree relatives of all our patients. Moreover, it is now well accepted that T-cell-mediated immunity to micro-organisms is governed by class II structures coded for in the major histocompatibility genes.

In children with chronically relapsing upper respiratory tract infections beneficial effects have been described of the drug levamisole (25). Levamisole treatment was also started in 13 of our patients with restricted dh defects to bacterial antigens. Two could not take the drug for longer than one to three months, due to severe adverse side effects. Eleven have, however, completed a half-year course and seven showed clear clinical improvement substantiated by a reversion of both the skin test and the MIF-assay from defective to improve/intact in four out of six tested cases. This indicates that therapeutical approaches to restore the defective T-cell mediated immunity might be feasible in our patients.

In conclusion our study indicates that defects in cell-mediated immunity form a likely basis for a considerable proportion of relapsing upper respiratory tract infections in adults. Such infections are often found in combination with other immune disorders such as atopy and thyroid autoimmunity, and are reminiscent of the T-cell disorders playing a role in chronic mucocutaneous candidiasis and pyogenic dermatosis.

REFERENCES

1. Arulanatham K., Dwyer, J., and Genel, M., 1979. Evidence for defective immunoregulation in the syndrome of familial candidiasis endocrinopathy. *N. Engl. J. Med.* 25:164.
2. Beard, L.J., Maxwell, G.M., Thong, Y.H., 1981. Immunocompetence of children with frequent respiratory infections. *Ach. Diseases in Childhood,* 56:101.
3. Berger, M.L., and Blanden, R.V., 1981. The T-lymphocyte in infectious pathology. *Path. Res. Pract.* 171:128.
4. Blomberg-vd Flier BME, Burg CKH v.d., Pos O., Plassche-Boers, E.M., v.d., Ketel, W.G., v., and Scheper, R.J. In vitro diagnosis of nickel allergy: the MMIT revisited. In: Experimental Contact Dermatitis (eds. C. Benezra, N., Hunziker, T., Maurer, R.J., Scheper, and J.L. Turk). *Roche Publications,* Basel.
5. Burns, M.W. and May, R.J., 1967. H. Influenzae precipitins in the serum of patients with chronic bronchial disorders. *Lancet i:* 354.
6. Burrows, B., Lebowitz, M.D., Knudson, R.J., 1977. Epidemiologic evidence that childhood problems predispose to airways disease in the adult (an association between adult and pediatric respiratory disorders). *Pediat. Res.* 11:218.
7. Canonica, G.W., Mingari, M.C. et al. 1979. Imbalances of T-cell subpopulations in patients with atopic diseases and effect of specific immunotherapy. *J. Immunol.* 123:2669.
8. De Haan, P., Boorsma, D.H., and Kalsbee, G.L. 1979. Penicillin hypersensitivity. Determination and classification of anti-penicillin antibodies by the ELISA. *Allergy* 34:111.
9. Denny, F.W., 1974. Effect of a toxin produced by H. influenzae on ciliated respiratory epithelium. *J. Inf. Dis.* 129:93.
10. Drexhage, H.A. and Oort, J., 1977. Skin test reactivity to H. influenzae antigens as an outcome of the antigen structure and the balance between humoral and cell mediated immunity in rats. *Clin. Exp. Immunol.,* 28:280.
11. Drexhage, H.A., Bottazzo, G.F., 1985. The thyroid and autoimmunity. *Pediatr. adolesc. Endocr.,* vol. 14, Karger, Basel (in press).
12. Editorial, 1982. How does influenza virus pave the way for bacteria. *Lancet i:* 485.

13. Editorial. March 30, 1985. Lower respiratory tract infections in childhood. *The Lancet,* pp. 734-735.
14. Hanifin, J.J.M., Lobitz, W.C. 1977. Review Article. New concepts of Atopic dermatitis. *Arch. Dermatol.* 113:663.
15. Hayward, A.R., 1977. Immunodeficiency. *Edward Arnold,* London.
16. Lehner, T., Wilton, J.M.A., Ivanyi. L., 1972. Immunodeficiencies in chronic mucutaneous candidiasis. *Immunology.* 22:775.
17. Palmer, S.H., 1976. Immunodeficiency and pulmonary disease. In: Lung biology in health and disease . (C.H., Kirkpatrick, H.Y., Reynolds, eds.), Vol. I, pp. 191-209. *Marcel Dekker,* New York.
18. Pauwels, R., Verschaegen, G. and Van der Straeten, M., 1980. IgE antibodies to bacteria in patients with bronchial asthma. *Allergy* 157:655.
19. Plassche-Boers, E.M., vd., Drexhage, H.A. and Kokjé-Kleingeld, M. The use of somatic antigen of H. influenzae for the monitoring of T-cell mediated skin test reactivity in man (submitted).
20. Plassche-Boers, E.M., vd, Drexhage, H.A. The dh skin test reactivity, the MIF-production and blastgenic responsiveness of T-cells to bacterial antigens in patients with relapsing purulent rhinosinusitis (submitted).
21. Rook, G.A.W., Stanford, J.L., 1979. The relevance to protection of three forms of delayed skin-test response evoked by M. leprae and other mycobacteria in mice. Correlation with the classical work in the guinea pig. *Parasite Immunology.* 1:111.
22. Turner-Warwick, M., and Cole, P. 1982. Lung disease. In: Clinical Aspects of Immunology. (P.J. Lachmann, and D.K. Peters, eds.), 4th ed., vol. II, pp. 822-852. *Blackwell Scientific,* Oxford.
23. Turk, D.C. and May, J.R., 1967. Haemophilus influenzae, its clinical importance. *English University Press,* London.
24. Valdimarsson, H., Higgs, J.M., Wells, R.S., Yamamura, M., Hobbs, J.R. and Holt, P.J.C., 1973. Immune abnormalities associated with chronic mucocutaneous candidiasis. *Cell. Immunol.* 6:348.
25. Van Eygen, M., Znamensky, P.Y. et al. 1976. Levamisole in prevention of recurrent upper respiratory tract infections in children. *Lancet i:* 38.
26. Zwan, J.C., vd, Kaufmann, H.K., Orie, N.M.G. and De Vries, K., 1977. Broncho-obstructive reactions with antigenic and toxic components of H. influenzae. *Acta Tuberc. Pneumol. Belg.* 68:281.

Participation of the Cellular Immunologic System in the Duchenne Muscular Dystrophy?

R. Beckmann[1], W. Pernice[1] and G. Löhr[2]

[1] *University Childrens hospital - Mathildenstr. 1 - D-7800 Feiburg*
[2] *Serono Pharmazeutische Präparate GmbH*
Merzhauser Str. 134 D-7800 Feriburg

INTRODUCTION

Immune-pathogenesis is incontestable in case of certain inflammatory myopathies like dermatomyositis and pseudomyopathic polymyositis; it is based on the detection of perivascular round-cell infilatrates, or on mononuclear cells without a visible relation to the vessels.

Also in case of muscular dystrophy one will find inflammatory reactions within the sceleton muscle, but this in a clearly smaller extension. Table 1 shows essential data of the important and numerous types of muscular dystrophy.

Assumptions that also in case of muscular dystrophy immune reactions caused by cells might be of importance remained unconfirmed. The existence of inflammatory infiltrates was explained by unspecific degrading processes.

In most types of muscular dystrophy a defect of the muscle cell membrane was demonstrated and an increased influx of calcium into not yet necrotic muscle cells is proved in Duchenne muscular dystrophy (DMD). Calcium is a lethal factor for the muscle cells and increases the muscle cell necrosis (1, 2).

The malignant Duchenne muscular dystrophy is to be found in males. Numerical statements world-wide refer to one boy with 1:3000/4000 new borns. The mother is transferring the pathophysiological gene having the same on one of the X-chromosomes. A causal treatment does not yet exist.

The myopathy is manifesting slowly and painless during the third and fifth year with the boys who seem to be healthy. In the age of 7-12 years the boys become hampered in walking and dependent on the invalid chair in consequence of slowly increasing necroses of the striated musculature and replacement of the same by connective tissue of no functional value.

TABLE 1. *Hereditary Muscular Dystrophy Forms*

Form	Sex Affected	Mode of Transmission	Age of Begin	Course and Prognosis
Pelvic-Girdle or infantile severe form (Duchenne)	Male	Sex-Linked, recessive	In the first 3 years of life	The ability to walk is lost between age 7-12 live expectency is shortened.
Benign (Becker) Type			Age 6-19	Slower, milder course with loss of walking ability after age 50.
Limb-Girdle Type (Leyden)	Male and female	Autosomal recessive	Age 2-40	The disease has a severe course with early onset, otherwise showing a mild course Live expectency is sometimes shortend.
Shoulder-Girdle or juvenile forms: Facio-Scapulo-humeral MD (ERB)	Male and female	Dominant	Age 7-25	Mild course with only rare loss of walking ability. Muscle function is not usually affected until after Age 30. Normal life-expectancy. This type of MD shows a descending (Distal) cause of affection.
Distal muscular dystrophy	Male and female	Dominant	Age 5-77	Mild course with normal life-expectency.
Oscular Muscular dystrophy	Male and female	Irregulary dominant?	Up to Age 60	Shows a slow lingering progress, usually over decades, limited to the outer eye-muscles.

Finally the **children become** completely invalide until death between the 18th and 22nd **year of life, scarcely later,** owing to a pulmonary affection and the dystrophic **cardiomyopathy (table 2 and 3).** Recent data in DMD-patients showed alterations of the **lymphocytes (3). Therefore, we** decided to differentiate lymphocyte subsets **in the peripheral blood of** patients with muscular dystrophies.

TABLE 2. *The clinical symptoms and progression of the malignant pelvic-girdle muscular dystrophies (Duchenne)*

1. A delayed statomotorical development or loss of the motor functions after a normal infancy. Clinical symptoms begin between age 7-12.
2. The muscle weakness begins in the pelvic girdle and in the thighs - increasing muscle atrophies are observed, thus leading to waddling, walking on one's tiptoes, difficulty in getting up from either a sitting or lying position, climbing up one's self to get to a standing position (Gower's sign) or using furniture as support.
3. Pseudohypertrophism is observed, especially affecting the calves or the tongue muscle.
4. If the disease remains untreated, the increasing loss of movement can lead to the development of contractures.
5. In the later course of the disease, the shoulder girdle becomes affected causing so-called scapulae alatae. The face muscles are rarely affected.
6. The spine and the skeleton itself can be affected (e.g. causing funnel breast) in a later stage of this disease.
7. Heart involvement.

Progression:
The progression is gradual, however at differing paces; long periods of standstill are possible. The patients lose their ability to walk between age 7-12 and most die of pulmonary or cardiac complications, before reaching age 25.

Diagnosis:
An early diagnosis is possible by examining the blood of the umbilical cord.

TABLE 3. *The clinical signs of muscular dystrophy*

1. *Progressive symmetrical wasting of the musculature.*
   On the trunk and the proximal extremeties, never showing even a spontaneous improvement. The chewing muscles as well as those of the tongue and soft palate are unaffected.
   In some cases (sub-forms) observed in the federal republic of germany, the musculature of the extremities was sometimes affected and the muscles of the eyes were mainly affected in the ocular muscular dystrophy.
2. Muscle weakness as well as hypotonia with symmetrical and functional impairment, eventually leading to flacid paralysis.
3. Decrease of the electrical muscular irritability, however no degeneration reaction or fibrillary and fascicular twitchings are observed; bladder, rectum as well as sensibility are all intact.
4. Pseudohyperthrophism is present, that is, an apparent increase of the muscle mass replaced by fatty- and connective tissue.
5. Inheritable disease with new mutations possible.
6. There is no involvement of either the central or peripheral nervous system.

MATERIALS AND METHODS

With help of a modern laser flow cytometry system (Spectrum III, Messrs. Ortho) the lymphocyte subsets of 20 DMD and limb-girdle patients were determined under standardized conditions:

1. OKT-11*   T-lymphocytes
2. OKT-4*   helper/inducer T-cells
3. OKT-8*   suppressor/cytotoxic T-cells
4. Anti-LEU-7**   LGL/NK-cells
4. Anti-LEU-10**   B cells, monocytes

As it is known that T-lymphocyte deficiencies appearing in different diseases can successfully be treated with thymic hormones (4, 5) we decided to treat the T-cell-deficiencies of 6 patients with muscular dystrophies with Thymostimulin (Tp-1 Serono®), a poly-peptide preparation with immuno-modulating activity.

Treatment scheme:
1st and 2nd week (5 times a week)
1 mg Thymostimulin ***/kg body weight/day i.m.
3rd and 4th week (3 times a week)
1 mg Thymostimulin/kg body weight/day i.m.
5th and 6th week (once a week)
1 mg Thymostimulin/kg body weight/day i.m.
The immunological parameters were followed over a period of 12 month.

RESULTS AND DISCUSSION

The present study examined the courses of various T-cell subpopulations in 20 patients suffering form Duchenne and limb-girdle muscular dystrophy. LGL/NK-cells (LEU-7-positive cells), suppressor cells (OKT-8-positive cells) and helper cells (OKT-4-positive cells) were completely within the norm. B-lymphocytes (LEU-10-positive cells) were elevated and didn't change during the observation time. In some of the patients (N = 6) the number of T-lymphocytes (OKT-11 positive cells) in the peripheral blood was decreased. Those patients were treated with the thymic hormone preparation Thyumostimulin (Tp-1 Serono®). This therapy led to an increase of the T-lymphocytes in the peripheral blood. (Fig. 1).

The course of the T-cell number in 14 patients with normal T-lymphocytes was followed for one year. In these patients a declining trend of T-cell-numbers was observed. (Fig. 2). However, at present the clinical efficacy of the trial cannot yet be evaluated, due to the slow and variously progressing course of muscular dystrophy. A two year observation period is required.

---

*   Ortho Diagnostic Systems Inc. Raritan, New Jersey 08869, USA
**   Becton Dickinson Laboratory Systems - 2800 Mechelen, Belgium
*** Tp-1 Serono® Serono GmbH - 7800 Feiburg, West Germany.

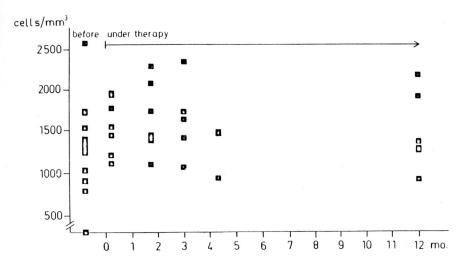

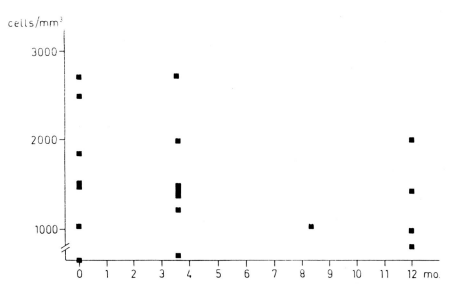

REFERENCES

1. Beckmann R. 1984. Klin. Wschr. 96, 599.
2. Beckmann R. 1983. Wissenschaftliche Zeitschrift der Friedirch-Schiller. Universität Jena, III. *Jenaer Myologie Kolloquium* 4/5, 673.
3. Pickard, N.A. et al. 1978. *New Engl. J. Med.* 299, 841.
4. Hobbs, J.R., Byrom, N.A., et al. 1985. Thymic Factor Therapy, *Raven Press*. 16, 175-187.
5. Fiorilli, M., Pivetti-Pezzi, P. et al. 1985. Thymic Factor Therapy, *Raven Press* 16, 205-210.

Improvement of T-Cell Percentage in Old People after Thymostimulin*-Therapy

J. Neumüller, A. Dunky, R. Eberl, G. Partsch

*Ludwig Boltzmann-Institute of Rheumatology and Balneology, Vienna-Oberlaa,
and 2nd Medical Department of the Municipal Hospital of Vienna-Lainz, Austria*

INTRODUCTION

Thymic hormones are known to improve T-lymphocyte dysregulations in primary or secondary immunodeficient syndromes and in several malignant disorders even after cytostatic therapy (1, 3, 9, 11, 12). The reasons for lymphocyte dysregulations are either a failure in lymphocyte maturation from pre-T-to helper or suppressor cells or the disappearance of those cells in the peripheral blood.

In old people the majority of immune functions is impaired leading to an increased suceptibility fo recurrent infections, predominantly of the urogenital system and the respiratory tract and a higher incidence for malignancies. (6, 7, 8, 10). In order to evaluate the influence of Thymostimulin-therapy in age-dependent cellular immunodeficiency, we investigated the T-cell subsets in peripheral blood before and during the treatment with this hormone.

PATIENTS AND METHODS

Patients and treatment scheme

14 out of 24 patients (71-84 years old) with recurrent infections of the urinary or respiratory tract were selected for this study. The selection criterion was a decreased T-lymphocyte percentage (OKT 3 pos cells < 60%, OKT 11 pos. cells < 70%). 7 of the selected patients were treated with Thymostimulin for 12 weeks. The hormone was administered i.m. as follows:

during the 1st week	50 mg daily,
during the 2nd week	50 mg every second day,
from the 3rd to the 12 th week	50 mg twice per week.

7 patients remained untreated and served as controls.

Determination of lymphocyte subsets was carried out before and after 1, 2, 4, 8 and 12 weeks from the begin of Thymostimulin-treatment.

Test procedure

Peripheral mononuclear cells (MNC) were isolated from 20 ml heparinized venous blood using a Ficoll-Paque separation medium according to the method of Byum (4, 5). Lymphocytes were washed twice in RPMI 1640 and supplemented with 5% fetal calf serum. The cell number was adjusted to 10^7/ml. The cell suspension was cooled to 4°C and separated in 9 wells a 100 µl in Seromat plates (Greiner) (total volume of one well: 200 µl). 10 respectively 5µl of monoclonal antibodies (MoAb) or antisera were mixed with the cell suspension of one well of the plate according to the scheme (Table 1). The percentage of fluorescent cells was determined using a Zeiss photomicroscope III with epifluorescence and compared with normal values (2).

TABLE 1.

MoAb	Producer	Lymphocyte subset	Volume
Leu M3 Phycoerythrin conjugated	Becton and Dickinson	Monocytes	5 µl
OKT 3 FITC conjug.		Pan T-cells	
OKT 11 FITC conjug.	Ortho Diagnostic Inc.	Pan T-cells	10 µl
OKT 4 FITC conjug.		T-helper/inducer cells	
OKT 8 FITC conjug.		T-suppressor/cytotoxic cells	
Leu 7 FITC conjug.	Becton and Dickinson	Natural killer cells	
Leu 10 FITC conjug.		B-lymphocytes	5 µl

Polyclonal Antisera	Producer	Lymphocyte subset	Volume
anti-human IgG, A, M F (ab)$_2$, FITC conjugated anti-human IgG, F (ab)$_2$, FITC conjugated	Behringwerke AG	B-cells activated B-cells	5 µl

RESULTS AND DISCUSSION

The median changes in the percentage of lymphocyte subpopulations in controls during this time are shown in Fig. 1. and the medians of the verum group are summarized in Fig. 2. The individual influence of Thymostimulin therapy for each patient is illustrated in Figs. 3-9. The percentage of MØ is calculated from the total amount of MNC's, - MØ's. The immune regulatory ratio (OKT4/OKT 8) is illustrated in Fig. 10.

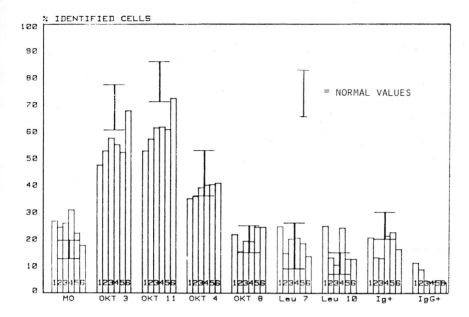

FIG. 1. Mononuclear cell-subpopulations medium values of control patients.

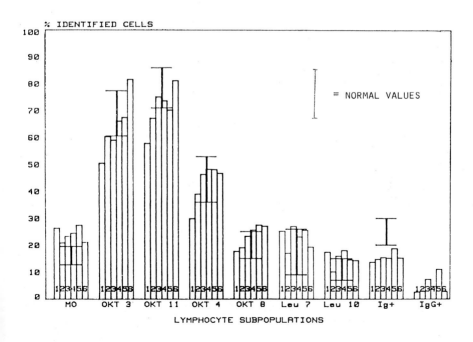

FIG. 2. Mononuclear cell-subpopulations medium values of thymostimulin-treated patients.

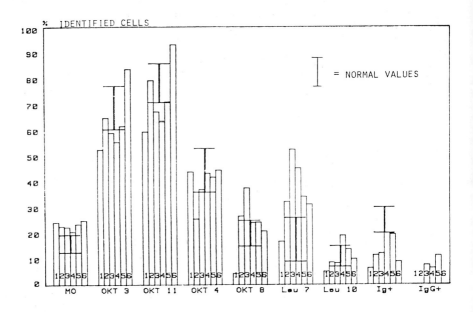

FIG. 3. Mononuclear cell-subpopulations in patient under thymostimulin-therapy.

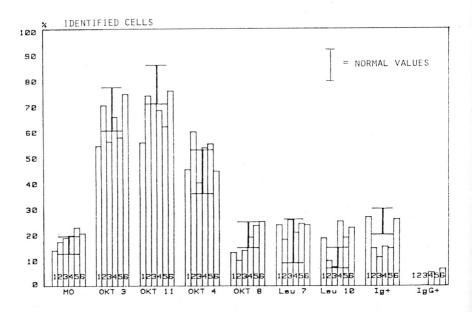

FIG. 4. Mononuclear cell-subpopulations in patient under thymostimulin-therapy.

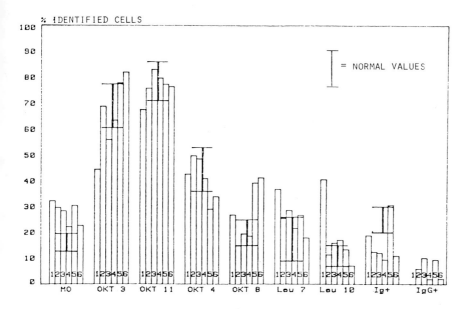

FIG. 5. Mononuclear cell-subpopulations in patient under thymostimulin-therapy.

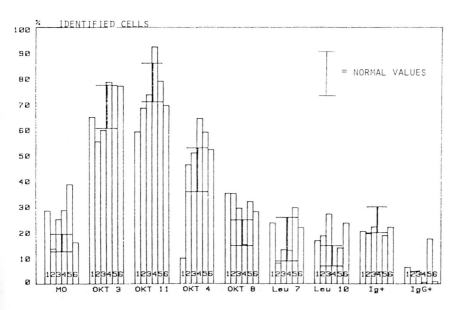

FIG. 6. Mononuclear cell-subpopulations in patient under thymostimulin-therapy.

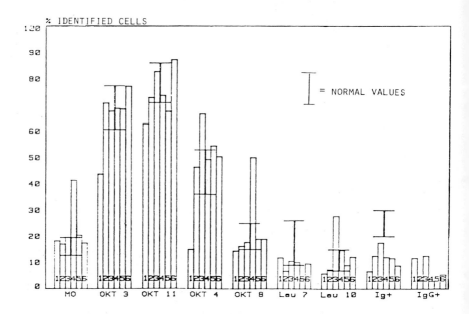

FIG. 7. Mononuclear cell-subpopulations in patient under thymostimulin-therapy.

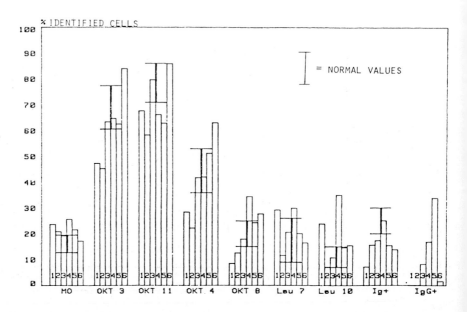

FIG. 8. Mononuclear cell-subpopulations in patient under thymostimulin-therapy.

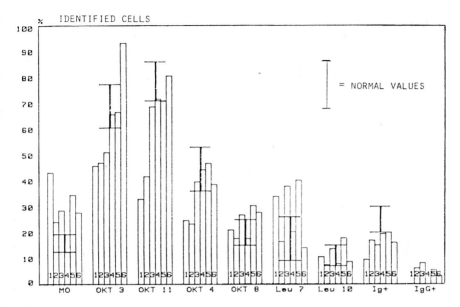

FIG. 9. Mononuclear cell-subpopulations in patient under thymostimulin-therapy.

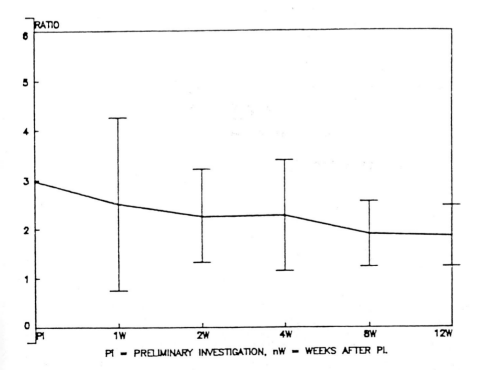

FIG. 10. T-helper/suppressor-cell ratio in thymostimulin-treated old patients.

The summarized results are:

a) In the percentage of T-cell subsets of the control patients variations of 20 to 30% are possible during a period of 3 months.

b) 4 out of 7 Thymostimulin treated patients reached normal T-cell values after 1 week (Figs. 3-6), 2 after 2 weeks (Figs. 7 and 8) and 1 after 4 weeks (Fig. 9) of therapy.

c) At the end of this study (12 weeks) 4 out of 7 controls reached also normal T-cell values.

d) An intermitting decrease below the normal values occured in 3 patients under therapy.

e) Variances in the OKT4/OKT8 ratio decreased during Thymostimulin-therapy.

f) In patients where OKT4 or OKT8 was below the normal range an improvement of these lymphocyte subsets occured after 1 to 4 weeks of Thymostimulin-therapy.

g) No significant influence of B-cell percentage could be demonstrated. Therefore the increase of T-cell percentage may be explained by an increase of maturation of immature lymphocyte subsets.

h) The U-test of MANN-WHITNEY was used to compare the two collectives. Beetween the control-group and the group of patients treated with Thymostimulin the following significant differences were found:

OKT3	OKT11
after 4 weeks: $p = 0,0253$	after 2 weeks: $p = 0,0060$
after 8 weeks: $p = 0,0040$	after 4 weeks: $p = 0,0476$
after 12 weeks: $p = 0,0474$	after 8 weeks: $p = 0,0350$

i) Patients unders Thymostimulin therapy showed remission of the chronic recurrent infection and indicate an amelioration of the subjective feeling.

REFERENCES

1. Aiuti, F. et al. (1979). Pediat. Res. 13, 792-802.
2. Behnken, L.J., et al. (1984). II. Freiburger Expertengespräch, *Editio Cantor.*
3. Bernengo, M.G., et al. (1983). Clinical Immunology and Immunopathology, 28, 311-324.
4. Boyum, A., (1964). Nature, 204, 793.
5. Boyum, A., (1968). Scand. J. Lab. Invest. 21 (Suppl.97), 77.
6. Casale, G. et al. (1983). Drug Res. 33, 889-890.
7. Erdmann, H., (2/1984). Onkologie 7, 112-117.
8. Lingetti, M. et al., Submitted for publication in: Gerontology.
9. Martelli, M.F. et al. (1982). Cancer 50, 490-497.
10. Rodeck, U., Kuwert, E., Keinecke, H.O., (1983). DMV, 198, 49.
11. Shoham, J. et al., (1980). Cancer Immunol. Immunother. 9, 173.
12. Tovo, P.A. et al. (1980). Thymus, Thymic Hormones and T-Lymphocytes 307-311. Eds. Aiuti, F. and Wigzell, H., Academic Press.

Longitudinal Assessment of Lymphocyte Subpopulations in Patients with Squamous Cell Carcinoma of Head and Neck

P. Schuff-Werner, G. Löhr, W. Rauschning, J.H. Beyer,
R. Golms, M. Schröder, H.W. v. Heyden and G.A. Nagel

University Clinics Department of Internal Medicine Division Hematology/Oncology
Robert-Koch-Str. 40 - D-3400 Göttingen FRG
Serono GmbH Pharmaceutical Products Research and Development Department
Merzhauser St. 134 - D-7800 Freiburg/Breisgau FRG
University Clinics Otorhinolaringology Geiststr. 10 - D-3400 Göttingen FRG

INTRODUCTION

Patients with malignancies are usually affected by secondary immunodeficiency concerning the T-cell compartment. The reduced immunocompetence in patients with advanced and multiple pre-treated malignancies results in a higher susceptibility to severe viral and fungal infections.

Thymostimulin (Tp-1 Serono®) is a soluble preparation of calf thymus, containing several polypeptides with molecular weight of approx. 6000 Daltons (2), that has been reported to induce lymphocyte maturation and to restore various immunological effector functions in vitro and in vivo (1, 3).

The aim of our current study is to investigate, if Thymostimulin may be of therapeutical value in avoiding secondary T-cell defects caused by chemotherapy.

Patients and Therapeutical Regime

20 patients with primarily inoperable squamous cell carcinoma (T3-T4/N1-N2/MO) have been treated with two cycles of chemotherapy (100 mg CIS-platinum/m at day 1 and 80 mg VP-16, day 3 to 5) to reduce the tumor size for further surgical treatment and/or radiation.

After the second cycle of chemotherapy 7 patients were treated additionally with Thymostimulin at a dosage of 1 mg/kg/day intramuscularly. In the first week after chemotherapy Thymostimulin was given daily and then twice weekly.

9 patients received no additional immunotherapy and served as controls.

4 patients had to be excluded from the study because the immunological examination was not performed in accordance with the protocol.

1 patient dropped out because of localized allergic skin reaction to Thymostimulin.

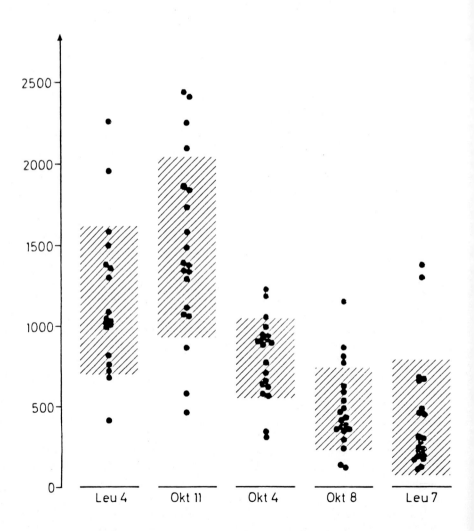

FIG. 1. Determination of Lymphocyte subpopulations in patients with squamous head an neck tumors (T_{3-4}, N_{1-2}, M_0) before first treatment with chemotherapy (absolute number of cells per μl).

Methods

Lymphocyte subpopulations were determined before (day 1), directly after (day 5) and three weeks after the first and the second chemotherapy (day 21).

For this, two different flow cytomtric technics were used in parallel.

The determination of OKT11, OKT4, LEU 7 and LEU 10 positive cells was done in whole blood specimens, using the spectrum III flow cytometer (Ortho Diagnostics, Heidelberg, FRG), whereas LEU 4, LEU 3 and LEU 2, B 1 and LEU 7 positive cells (not all data shown in this paper) were measured in Ficoll/Hypaque isolated mononuclear cell suspensions using a Facs-analyzer (Becton Dickinson Laboratory Systems, Heidelberg, FRG).

CONCLUSIONS

Prior to first treatment there is no detectable defect in the distribution of lymphocyte subsets in patients with primarily inoperable squamous cell carcinoma of head and neck (Fig. 1.).

Under treatment with CIS-platinum and VP-16 the absolute number of OKT11 and LEU 4 positive T-lyphocytes decreases slightly as do the T-helper/inducer (OKT4 pos.) and the T-suppressor/cytotoxic (OKT8 pos.) subsets. The decrease of OKT4 and OKT8 positive T-lymphocytes does not result in a significant alteration of the T4/T8 ratio.

In contrast, additional treatment with Thymostimulin directly after the chemotherapeutic regimen results in a marked increase of T-lymphocytes (Fig. 2) and their subsets as compared to the untreated controls (Fig. 3-5).

The increase of OKT8 positive cells under Thymostimulin treatment is more pronounced than the increase of OKT4 pos cells. This results in a decrease of the T4/T8 ratio. It is still unclear if these remarkable changes of mature peripheral lymphocytes is of benefit for the clinical outcome of the patients.

It might be possible that additional treatment with Thymostimulin prevents chemotherapy-induced (seconday) immunosuppression.

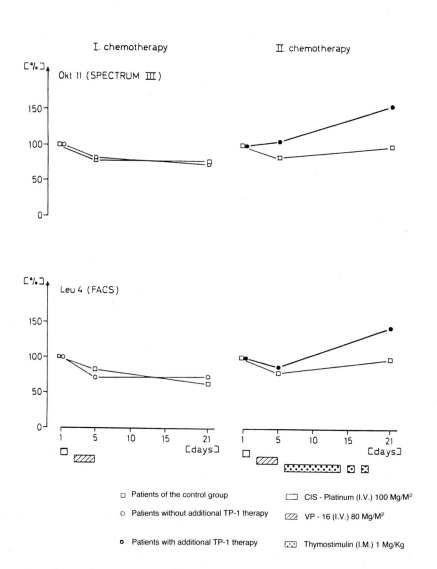

FIG. 2. Influence of chemotherapy and chemoimmunotherapy on OKT11 positive lymphocytes as determined by spectrum III analysis and on LEU 4 positive lymphocytes as determined by FACS analysis. The absolute number of cells per μl is expressed in percent as compared with the number of positive cells before starting therapy (100%).

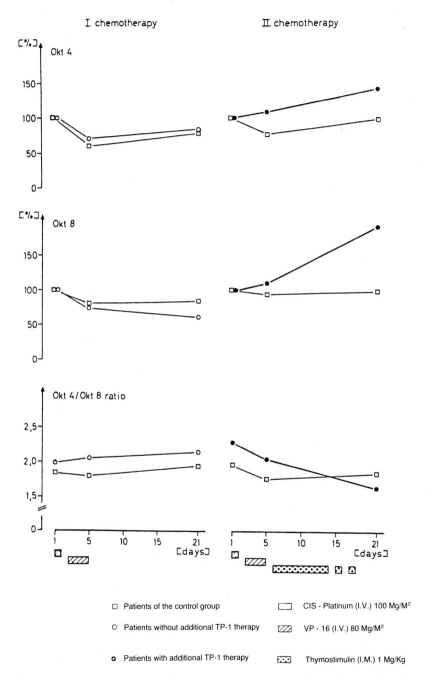

FIG. 3. Influence of chemotherapy and chemoimmunotherapy on OKT8 and OKT4 positive Lymphocytes. The absolute number of cells per µl is expressed in percent as compared with the number of positive cells before starting therapy (100%).

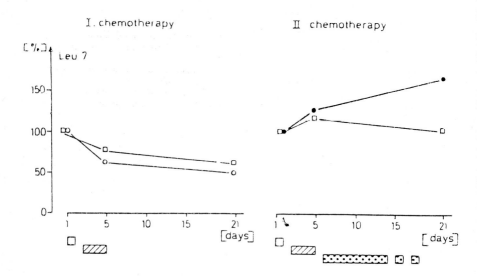

FIG. 4. Influence of chemotherapy and chemoimmunotherapy on LEU 7 positive lympocytes. The absolute number of cells per μl is expressed in percent as compared with the number of positive cells before starting therapy (100%).

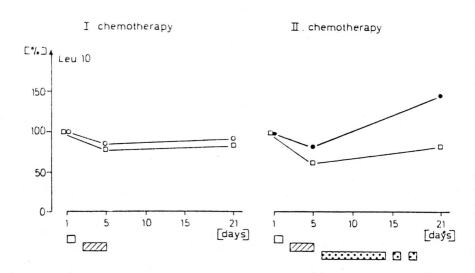

FIG. 5. Influence of chemotherapy and chemoimmunotherapy on LEU 10 positive lympocytes. The absolute number of cells per μl is expressed in percent as compared with the number of positive cells before starting therapy (100%).

REFERENCES

1. Byrom, N.A., Nagbekar, N.M., Hobbs, J.R., 1984., Thymic factor modulation of lymphocyte surface markers. in N.A. Byrom and J.R. Hobbs (eds.): Thymic Factor Therapy, *Raven Press*, N.Y. pp. 53-61.
2. Falchetti, R., Bergesi, G., Eshkol, A. et al. 1977. Pharmacological and biological properties of a calf thymus extract (Tp-1). *Drugs. exp. Clin. Res.* 3, 39-47.
3. Shoham, J., Theodor, E., Brenner, H.J. et al. 1980. Enhancement of the immune system of chemotherapy-treated cancer patients by simultaneous treatment with thymic extract (Tp-1). *Cancer Immunol. Immunother.* 9, 173-180.

Concluding Remarks

Maxime Seligmann

One of the nice things in this meeting is that we heard several excellent talks about basic immunology in mice or men, describing some new findings that are important for our understanding of immunodeficiency diseases or for their handling. However, since we are late, I wish to concentrate on primary immunodeficiency diseases where it is obvious that recent progress and future avenues mainly pertain at present to two fields, the membrane defects and the studies in molecular biology.

Several syndromes featured by membrane defects have been described and discussed yesterday. Their mechanisms and etiology are however still poorly understood. For instance, the diagnosis of the interesting syndrome featured by the lack of IL_1 receptor presently relies only on absorption experiments and this disease should help to identify this receptor. The Gp 115 defect described in the Wiskott-Aldrich syndrome appears to be linked to instability and increased shedding of a group of membrane glycoproteins whose synthesis is apprently normal. On the opposite, the genetic deficiency in LFA_1 and CR_3 membrane proteins is featured by the absence of production of the β chain that they have in common. We do however not yet know what happens at the gene level. The study of these patients should also help to understand the functions of the third affected membrane protein, p150,95, that is presently characterized only by its biochemical structure.

As far as the so-called bare lymphocyte syndrome is concerned, we do not yet know the genetic basis for the lack of production of HLA class II molecules since the messenger RNA is absent but allogenotypes are normal at the DNA level. A striking finding is the difference in phenotypic expression of this syndrome, according to the left or right bank of the Rhine river, although on both sides, many patients are of North African origin...

As far as the data in molecular biology are concerned, the Schwaber and Rosen findings in X-linked agammaglobulinemia, showing that the B cells of some patients produce incomplete μ chains devoid of V_H and a short mRNA with absent VDJ region, are most difficult to reconcile with those of Kubagawa and Cooper who showed in EBV lines of 3 patients normal entire intracytoplasmic μ chains with VH determinants and normal DNA rearrangements. This discrepancy opens the possibility that X-linked agammaglobulinemia is heterogeneous and not a single disease. Although the X-linked hyper IgM immunodeficiency appeared most promising for DNA studies aiming to demonstrate a switch element deficiency, the possibility is presently open that this disease may not be an intrinsic B cell defect but rather a defect in switch T cells. The mapping on the X chromosome of the gene(s) responsible for X-linked primary immunodeficiency diseases, and specially X-linked agammaglobulinemia, is presently actively pursued in several laboratories. Definite results are however not a hand since we heard nothing about it during this meeting. However, we heard new and interesting DNA data, which may be relevant to this problem, about an experimental model, namely the Xid mutation in CBA/N mice. Most intriguing is the finding that the XLR gene family, that is closely linked with this defect, is only expressed in late B cells and is also expressed in peripheral T cells.

Of great interest is the finding that the chromosomal translocations and breaks in ataxia telangectasia do mainly occur at those precise sites where the $T\alpha$, $T\beta$ and $T\gamma$ chains of the T cell receptor are encoded. However, this may be merely the consequence of the basic genomic abnormality in this disease.

Finally, the only immunoglobulin deficiencies where the occurence of a genomic deletion has been strongly suggested, are those of the two patients studied by Carbonara with lack of IgA_1 IgG_2 and IgG_4 (and also IgE in one of the cases). In summary, we can state that genomic deletions are much more scarce in immunodeficiency diseases than our own gaps in the present understanding of the genetic mechanism underlying this group of diseases.

As far as AIDS is concerned, I believe that what we heard this morning about the genomic variations of the LAV/HTLV III virus, about this small fraction of surviving lymphocytes that harbour integrated provirus and can transmit it and about the infection by the virus of activated B cells and monocytes that constitute potential reservoirs does not make us optimistic about the possibilities of preventive and curative treatment in a rather near future. Since I am the last speaker, I would like to thank on behalf of all guests and participants, Dr. Fernando Aiuti and the Serono organization for their efforts and arrangements that brought us together at this successful meeting.